BEFORE
YOU TAKE
THAT PILL

BEFORE
YOU TAKE
THAT PILL

Why the Drug Industry
May Be Bad for Your Health

J. DOUGLAS BREMNER

AVERY

a member of Penguin Group (USA) Inc.

New York

AVERY

Published by the Penguin Group
Penguin Group (USA) Inc., 375 Hudson Street, New York, New York 10014, USA •
Penguin Group (Canada), 90 Eglinton Avenue East, Suite 700, Toronto, Ontario
M4P 2Y3 Canada (a division of Pearson Canada Inc.) • Penguin Books Ltd,
80 Strand, London WC2R 0RL, England • Penguin Ireland, 25 St Stephen's Green,
Dublin 2, Ireland (a division of Penguin Books Ltd) • Penguin Books (Australia),
250 Camberwell Road, Camberwell, Victoria 3124, Australia (a division of Pearson
Australia Group Pty Ltd) • Penguin Books India Pvt Ltd, 11 Community Centre,
Panchsheel Park, New Delhi–110 017, India • Penguin Group (NZ), 67 Apollo Drive,
Rosedale, North Shore 0632, New Zealand (a division of Pearson New Zealand Ltd) •
Penguin Books (South Africa) (Pty) Ltd, 24 Sturdee Avenue,
Rosebank, Johannesburg 2196, South Africa

Penguin Books Ltd, Registered Offices: 80 Strand, London WC2R 0RL, England

Most Avery books are available at special quantity discounts for bulk purchase for sales promotions, premiums, fund-raising, and educational needs. Special books or book excerpts also can be created to fit specific needs. For details, write Penguin Group (USA) Inc. Special Markets, 375 Hudson Street, New York, NY 10014.

Library of Congress Cataloging-in-Publication Data

Bremner, J. Douglas, date.
Before you take that pill : why the drug industry may be bad for your health /
J. Douglas Bremner.
p.   cm.
Includes bibliographical references.
ISBN 978-1-58333-295-5
1. Drugs—Side effects—Popular works.   2. Dietary supplements—Side effects—Popular
works.   I. Title.
RM302.5.B74   2008   2007044792
615'.7042—dc22

Printed in the United States of America
1   3   5   7   9   10   8   6   4   2

BOOK DESIGN BY MEIGHAN CAVANAUGH

While the author has made every effort to provide accurate telephone numbers and Internet addresses at the time of publication, neither the publisher nor the author assumes any responsibility for errors or for changes that occur after publication. Further, the publisher does not have any control over and does not assume any responsibility for author or third-party websites or their content.

Neither the publisher nor the author is engaged in rendering professional advice or services to the individual reader. The ideas, procedures, and suggestions contained in this book are not intended as a substitute for consulting with your physician. All matters regarding your health require medical supervision. Neither the author nor the publisher shall be liable or responsible for any loss or damage allegedly arising from any information or suggestion in this book.

*I would like to dedicate
this book to my wife, Viola,
and my two children,
Dylan and Sabina.
May they have many years of
health and happiness.*

CONTENTS

Introduction

We see it on TV and read it in the paper every day: Medications save lives. New breakthroughs in medicine are bringing new drugs to the market every day. The American medical system will soon eliminate disease and discomfort and allow us to live a hundred years. Right?

Not exactly. In fact, one hundred thousand Americans die every year from medications that they didn't need or that were prescribed in the wrong way. A million people have serious side effects that require hospitalization. Doctors don't always have all the information they need to balance the risks and benefits of medication. Drug companies whose primary motivation is to sell medication are aggressively promoting their products. Now, more than half of *all* Americans are taking a prescription drug.

Why do I say this? I am a doctor. Like other doctors, I was trained at a medical school and adapted practices taught to me, mainly focused on treating disease with medications and surgery, with little on nutrition, behavior, spirituality, or disease prevention through lifestyle changes. After that I attended lectures at the annual medical meetings and got updates on new treatments from the leading doctors in my field. Like my peers, I believed that medications were a good thing, that any risks and undesirable

1

side effects would be solved through future medical breakthroughs, continuous research, and newer drugs. I accepted that the high price of drugs was justified by the need to pay for the research to develop new ones, and that generic drugs were bad because they drained money away from research for new life-saving drugs.

However, being a physician scientist, I am naturally inclined to question the evidence for any particular statement of fact. For most of my career this has been limited to specific questions related to my area of research, which is mainly focused on the brain and, more recently, heart disease.

Probably the first time this curiosity bumped up against the American medical and pharmaceutical behemoth was about eight years ago, when I was an assistant professor of radiology and psychiatry at Yale University School of Medicine. We were interested in studies of monkeys showing that exposure during pregnancy to dexamethasone, a drug used to prevent bleeding in the brain in premature babies, caused brain damage. No one had as yet considered the possibility that it could have such a side effect in human newborns, but I couldn't get any of the doctors working with the babies to collaborate with me on the research. Could it be that they didn't want to be associated with research that might reveal that a drug they had been using for years was actually causing brain damage? As for the effects of dexamethasone on the brain, we still don't know, since that research was never done.

About a year ago, out of idle curiosity, I began to question the available evidence on the effectiveness of many of the medications that were being heavily promoted for the "prevention" of various diseases. I asked my wife, who is a professor of cardiology at Emory University, what evidence there was to substantiate the claim that cholesterol causes heart disease and that taking medication to lower cholesterol actually works. She said there was "lots" of evidence. I asked her where it was. She referred me to the Web site of the American Heart Association, whose expert panel profiled who was at risk for heart disease and who should be taking medications like Lipitor to lower their cholesterol as a preventative. There was a series of "points" supposedly related to a person's risk of heart disease that were based on "risk factors" like age, diabetes, hypertension, family medical history, smoking, and history of heart disease. If the sum of these points was great enough, you were counseled to "talk to your doctor," and we all know what that means. Although the panel didn't provide any evidence for its assertions (I later learned that for many of its recommendations there wasn't any), being a typical physician and the fact that this wasn't my area of expertise, I took its "authority" at face value and didn't pursue it further.

If nothing else had happened, that probably would have been the end of it. However, other flukes of history pushed me to look at things in a different way. My main area of research has involved imaging the brain of patients who suffer from depression and other mental disorders. Several years ago I was contacted by the families of some young people who had killed themselves while taking a medication for acne called Accutane. They asked if brain imaging would show similar changes in the same area of the brain of all those who were so adversely affected by Accutane. I spoke with the company that made the drug about supporting research, but it wasn't interested. With private donations my colleagues and I eventually performed a study showing that Accutane affected brain function, suggesting how it could cause depression and suicide.[1]

You might think that people would be happy to learn more about a potentially dangerous side effect, but they weren't. Dermatologists who prescribe Accutane told me that I shouldn't do this research, because Accutane was a "good" drug that helped a lot of people with severe acne. I asked the FDA and the NIH to support clinical trials investigating the relationship between Accutane and depression. Staff at the FDA said they were "watching Accutane closely," but "they couldn't require the manufacturer to cooperate in trials of drug safety." One doctor at the NIH told me that the relationship between Accutane and depression "wasn't clinically relevant for dermatology." Based on my interactions with Roche, the manufacturer of Accutane, I did not get the feeling that it was encouraging doctors to research the Accutane and depression issue.

As reported in *USA Today* (Kevin McCoy, December 7, 2004, "Drug Maker Rebuffed Call to Monitor Users"), scientists at Roche had written a report in 1999 in which they expressed the opinion that Accutane could cause depression. However, a Roche official testified in 2004 that the Roche marketing team argued against the report, stating that it could "impact on marketing strategy and product liability." What was going on here? Was selling a drug more important than helping people?

My experience and my reading led me to the conclusion that it wasn't always about saving lives. It was also about making money, a lot of money, meaning billions of dollars. Behind that was millions of dollars of marketing to doctors and patients to convince them they needed the drug. And sometimes that corporate greed led to a lot of harm.

The more I looked at different drugs, the more I worried about whether the appropriate balance of safety and efficacy was being achieved. I also worried about whether too many people were taking these drugs and whether people for whom there was no hope of benefit were being harmed by drugs. I began to question assumptions that all doctors make. Were medications for cholesterol really that helpful for people without heart disease? Or for women? Should you really take a pill for something like diabetes, which is caused by eating too much? Do you need to take a pill to go to sleep? Do you need to take vitamins and supplements to meet that USDA requirement, and who came up with those requirements anyway? Do you need a pill to have sex? Are those things helping you, or are they hurting or even killing you?

The material in this book is derived from information in books and the medical literature, much of it, including papers from prominent journals, never widely disseminated or otherwise buried in tables of incomprehensible numbers, or lost in the medical literature because of a lack of citation by other doctors.

You have the right to know the risks and benefits of the pills that you take and to make your own decisions about what is right for you.

This book is for anyone who is on medication, is thinking about taking a medication, knows someone on medication, or is taking a vitamin, herb, or supplement. It is also for people not on medication, since a doctor or a drug company is bound to eventually recommend a drug to them as well.

This book covers more than three hundred of the most commonly prescribed drugs, the fifty top-selling prescription drugs, all of the vitamins, and the best-selling herbs and supplements. Some of the drugs that are covered include some particularly unsafe ones that aren't used much anymore, but that you should watch out for (even though they haven't been taken off the market by the FDA) or that illustrate a particular point. This book does not cover cancer, medical emergencies, or rare and life-threatening disorders. This book is meant to be read. It is not a reference or a comprehensive list of any possible side effects and drug interactions. You should use other books to check the possible interactions of drugs you are taking, including drug-herb interactions, or unusual side effects. I list some of these at the end of this book.

Life is important to us. We all want to live as long as possible and want the same for our loved ones. If this book enables you to use medications safely and convinces you to change your diet and lifestyle to prevent disease, I will consider it a success.

May you and your family enjoy many years of good health.

1.

The Drug Problem

Today we are faced with what may be the single greatest drug safety catastrophe in the history of this country or the history of the world. . . . In my opinion, the FDA has let the American people down and, sadly, betrayed a public trust.

Those ominous words, spoken by David J. Graham, M.D., MPH, associate director of drug safety for the U.S. Food and Drug Administration (FDA), on November 18, 2004, were part of congressional testimony concerning the dangers of the arthritis medication Vioxx, which had just been taken off the market because of evidence that it increased the risk of heart attack. Yet he could have been talking about the prescription-drug industry in general, especially since he mentioned that Vioxx was not the only medication that posed serious health threats. It was only the tip of the iceberg. Graham identified five widely prescribed drugs still on the market that are particularly dangerous, including Accutane, Bextra, Crestor, Meridia, and Serevent. (In 2005 Bextra was taken off the market.)

While it's true that many drugs help people live longer and better lives, myriad others may be harmful in ways you're unaware of. Dr. Graham's testimony provided the public a fleeting glimpse of the knowledge that is normally hidden from view or frustratingly difficult for the average person to access. Pharmaceutical and supplement manufacturers have to increase sales and profits, as all businesses must, and they do so in part by developing drugs to treat disease and also by convincing people they need meds to prevent disease or lessen the perceived risk of future illness. The result is that nondisclosure of potentially harmful side effects of the drugs they make has become routine. Unearthing and compiling that veiled or hidden information is the mission of this book.

How We Got Here

The latest drive to get new pills on the shelves and into people's mouths began when government deregulation and an earnest attempt to help HIV-AIDS patients access important life-extending drugs collided. In the 1980s there was a strong movement to decrease the role of government regulation in all businesses, and budgets of regulatory agencies like the FDA were slashed as part of that effort. The Reagan administration painted the FDA as a bloated bureaucracy that was slowing down the approval of drugs and getting in the way of business.

There was some truth to that claim. At that time it could take up to two years to gain drug approval, two years too long if you were suffering from HIV-AIDS. Throughout the 1980s, AIDS activists and patients echoed the drug companies' sentiments, complaining that it was taking too long to bring disease-fighting drugs to market. The pharmaceutical industry lent a sympathetic ear and a loud voice to calls for speeding up the approval of AIDS drugs such as Agenerase (amprenavir). Since drugs are on patent for a limited number of years, every year spent waiting for approval from the FDA means losing a year of profits.

Couple that with the fact that the FDA could now honestly say that, because of cuts, it was understaffed. The answer was essentially legislation allowing pharmaceutical companies to pay the salaries of the staff at the FDA. In 1992, the Prescription Drug User Fee Act (PDUFA) stipulated that a fee (now $576,000) be paid to the FDA by the pharmaceutical companies for each new drug application. The number of staff at the Center for Drug Evaluation and Research (CDER) doubled overnight. Today, the FDA receives about $260 million a year from these fees. Part of the bill stipulated that funding by Congress for new drug evaluations had to increase by 3% per year. Since the overall funding for the FDA did not increase at 3% per year, the FDA had to actually cut funding for surveillance and research of approved drugs.

The change in law had another interesting result: The boundaries among the drug companies, the FDA, and doctors became increasingly blurred. FDA officials sometimes move to jobs in the pharmaceutical industry, which means they may not want to burn their bridges with industry. The same FDA officials who approve the drugs are responsible for monitoring them after they are on the market, which gives them an obvious disincentive to say that the drugs they earlier certified as safe were now unsafe. Finally, the FDA gets input from outside advisory panels made up of doctors who are experts in their fields. Most of these doctors receive payments as consultants, research grants, and support for travel to conferences from drug companies. In some cases, the doctors are working as paid consultants to the same companies whose drugs are coming up for approval by their advisory committees.

For instance, as reported by *USA Today* on October 16, 2004 ("Cholesterol Guidelines Become a Morality Play") eight of the nine doctors who formed a committee in 2001 to advise the government on cholesterol guidelines for the public were making money from the very same companies that made the cholesterol-lowering drugs that the doctors were urging millions of Americans to take. For example, one of the committee members, Dr. H. Bryan Brewer, chief of the Molecular Disease Branch at the National Institutes of Health, worked as a consultant or speaker for ten different pharmaceutical companies and made more than $100,000 over three years while he was on the committee and at the same time sat on the board of one of these companies. (*Los Angeles Times,* December 22, 2004, "The National Institutes of Health: Public Servant or Private Marketer?"). Dr. Brewer left the NIH in 2005 in the midst of adverse publicity about potential conflicts of interest. Nassir Ghaemi, M.D., a psychiatrist at Emory University, was quoted in the *Emory Academic Exchange* (February 2007) as having said, "Critics say we are being influenced and don't realize it—that drug companies are smarter than we are and know a lot more about human psychology than we think, and they're probably right about that to some extent."

Expert consensus guidelines have a potent effect on doctors; they can be held liable if they do not adhere to accepted standards of care. Dr. Curt D. Furberg, a former head of clinical trials at the National Heart, Lung, and Blood Institute and now a professor at Wake Forest University in North Carolina, explained how such information reaches physicians: "The [company] reps tell the doctors, 'You should follow these guidelines,' implying that you're not a good doctor if you don't follow these guidelines" (*Los Angeles Times*, December 22, 2004, "The National Institutes of Health: Public Servant or Private Marketer?").

The result of this comingling was a boon for drug makers: Approval time of their products decreased from twenty months to six months right after the law changed. However, the number of drugs that had to be later withdrawn also increased from 2% to 5% of drugs.

There is another troubling dichotomy that could have terrible repercussions for our health: While the number of people with disease is not growing, the number of adult Americans taking medication *is* increasing: Half of us take prescription drugs and 81% of us take at least one kind of pill every day, and that percentage is expected to rise in the coming years. To gain the most market share, companies have to invent drugs for diseases that previously had no treatment (or treat problems that may not necessarily require drug treatment, such as "restless leg syndrome"), or create preventative medications for alleged risks (like the risk of fracture in the elderly) to expand the potential pool of medication takers. That meant moving from the realm of giving medications to sick people to giving medications to people who looked well but might be at an increased risk based on the result of a blood test or some other hidden marker of disease. Thus the era of disease prevention and risk-factor modification was born.

To promote this shift, for the past two decades the pharmaceutical industry has pushed educational programs, which it claims are designed to identify people in need of treatment or prevention with medication. It usually does this by donating money to organizations that advocate on behalf of a specific disease, whose members will in turn "get the word out" to increase public awareness and screening, and thereby expand the number of individuals who will potentially take the medication. This is fine for identifying individuals with undiagnosed high blood pressure or for detecting the early stages of colon cancer. But awareness campaigns are not always meant to be purely, altruistically educational; most are linked to a drug company's marketing campaign.

There are a number of conditions for which we are now urged to obtain screening and potential treatment, including high cholesterol, osteoporosis, hypertension, diabetes, and heart disease. However, the potential benefit of medications to treat these conditions is often exaggerated, side effects are minimized, and in some cases recommendations are based on evidence from groups of people unrelated to the person being treated (e.g., women with risk factors for heart disease are urged to take cholesterol-lowering medications that are based on studies of men). In addition, doctors who work as paid consultants to the pharmaceutical industry often write the guidelines used to assess who should take the drugs, so it is unclear how unbiased their recommendations really are.

Another factor that has expanded use of prescription medications happened in 1997, when the FDA lifted the ban on direct advertising to consumers along with a law that required ads to list every possible side effect. Soon after, Americans were bombarded daily with commercials for prescription drugs. The U.S. is the only country in the world where you can turn on the TV and hear an announcer tell you to go 'ask your doctor' for a drug. Doctors often will prescribe medications for patients even if they don't think their patients need them. For example, one study showed that 54% of the time doctors will prescribe a specific brand and type of medication if patients ask for it.

A Bleak Diagnosis

With so many of us popping pills or gulping down spoonfuls of medicine, it's not surprising that more of us report related adverse effects. One hundred thousand Americans die every year from the effects of prescription medications. More than a million Americans a year are admitted to the hospital because they have had a bad reaction to a medication. About a quarter of the prescriptions that doctors write for the elderly have a potentially life-threatening error. Many of these people are getting medications that they don't need, or are being medicated for problems that can be appropriately and safely addressed without drugs. For example, most cases of adult-onset diabetes can be prevented and possibly cured with a change in diet alone—and with considerably fewer negative side effects and numerous healthy ones, like weight loss and lower blood pressure and cholesterol.

In 2005 in the aftermath of the Vioxx debacle and its withdrawal from the market, the Institute of Medicine was asked to provide recommendations for improving drug safety. As part of this process they interviewed Janet Woodcock, deputy commissioner of operations at the FDA. As reported by the *New York Times* on June 9, 2005 ("Drug Safety System is Broken, Top FDA Official Says"), she told the Institute that the nation's drug-safety system had ". . . pretty much broken down." She went on to say that ". . . the keystone of the current system is the prescriber, and that person is the one who decides if the benefits of a drug outweigh the risks for that patient. This system has obviously broken down to some extent as far as the fully informed provider and the fully informed patients." She charged that neither doctors nor patients had enough information about the side effects of drugs to make informed decisions about taking them. Dr. Woodcock went on to say that ". . . the bottom line is that a lot of drug safety problems are actually preventable, [because] most adverse events are from known side effects."

Unfortunately, doctors may not be able to provide their patients with all the details on side effects. They aren't hiding anything; they just can't keep up with new information. There are more than five thousand medical journals, each of which publishes twenty articles a month, meaning that there are more than 1 million articles published each year. It's impossible for anyone to read all of this, let alone a busy general practitioner or internist, or even a specialist, all of whom are often buried by insurance forms and HMO paperwork. Most of the information doctors receive consists of distilled versions of research results that are assembled by the pharmaceutical industry and distributed through promotional materials and the product representatives who visit doctors' offices. Legitimate publications *are* distributed, but papers that are not favorable are ignored, and favorable data within papers are highlighted to the exclusion of less-favorable data.

In addition, drug companies hire academic physicians to give lectures but require that they show only slides that have been approved by the company. The companies support "grand-rounds" lectures (traditional lectures given by outside speakers to the entire department) at universities but have the right to accept or reject the speakers.

Marcia Angell wrote about other ways drug companies distort the flow of information to doctors about the risks and benefits of medications in her excellent book *The Truth About the Drug Companies,* in which she contends that doctors get most of their information about drugs during weekly visits from drug-company product representatives, who are typically young, attractive women with no background in health or science. In fact, as reported by the *New York Times* on November 28, 2005, drug companies often recruit former college cheerleaders for this job ("Gimme an Rx! Cheerleaders Pump Up Drug Sales").

Reps are sent into the field with a list of talking points to help them answer questions as well as packets of product-favorable articles and other material such as copies of expert consensus guidelines (created by their paid consultants) to leave with doctors. The critical information contained in these articles is often buried in tables without comment, and there are often conclusions that are not supported by the data in the papers, and I cite several examples of this throughout this book.

Drug companies also buy information about the medications that doctors prescribe from major drugstore chains like CVS and then use this information to reward doctors who frequently prescribe their drugs with trips to resorts and other perks. Drug companies also lavish dinners, gifts, and paid trips to conferences on doctors. Research studies show that, although doctors deny that the perks have any effect on their prescribing practices, there are changes in objective measures, like how often a doctor will try to have a drug from a particular company put on his hospital's formulary.

Do We Get Our Money's Worth?

I'm not saying that some drugs don't ever successfully prevent disease or that newly described diseases and syndromes are necessarily invalid, but the fact is that no matter how you look at it, the U.S. (and to a lesser extent other industrialized countries) has a prescription-drug problem. Americans spend twice as much on drugs and take twice as many drugs as those in other industrialized countries yet have the worst health. That means we are paying money for drugs that are not working for us.

Despite the fact that Americans spend twice as much on health care as those of any other country in the world, we have some of the most negative health-care outcomes in the industrialized world, including total life expectancy and survival of children to their fifth birthday. In a survey of thirteen industrialized nations, the U.S. was found to be last in many health-related measures and second to last overall. Countries with the best health care included Japan, Sweden, and Canada, in that order. Factors that were thought to explain the negative health-care outcomes in the U.S. included the lack of a developed and effective primary-care system and higher rates of poverty. Even in England, where there are higher rates of smoking and drinking and a fattier diet, people have better health than we Americans.

It is no accident that we are paying the most money and getting the worst health care. In *Overdosed America: The Broken Promise of American Medicine,* author John Abramson, M.D., says we are pouring money into expensive drugs and medical devices that have marginal value compared to more economical alternatives. Meanwhile we neglect the development of things like primary care, which can have a real impact on health. Forty-three million Americans go without health insurance, and that number is growing. We are also paying a lot of money for health care we may never even receive, as a result of the rising costs of individual health insurance, health-care benefits that drive companies into the ground, expensive Medicare drug benefits, and uncontrollable Medicaid costs.

Many of the aforementioned expenses are related to expensive drugs that we often don't need, that are no more effective than older alternatives, or that are simply not as valuable as drug companies make them out to be. For example, studies have shown that peasants in Indian villages who have been diagnosed as schizophrenic and are treated with chlorpromazine, the original antipsychotic, which is dirt cheap, and receive family support actually do *better* in terms of having fewer psychotic symptoms than Americans who get expensive new-generation antipsychotics and traditional Western psychiatric care. Another example is Nexium, "the purple pill," which works no better for gastric reflux than older medications like Prilosec, even though it costs much more.

Drugs cost twice as much in the U.S. as in Canada or Europe. A year of treatment with many medications can cost up to $3,000. In response to efforts to regulate the content of TV ads for drugs, Billy Tauzin, president of the Pharmaceutical Research Manufacturers of America (PhRMA), the lobbying organization for the drug companies, was quoted by the *New York Times* (May 17, 2005) as having said, "We don't make ice cream or handbags or automobiles, we make products that save lives" ("Drug Industry Is Said to Work on Ad Code").

The argument drug manufacturers make for the high cost of their products, which has become an old saw by now, is that the money supports research and development of new life-saving meds. They also say that expensive advertising is needed not to sell drugs but to educate doctors and patients. Indeed, a whopping 80% of their budgets is used for marketing.

The major drug companies don't develop a lot of new drugs. The truth is, most new drugs are developed through basic science research conducted in universities and not in drug-company laboratories. University scientists receive research grants from the National Institutes of Health (NIH). The NIH is supported by money from taxes. Take the case of the COX-2 inhibitors, like Vioxx. The mechanisms of COX-2 inhibition that led to the development of the COX-2 inhibitors were discovered at a university by researchers supported by taxpayers' dollars.

In order to keep making money, drug companies are under enormous pressure to create new drugs they can patent and sell without competition for twenty years, after which patents run out and generic (cheaper) versions go to market. In fact, there really aren't a lot of truly new drugs being developed these days. Most pharmaceuticals touted as new are essentially the same as other drugs in their class, with a slight chemical modification that allows the company to have a unique patent. These are called "me-too" drugs.

Once the drug companies have developed a "new" drug, they patent it and begin clinical trials in the hopes of gaining FDA approval for its use. In order to get approval, they must perform two multicenter randomized placebo, or sugar-pill–controlled, studies demonstrating that their drug is better than nothing. This means that patients get randomly assigned to either the drug or placebo for, say, three months, and neither the doctors nor the patients know what they are on. This is the gold standard for evaluating the risks and benefits of drugs, and it is required to definitively evaluate drugs as well as alternative treatments.

The placebo response is essentially how much better you do if you take a pill that you *believe* helps you, even if it really does nothing in terms of its actual effect on your body. At the end of the study the "blind" is removed, and the doctors look to see if the drug was better than the placebo in improving the symptoms of the disease or preventing some predefined event, like a heart attack. The company must conduct at least two studies showing that the drug is better than the placebo. If they complete eight studies, only two of which show that the drug is better than the placebo, the drug has fulfilled the requirement, notwithstanding the six failures.

Because the drug companies are required to show only that a drug is more effective than no medication at all, we usually never know whether it is better than an older drug that the new version seeks to replace. It is usually left to marketing people to generate enthusiasm through TV ads, product-representative visits to doctors' offices, and sponsored lectures, and to convince practitioners and their patients that the new drug is safer or better than the old drug. They do this by picking some aspect of the drug's properties that theoretically makes it better.

For example, when tricyclic antidepressants went off patent, they were replaced by a new generation of drugs called selective serotonin reuptake inhibitors (SSRIs). Even though SSRIs were never shown to be better at treating depression than the old drugs, it was argued that because the SSRIs were more specific in blocking serotonin uptake, as opposed to nonspecific blockage of serotonin, norepinephrine, and other chemicals, they would be more effective and have fewer side effects. The same argument was made for the COX-2 inhibitors, like Vioxx, which were said to more specifically inhibit the COX receptor involved in pain, unlike the nonspecific nonsteroidal anti-inflammatory drugs (NSAIDs).

In his book, *The $800 Million Pill: The Truth Behind the Cost of New Drugs,* Merrill Goozner, M.D., says that charging a lot for patented medications to pay for developing future drugs is unnecessary. The second-generation drugs for a particular disorder often will cost up to ten times as much as the old drugs that have gone off patent. The few studies that have made direct comparisons have for the most part not shown any significant increase in efficacy over the old drugs. For example, the newer antidepressant drugs, like Prozac, have never been shown to work any better than the older tricyclic antidepressant drugs.

Sometimes new drugs are found to have side effects that are far more dangerous than those of the older alternatives, but typically when this happens, companies resist admitting it for as long as possible. For instance, the painkiller Vioxx was a second-generation drug that was never shown to be a more effective pain reliever than the old painkiller, Advil, which could be purchased for a fraction of what Vioxx cost and over the counter. However, Vioxx was marketed as having a lower risk of gastrointestinal bleeding. It was only after the drug had been on the market for many years that it was discovered that it increased the risk of heart attack severalfold (see Chapter 2). Tens of thousands of people had died unnecessarily as a result of taking Vioxx, and to make matters worse, they had to pay a lot more money for the privilege. What this shows is that the FDA should require companies to test new drugs against old ones and to compare the two on the basis of their efficacy and side effects.

Given medical scares like Vioxx, it's not surprising that the public image of the FDA and the drug companies has begun to suffer and that Americans have become wary of both. *The Economist* reported November 24, 2004 ("Lessons for Pharma from Tobacco"), that less than 50% of us perceive drug companies as "favorable." That's only slightly above the low ratings we give oil and tobacco companies.

Another reason why our confidence has been shaken is the common defense drug companies use against charges of drug toxicity: "It was approved by the FDA." Congress has even proposed legislation relieving drug companies of liability in cases that involve drug-safety problems if the drug has been approved by the FDA. The FDA is so paralyzed by politics and its desire to balance scientific advancement, commerce, and safety that it could be letting down its guard. For instance, Daniel Troy, the chief counsel for the FDA under George W. Bush in 2004, was a political appointee who formerly worked in a Washington law firm that defended the interests of pharmaceutical companies. As reported by *Drug Store News* (December 22, 2004, "FDA Chief Counsel Resigns"), he worked as a "friend of the court" on cases in which pharmaceutical companies had been sued for drug-safety problems. The logic was that the FDA had approved the drug and therefore had an interest in the outcome.

Finding Answers

If you are like many Americans who are prescribed a drug or who love someone who has been, you hop online to research and read about it (and the circumstances that warranted the prescription in the first place) and spend many frustrating hours coming up with little useful information. Worse, you may unwittingly be accessing information on the Internet that is not medically sound or that is just anecdotal. In fact, research shows that one out of four medical-information Web sites offers information that is inaccurate or misleading, and only one out of five is authored by identifiable medical experts.

The book on every doctor's shelf, the *Physicians' Desk Reference (PDR)*, provides detailed information about drug side effects and drug interactions, but it is based on product inserts that go into packages of drugs the FDA has approved. New information obtained on the millions of patients treated with drugs after they have reached the market is *not* incorporated into annual versions of the *PDR*. Since most of the consumer reference books on drugs are simply over-the-counter versions of the *PDR*, these books also do not include data on the millions of people who take the drug after it has reached the market.

Before You Take That Pill provides more information about side effects than other books because I have included information that was collected *after* a drug was put on the market as well as before the drug came to market but that was not widely reported. In addition, for each of the most commonly prescribed drugs, this book provides a short history of how it came to market so that you can learn as much as possible about it.

My book also includes information on the safety of certain vitamins and supplements, since research has shown that some vitamins and supplements pose serious safety hazards that you may be unaware of. We have been overindulgent in our endorsement of the makers of vitamins and supplements, especially those companies that promote their products as healthy alternatives to prescription medications. Many doctors take a hands-off approach to vitamins in the belief that if they don't do any harm, it's okay to take them.

However, vitamins and supplements can and do indeed cause harm. Unfortunately, the government has contributed to the misinformation concerning vitamins and supplements. The U.S. Department of Agriculture (USDA), whose job it is to promote the interests of agriculture (i.e., producers of food) and not health, regulates foods and beverages. Vitamins and supplements are classified as foods, not drugs. Lobbyists for the vitamin and supplement industry have blocked efforts by the Department of Health and Human Services (DHHS), the federal agency responsible for health, to get involved.

The USDA's Recommended Daily Allowance (RDA) of vitamins and minerals has been great for the vitamin and supplement industry as well as for cereal makers, who supercharge their sales by adding vitamins and minerals to breakfast foods and then convincing customers they need to eat these fortified products to get their minimal daily requirements of vitamins and minerals. This is despite the fact that there is no way to get enough of the recommended vitamins and minerals from normal food without overeating. Government recommendations are actually four times higher than what a person really needs. I will tell you later why you *don't* need extra vitamins and that if you stick with fresh fruit and vegetables and other whole foods, you will stay healthy. I will tell you why those making big money on vitamins and supplements are doing so at the expense of your pocketbook—and sometimes your life.

All this is not to say that many medications have not changed life for the better, particularly those that treat infections. However, ironically, most recent health gains have come through increased knowledge of health risks and better health practices (i.e. prevention). We smoke less, have better access to nutritious fruits and vegetables year-round, pay more attention to cleanliness and hygiene, and have improved safety in general. For instance, in the nineteenth century it was not known that dirty water and shared cups could spread disease. Hand washing is still the single most powerful way to prevent the spread of communicable disease, but this was not discovered until 1847, when Ignaz Semmelweis, a young Viennese doctor in an obstetrics ward, observed that midwives who washed their hands had lower mortality rates among their patients than did doctors, who often went from autopsy room to delivery ward without so much as a hand wipe.

Future advances in health will likely come more from changes in lifestyle, diet, and exercise than from medications. Almost all of the conditions for which pills are prescribed that I discuss here are preventable through such changes. Other conditions, like cancer, are partially preventable. However, cancer medications and those for acutely life-threatening conditions like heart attacks are beyond the scope of this book. Instead I have focused on those drugs that are used by the largest number of people and thus have the most potential to cause unnecessary harm.

My Research Approach

Rather than take a random approach to drug safety, I have systematically reviewed information found in hundreds of articles in the medical literature with a very critical and keen eye. I have focused on the major and most respected and reliable journals, including *The New England Journal of Medicine*, *The Journal of the American Medical Association*, *British Medical Journal*, and *The Lancet*.

I have read and analyzed all of the articles in these journals as well as editorials and news articles (*British Medical Journal* is the best for medical news reporting) for information relevant to drug safety. Following footnotes and leads from articles in these journals to other research and reports, I have drilled deeply into drug research and outcomes. In addition, I have reviewed investigative reporting in the *New York Times* and the *Los Angeles Times* relevant to drug-safety issues. Where appropriate, I have consulted colleagues in specific areas of expertise. I have also reviewed five hundred of the most commonly prescribed medications to make sure that I have included all the medications that will be most relevant to the vast majority of medication users. I have synthesized and described research results in detail in this book, and I have tried to be as straightforward as possible so that you can understand what credible research says about drug risks.

The drugs in this book represent the most treated conditions in the country. I have organized this book by the number of drug prescriptions written, starting with the most frequent and ending with the least prescribed of those drugs that are most commonly used. Vitamins and supplements are included at the end, and I have also covered the topic of children and medicine. The chapters themselves have been organized by classes of drugs (which have similar risk factors) prescribed for certain health conditions. Organizing material by drugs typically prescribed for these conditions will help you compare different drugs prescribed for the same condition.

Understand that my goal is not to warn you off taking drugs, vitamins, or supplements but rather to give you all the information you need but cannot necessarily acquire from reading the package or from talking to your doctor so you can make an informed decision. There may be some drugs that are risky, and at the end of each chapter I summarize the medications discussed in order of risk, from lowest to highest. You and your doctor may decide that some risks are worth the benefits in your case.

My hope is that this book causes you to rethink the role of medications and other pills in your life in relation to other actions you can take to maximize your health, such as making changes in your diet; incorporating exercise into your daily routine; learning and using stress-reduction techniques; and changing other behaviors like quitting smoking. The most common disorders, like diabetes and heart disease, are often better treated and prevented through changes in diet, exercise, and lifestyle than they are with medication. Pharmaceuticals can be lifesaving for some conditions, such as insulin for type I diabetes, thyroid hormone for hypothyroidism, and antibiotics for life-threatening infections. All of this has been illustrated by several scientific studies that I discuss in this book. Before you take that pill, consider taking charge of your health by making informed decisions and smart changes in your lifestyle. In some cases, however, you may need medications to prevent or treat a disease or to help you with troubling symptoms or disabilities. In those cases I want you to know as much as you can about the risks and benefits. I hope this book helps you do that.

To your health!

2.

Arthritis Medications

One night a few years ago I was watching television when a commercial came on that caught my attention. An older but very attractive woman pirouetted across a skating rink as cheerful, up-tempo music swelled around her. Three Dog Night's rock classic "Celebrate, Celebrate!" urged her on to ever more acrobatic moves. Next, the words *Celebrex* and *Ask your doctor* appeared on the screen, and with them the promise of the happiness and vitality that I, along with millions of baby boomers, fantasize about. The ad conjured up a lovely picture. Unfortunately, it turned out that the side effects of Celebrex (celecoxib) and those of similar drugs—Vioxx (rofecoxib) and Bextra (valdecoxib)—called COX-2 inhibitors left many osteoarthritis sufferers who took them skating on thin ice.

COX-2 inhibitors are prescribed primarily to fight the pain and stiffness that accompanies osteoarthritis, a painful and disabling condition that affects 20 million people in the U.S. Osteoarthritis is caused by the destruction of cartilage in the joints that increases with age and is exacerbated or triggered by physical injury or wear and tear. It's a dreadful ailment that truly does limit sufferers from the potential joys of activities like knitting, walking, or golf, let alone gliding across a frozen pond on razor-thin blades.

So I can't blame anyone who has joint disease from seeking pharmaceutical solutions, which do exist but must be used and chosen with caution.

Vioxx and Friends

It's worth spending some time looking at the stories of two COX-2 inhibitors that have been taken off the market, Vioxx and Bextra, as they help put in perspective the drugs still available (Celebrex, which I discuss later, is still available.) The stories of these drugs are also prime examples of why and how a rush to market can have devastating effects on the consumer.

Before Vioxx and its sister medications were developed, many people suffering from joint disease managed the accompanying pain and other symptoms by taking one of several nonsteroidal anti-inflammatory drugs (NSAIDS—pronounced *en*-saids) with familiar names like ibuprofen (Advil, Motrin), indomethacin (Indocin), meloxicam (Mobic), diclofenac (Cataflam, Voltaren), nabumetone (Relafen), and naproxen (Aleve, Naprosyn, Naprelan, Anaprox). These first NSAIDS inhibit the cyclo-oxygenase-1 (COX-1) and cyclooxygenase-2 (COX-2) enzymes that are responsible for the synthesis of prostaglandins, which promote inflammation and can exacerbate conditions like rheumatoid arthritis.

Vioxx and Celebrex, also NSAIDS but ones that target the COX-2 enzymes more specifically, were developed for two reasons. The first was to create a new group of (expensive) patented drugs to replace the older NSAIDS that had gone off patent and became available inexpensively and over the counter. As I outlined in Chapter 1, pharmaceutical companies do not make a lot of money from a drug once it becomes generic; they stay in business, keep market share, and grow profits by constantly developing new drugs that can be sold at significantly higher prices while under patent.

The second reason for developing these medications was that the drug companies wanted to find medications that eliminated the gastrointestinal bleeding, a serious complication for many patients, associated with the older NSAIDS. Ironically, the first group of nonspecific NSAIDS was thought to be a better alternative to drugs like aspirin, which fell out of a favor as a treatment because they too are associated with gastrointestinal bleeding. Numerous studies have shown that regular, long-term use of the older NSAIDS not only can cause bleeding but also may lead to a host of other unpleasant side effects such as diarrhea, nausea, vomiting, stomach upset, and loss of appetite. Less commonly, they can affect kidney or liver function.

So when the specific COX-2 inhibitors hit the market, it looked like they had none of the negatives of ibuprofen and naproxen and would be more effective at reducing discomfort and pain. Well, it turned out that these "cutting edge" medications had three significant downsides.

- *Cost:* About $3,000 per year, ten times as much as over-the-counter naproxen.
- *Efficacy:* COX-2 inhibitors are no more effective for pain relief than nonspecific NSAIDS *or* aspirin.
- *Side effects:* COX-2s have even nastier (and in some cases fatal) side effects than those listed for older NSAIDS. While they may not cause stomach bleeding, they do seem to cause the most heart attacks, probably by increasing blood clotting. People with preexisting heart disease are most at risk.

Despite these facts, early enthusiasm from drug companies for these drugs and the apparent low risk of taking them got them pushed through the FDA approval process and onto the market quickly and with little information about their long-term risks. Study results published after the drugs were made available to the public, however, showed that more careful attention should have been given to them before approval was given.

Consider the results of the Vioxx GI Outcomes Research study (VIGOR; 2000), which was completed after Vioxx was approved by the FDA.[1] Eight thousand seventy-six patients with osteoarthritis over the age of fifty were randomly given either Vioxx or naproxen. Though there was half as much gastrointestinal bleeding in the Vioxx patients as there was in the naproxen group, there was a fourfold increased risk of heart attack in the Vioxx users.

The study's authors argued that the increase in heart attacks among the Vioxx patients was attributable to the fact that naproxen had heart-protective effects. The study rationalized these findings by saying that if the Vioxx test subjects had taken aspirin as a preventative measure, they wouldn't have had a heart attack. However, the authors neglected to point out that by taking aspirin, the patients would have lost the protection against stomach bleeding, Vioxx's chief selling point!

It was four years later, in 2004, when a study was conducted to see if Vioxx (rofecoxib) could prevent the recurrence of colon cancers, that the drug's associated risk of heart attack attracted the attention of researchers and the media. The Adenomatous Polyp Prevention on Vioxx (APPROVe) trial studied 2,586 patients with a history of colorectal adenomas who randomly received either rofecoxib or a placebo for three years.

Forty-six patients on rofecoxib had a thrombotic event (i.e., stroke or heart attack) vs. twenty-six patients in the placebo group—twice as many.[2] The risk became apparent after only eighteen months of treatment. There was also a fourfold increase in heart failure in the Vioxx subjects, most likely related to a Vioxx-caused increase in their blood pressure. It turns out that COX-2 inhibitors block the production of prostacyclin (a member of the family of lipid molecules known as eicosanoids) without affecting synthesis of another compound called thromboxane A-2. This in turn leads to a depression of prostaglandin I-2, a compound that increases blood pressure as well as the ability of blood to clot, which leads to more heart attacks and strokes.

The ADVANTAGE study (Assessment of Differences between Vioxx and Naproxen to Ascertain Gastrointestinal Tolerability and Effectiveness) randomized 5,557 patients with arthritis to Vioxx or naproxyn.[3] As reported in the *New York Times* on April 24, 2005, by Alex Berenson ("Evidence in Vioxx Suits Shows Intervention by Merck Officials"), the publication of the study results in 2003 reported five cardiac deaths in patients taking Vioxx vs. one in patients taking naproxen. The article reported that in an e-mail exchange from 2000, Merck officials pressured a company scientist to not determine that the death of a patient was cardiac related "so that we don't raise concerns." However, the FDA had reviewed the study results in 2001 and determined that in this case (and those of two others reported in the paper) the deaths were cardiac related, making the increase in cardiac deaths a statistically significant increase of eight with Vioxx compared to one with naproxen. The fact that none of the patients in the study had preexisting heart disease (unlike many people in the real world who suffer from arthritis) makes the increase in cardiac events with Vioxx all the more remarkable. Why the FDA did not release its conclusions about Vioxx and the risk of heart attacks until 2005 is unclear.

Following the publication of the APPROVe trial and the belated admission of increased heart attacks in ADVANTAGE, Merck announced in September 2004 that it would pull Vioxx from the market, but not before considerable damage had been done. It has been estimated that Vioxx caused 88,000 to 139,000 heart attacks, with 30% to 40% of them fatal.[4]

The COX-2 inhibitor Bextra was supposed to have more advantages than Vioxx in the treatment of osteoarthritis. The drug's manufacturer, Pfizer, argued that Bextra should have a lower risk of heart attacks than Vioxx. This claim has not been supported by research. In fact, Nussmeier and colleagues studied 1,671 patients randomized to parecoxib (Dynastat, a COX-2 inhibitor that is given intravenously to surgical patients) or valdecoxib (i.e., Bextra). Patients with parecoxib or valdecoxib showed a 3.7-fold increase in heart attack or stroke.[5] Curt Furberg, Bruce Patsy, and Garret Fitzgerald analyzed data from this study along with data made available by the FDA and also found a greater than threefold increased risk of heart attack and stroke.[6] After these studies were published, Pfizer initially argued with the results. Nevertheless, on October 14, 2004, as reported in the *New York Times* on October 16, 2004 (Reed Abelson, "Pfizer Warns of Risks from Its Painkiller"), it sent a 'Dear Doctor' letter to health-care professionals warning of the possible risk of heart attack with Bextra.

Bextra also has been associated with rare occurrences of Stevens-Johnson syndrome, a potentially fatal condition involving blistering all over the skin, mouth, and eyes. This and other problems led FDA whistle-blower Dr. David Graham to cite Bextra as one of the five most dangerous drugs on the market in November 2004. In January 2005 insurer Kaiser Permanente took Bextra off its formulary, reasoning that the risks of the drug outweighed the benefits. Under a storm of controversy Pfizer finally pulled the drug from the market in April 2005.

Celebrex (or celecoxib, the generic name), marketed by Pfizer and Pharmacia, is a COX-2 inhibitor still on the market in the U.S. In 2000, a large review of the drug, called the Celecoxib Long-term Arthritis Safety Study (CLASS), which was published in the *Journal of the American Medical Association*, reported a 50% reduction of ulcers and stomach bleeding with celecoxib as compared to NSAIDS.[7] Patients taking aspirin lost the protection afforded by Celebrex. This study looked at one year of treatment, but only the results found after six months were published. Based on data released to the FDA, it was later discovered that in the second six months there had been an increase in heart attack risk. The editor of the journal, Catherine DeAngelis, M.D., was understandably perturbed when she learned after the fact about this deliberate attempt to withhold such important information and expressed her disapproval in an editorial in her journal.

Findings that suggested an increased risk of heart attack with COX-2 inhibitors brought more attention to this question and prompted further research. Scientists working on the Adenoma Prevention with Celecoxib (APC) study, which was designed to see if Celebrex (celecoxib) could prevent recurrent adenomas of the colon in patients with a history of colonic adenomas at high risk for the development of colon cancer, looked at the safety of Celebrex in relation to heart attacks. For this study, published in 2005, 2,035 patients with a history of colorectal adenomas were examined. Patients were randomized to two doses of celecoxib or placebo in order to assess the ability of celecoxib to prevent cancer. Patients on celecoxib showed a 2.3-fold increased risk of stroke, heart attack, or heart failure with 400 mg of Celebrex a day and a 3.4-fold increase with 800 mg of

Celebrex a day.[8] There was also a threefold increase in death from heart disease or stroke at the highest dose. This study suggested that there was a dose-response effect, i.e., the higher the dose, the greater the risk. Celebrex was effective, however, in reducing the recurrence of adenomas.[9]

Another cancer-prevention trial, published in 2006, was the Prevention of Colorectal Sporadic Adenomatous Polyps (PreSAP). In this study 1,561 patients who had had an adenoma removed from their colon and were at high risk of recurrence were assigned to celecoxib or placebo for three years. At three years, there was a significant reduction in the recurrence of polyps in the celecoxib group vs. placebo (34% vs. 49%) as well as 30% more cardiovascular events with celecoxib, an increase that was not considered statistically significant. However, there was a significant doubling of cardiovascular events in patients on celecoxib who were not taking aspirin.[10]

Overall, COX-2 inhibitors are not recommended for cancer prevention in patients who do not have familial polyposis (even those with polyps found on routine colonoscopy) since polyps do not necessarily proceed to gastrointestinal cancer, and people on a coxib are five times more likely to have a cardiac event as they are to develop gastrointestinal cancer if they don't take a coxib.

A study completed by Pfizer in 1999 that was never published and was not posted on the Internet until 2004 randomized 425 patients to 400 mg of Celebrex a day or a placebo for one year for the prevention of Alzheimer's disease. Thirteen out of 285 (4.6%) patients on Celebrex died compared to 4 out of 140 (2.9%) on placebo. There was a greater than twofold increase in heart attacks, arrhythmias, heart failure, and/or cerebrovascular events with Celebrex.[11]

Despite the known problems and risks associated with COX-2 inhibitors and the fact that several have been pulled from the market, drug companies continue to develop new versions. One of the most recent is lumiracoxib (Prexige) (which is likely to have been approved by the FDA and to have reached the shelves by the time you are reading this book), a drug developed by Novartis that has been specifically assessed for heart-attack risk in comparison to naproxen and ibuprofen in the Therapeutic

Arthritis Research and Gastrointestinal Event Trial (TARGET). In this study, 18,325 patients over the age of fifty who had osteoarthritis were randomly given lumiracoxib, ibuprofen, or naproxen for one year. Sixty-four patients on NSAIDS had gastrointestinal bleeding vs. fourteen on lumiracoxib, a significant reduction.[12]

The lumiracoxib patients were twice as likely to experience a heart attack as those on naproxen (but not ibuprofen) who were not taking aspirin.[13] Overall there was a 35% increase in heart attacks with lumiracoxib as compared to naproxen and ibuprofen, which was not statistically significant. Remember, however, that the study lasted only twelve months. It took 18 months of Vioxx treatment for the increased risk of heart attack to emerge. Most patients with heart disease were excluded from this study of Prexige, which is unlike the real world, where up to 40% of patients with arthritis also have heart disease or other significant risk factors. Lumiracoxib (Prexige) was also associated with a fourfold increase in elevated liver enzymes, indicating liver damage.

In 2006 a review of COX-2 inhibitor safety from studies performed up to that time found a significant risk of cardiac events across the spectrum of COX-2 drugs.[14] Overall there was a statistically significant 42% increase in vascular events and an 86% increase in heart attacks. The risks of taking COX-2 drugs were double that of taking naproxen. Diclofenac was also associated with a statistically significant 63% increase in the risk of vascular events. Naproxen had no risk, and ibuprofen had a 51% increase, which was not statistically significant.

Problems with the COX-2 inhibitors have led many physicians to conclude that they shouldn't be used at all.[15] Many have gone back to recommending tried-and-true remedies such as NSAIDS. As I explained earlier in the chapter, these medications, including ibuprofen (Motrin, Advil) and naproxen (Naprosyn, Aleve), are sold over the counter and therefore don't need a doctor's prescription. They are, however, associated with stomach bleeding, which is why it may be good to take a medication like Prilosec with them (see Chapter 9). Another alternative to COX-2 inhibitors for pain relief is enteric-coated aspirin or acetaminophen (Tylenol). Given the risk of heart attack and the lack of superior reduction of pain with the COX-2 inhibitors, I do not recommend them for use in most cases; I recommend aspirin or the over-the-counter (OTC) NSAIDS combined with OTC Prilosec.

Alternatives

At this point you may be thinking that there's little that can be done to keep the pain of osteoarthritis at bay. That's not true; for some people aspirin, acetaminophen (Tylenol), and NSAIDS are very effective in treating the acute pain of osteoarthritis over short periods of time. What follows is a discussion of alternative treatments and my assessment of their efficacy. Discuss these options with your health-care provider.

CORTICOSTEROID INJECTIONS

Other traditional treatments, such as corticosteroid injections, can reduce pain and increase function in those suffering from joint disease. Corticosteroids (glucocorticoids) are drugs related to cortisol and include betamethasone (Celestone), budesonide (Entocort, EC), cortisone (Cortone), dexamethasone (Decadron), hydrocortisone (Cortef), methylprednisolone (Medrol), prednisolone (Prelone), prednisone (Deltasone), and triamcinolone (Kenalog). Cortisol, a hormone naturally produced in the adrenal cortex, has a number of effects, including the inhibition of inflammation. Corticosteroids have side effects of their own, and injections should not be administered more than twice a year to prevent damage to cartilage. For example, injection of corticosteroids can produce symptoms that are similar to those of Cushing's disease (overproduction of cortisol). These include deposits of fat on the upper back and face, high blood pressure, diabetes, slow wound healing, osteoporosis, cataracts, acne, muscle weakness, ulcers, thinning of the skin, and mood changes. All commercial preparations of corticosteroids potentially have these side effects.

NATURAL ALTERNATIVES

There are several natural remedies available for arthritis; some work better than others. If you have rheumatoid arthritis (RA) or other types of arthritis besides osteoarthritis, natural remedies are limited in their ability to halt the progression of the disease, and pharmacological solutions may be the most effective.

However, for those of you who have been diagnosed with osteoarthritis, two popular natural arthritis remedies, glucosamine and chondroitin, may help. But if you don't have osteoarthritis there is no evidence that these over-the-counter products prevent the development of osteoarthritis or reduce aches and pains unrelated to osteoarthritis, in spite of the claims of the manufacturers of vitamins and supplements.

Glucosamine is derived from the shells of crabs and oysters and is widely promoted as a natural substance for the treatment of arthritis and joint pain. Glucosamine is considered a precursor of proteoglycans, which are thought to be instrumental in helping cartilage retain water and in promoting formation of an elastic layer that may improve the functional characteristics of cartilage.

Chondroitin is a product derived from the cartilage of sharks and cows that is promoted for use in the prevention of arthritis and the treatment of joint pain. Often combined with glucosamine, it is sold in health-food stores. Chondroitin stimulates the production of proteoglycans and hyaluronic acid and inhibits proteolytic enzymes, which destroy cartilage. Chondroitin and glucosamine are often given in combination for osteoarthritis.

Most of the earlier studies of glucosamine and chondroitin were performed by manufacturers and were not well controlled.[16] In 2000 a meta-analysis of studies of glucosamine and chondroitin found that the studies that were funded by supplement manufacturers resulted in more favorable results for the supplement combo than did independent studies; few of the manufacturers' studies were properly controlled. Overall there was a moderate effect for both, and the authors concluded that some degree of efficacy was probable.[17]

Only one of the studies reviewed in 2000 reported that patients definitely did not know whether they were being given a supplement or a placebo. In that study, 252 patients with osteoarthritis of the knee were randomly assigned to receive four weeks of glucosamine or placebo. Glucosamine was associated with a drop in pain ratings from 10.6 to 7.5 vs. 10.6 to 8.4 with placebo, and 52% of glucosamine patients had a clinically significant change as measured by a 3-point drop on an index of arthritis severity compared to 37% of those on placebo, differences that were statistically significant.

More recently several randomized placebo-controlled trials have been performed. In one study 212 patients with osteoarthritis of the knee were assigned to placebo or glucosamine for three years of treatment. Patients on placebo had a greater narrowing of the disk space in the knee than did those on glucosamine as measured by X-ray (– .31 mm vs. – .06 mm). Glucosamine patients experienced an improvement in pain ratings significantly greater than that of those on placebo. Glucosamine produced no increase in side effects compared to placebo.[18]

In another study 98 males with osteoarthritis of the knee were assigned to glucosamine or placebo for two months of treatment. There was no difference in pain ratings between patients treated with glucosamine (3.3) and those with placebo (3.5).[19] Glucosamine was also associated with more side effects, including loose stools, nausea, heartburn, and headache.

Another study randomized 202 patients with osteoarthritis of the knee to three years of treatment with glucosamine or placebo. Placebo-treated patients had a greater degree of joint-space narrowing as measured by X-ray than those treated with glucosamine (– .19 mm vs. + .04 mm). There were statistically significant greater reductions in measures of pain self-ratings (– 2 vs. – 1.3) as well as measures of stiffness and function for the glucosamine group. One randomized placebo-controlled study showed a glucosamine-chondroitin combination to be more effective than placebo.[20]

In 2006 a large, well-controlled study assigned 1,583 patients with osteoarthritis of the knee to glucosamine, chondroitin, a glucosamine/chondroitin combination, celecoxib, or placebo for six months of treatment. A positive treatment outcome was defined as a 20% change in knee-pain severity. Sixty percent of placebo patients responded to treatment vs. 67% of glucosamine/chondroitin patients, a difference that was not statistically significant. Celecoxib had a 70% response, which was statistically significantly better than that of placebo. A subgroup of patients with moderate to severe pain at baseline did significantly better with glucosamine/chondroitin than with placebo (79% response vs. 54%).[21] In summary, the glucosamine/chondroitin combination shows some efficacy for treatment of osteoarthritis.

Ginger (*Zingiber officinale*), a natural remedy obtained from the root of the ginger flower that is used in Ayurvedic medicine for the treatment of inflammation and rheumatism, is thought to have anti-inflammatory properties. There is no evidence that the ginger contained in supplements is superior to fresh ginger from the grocery store or ginger tea. Ginger has no side effects, so if you want to use it there are no reasons not to. A recent treatment study of patients with osteoarthritis showed that ginger actually worked better at reducing inflammation than ibuprofen, but there was no difference when it was tested against a placebo.[22]

DIET AND BEHAVIOR

One of the most common causes of osteoarthritis is obesity. Another common cause is a history of joint injury. Carrying around unnaturally large amounts of weight puts undue strain on the joints and cartilage of the body. The most important thing you can do for your joint pain if you are overweight is to lose weight. Also sports injuries early in life have a tendency to spur osteoarthritis in later life. Based on this information you should think twice about pushing kids, especially reluctant ones, onto the playing field. In spite of popular myths to the contrary, there is no evidence that sports like running increase the risk for osteoarthritis.

Rheumatoid Arthritis

Rheumatoid arthritis (RA) is an autoimmune disease that causes chronic inflammation of the joints in people both young and old. RA can also cause inflammation of the tissue around the joints and organs in the body. RA is a chronic illness, meaning it can last for years, and people with RA may go for long periods without any symptoms. However, RA is a progressive illness with the potential to cause joint destruction and functional disability. Aspirin and NSAIDs are the safest medications for treating the symptoms of RA if it is not aggressively progressing. Acetaminophen (Tylenol) is antifever and antipain but not anti-inflammatory, and will not battle the inflammation of RA (although it is an effective first line of treatment for osteoarthritis, which does not involve as much inflammation as RA).

DISEASE-MODIFYING ANTIRHEUMATIC DRUGS

If aspirin or NSAIDs fail to control the pain of RA, additional medication therapy may be required. This may involve disease-modifying antirheumatic drugs (DMARDs), very powerful medications that have potentially dangerous side effects. DMARDs should be used with great caution and under medical supervision, and only if aspirin and NSAIDs have failed to help and the RA is definitely progressing. DMARDs have many potentially toxic side effects that have not been highlighted by their manufacturers relative to their reputed benefits. You need to understand the true potential toxicity of these medications before you start to take them. As always, it is a question of balancing the risks and benefits.

Methotrexate (Rheumatrex), a DMARD that is a powerful cancer drug approved for RA, inhibits all cellular processes, including the inflammatory processes that underlie RA progression. Methotrexate can therefore result in suppression of the bone marrow. Because of this risk, patients need to undergo frequent monitoring with blood tests; patients who are unwilling to do so should not take this drug. It should be understood that methotrexate is a major toxin that is used primarily for cancer patients as a last resort.

Penicillamine (Cuprimine), a derivative of penicillin that is also used to treat RA, acts by inhibiting the immune system. It can cause skin lesions and, like the other RA drugs, bone-marrow suppression. Any drug that inhibits the immune system can be very dangerous, since we need our immune system to fight off infections. There are some contraindications with this medication, including penicillin allergy, pregnancy, breast-feeding, liver or kidney disorder, or gold-salt treatment. Another drug, leflunomide (Arava), also acts to inhibit the immune system. Side effects include rash, nausea, hair loss, hypertension, stomach upset, and, more rarely, liver dysfunction.

Auranofin (Ridaura), gold salts taken orally or injected, inhibit inflammation and thus delay the progression of RA by a poorly understood mechanism. Because gold salts have a number of noxious effects, including skin pigmentation and a rare but potentially fatal possibility of bone-marrow suppression, in which counts of red blood cells, white blood cells, and platelets decrease, they should be considered a last resort. Gold salts should never be used by patients with kidney disease, Sjogren's syndrome, systemic lupus erythematosis (SLE), congestive heart failure (CHF), hypertension (HTN), urticaria, colitis, or gold sensitivity or by women who are pregnant or breast-feeding.

TUMOR NECROSIS FACTOR (TNF) INHIBITORS

Tumor necrosis factor (TNF) inhibitors, including etanercept (Enbrel), have more recently reached the market as a gentler alternative to DMARDs in treating RA. For instance, they do not have as much potential for extreme toxicity as methotrexate, which can cause bone-marrow suppression, shutting off production of blood cells, a potentially fatal side effect. They act by suppressing the immune system and thus can increase susceptibility to cancer and infections. Other side effects include headache and abdominal pain.

The bottom line is that, as it currently stands, RA is a disease that is relentlessly progressive and that can be slowed but not stopped with currently available medications. The medications that are effective in slowing the advance of RA have a number of potentially toxic side effects. I can't give specific advice about what to take, but you should be aware of the potential toxicities of these drugs and work with your doctor to find the best path forward.

Medications for Low-Back Pain

Low-back pain is a disabling condition that affects a large number of people in the U.S. Causes of low-back pain can include but are not limited to dislocation of the vertebral discs. The so-called muscle-relaxing drugs used in the treatment of low-back pain, which include carisoprodol (Soma), chlorzoxazone (Parafon), cyclobenzaprine (Flexeril), methocarbamol (Robaxin), and orphenadrine (Norflex), can cause drowsiness, dizziness, loss of appetite, vomiting, and diarrhea. Muscle relaxants have not been shown to be superior to NSAIDs for the relief of low-back pain. These drugs are promoted as medications that relax the back muscles that contribute to low-back pain. However, these medications act on the brain rather than the muscles to cause relaxation. In other words, they are sedatives. Since they do not do what they purport to do, I don't recommend using them.

The Bottom Line

I do not recommend that anyone use COX-2 inhibitors ever. If you have arthritis pain I recommend medications that are sold over the counter and therefore don't require a doctor's prescription, including ibuprofen (Motrin,

Advil) and naproxen (Naprosyn, Aleve). Because these medications can be associated with stomach bleeding, it is advisable to take a medication like Prilosec with them (see Chapter 9). Another alternative to COX-2 inhibitors for pain relief is enteric-coated aspirin or acetaminophen (Tylenol). For rheumatoid arthritis there are unfortunately no silver bullets. You will have to see what medication treatment strategy works for you. For low-back pain I do not recommend using medication. And remember that the best treatment for arthritis is prevention. Exercise regularly but avoid contact sports like football that lead to injuries that can cause osteoarthritis to develop in later years.

Drug	Use	Common, Benign Side Effects	Serious Side Effects	Life-threatening Side Effects	Reasons Not to Take
Osteoarthritis Medications					
Salicylates					
Moderate Risk					
Acetylsalicylic Acid (Aspirin)	Pain, fever	Nausea, vomiting, diarrhea, loss of appetite, headache, dizziness	Stomach upset, edema	Stomach bleeding, liver damage, kidney damage	Children with febrile illness; history of stomach ulcers, liver or kidney disease, pregnancy
Para-Amenophinol Derivatives					
Low Risk					
Acetaminophen (Tylenol)	Pain, fever	Nausea, vomiting, diarrhea, loss of appetite, headache, dizziness	Stomach upset, edema	Stomach bleeding, liver damage, kidney damage	History of stomach ulcers, liver or kidney disease, pregnancy

Drug	Use	Common, Benign Side Effects	Serious Side Effects	Life-threatening Side Effects	Reasons Not to Take
Nonsteroidal Anti-Inflammatory Drugs (NSAIDs)					
Moderate Risk					
Ibuprofen (Advil, Motrin)	Arthritis pain	Nausea, vomiting, diarrhea, loss of appetite, headache, dizziness	Stomach upset, edema	Stomach bleeding, liver damage, kidney damage, heart attack, stroke, severe rash (SJS)	History of stomach ulcers, liver or kidney disease, heart disease, pregnancy
Indomethacin (Indocin)	Arthritis pain	Nausea, vomiting, diarrhea, loss of appetite, headache, dizziness	Stomach upset	Stomach bleeding, liver damage, kidney damage	History of stomach ulcers, liver or kidney disease
Meloxicam (Mobic)	Arthritis pain	Nausea, vomiting, diarrhea, loss of appetite, headache, dizziness	Stomach upset	Stomach bleeding, liver damage, kidney damage	History of stomach ulcers, liver or kidney disease
Diclofenac (Cataflam, Voltaren)	Arthritis pain	Nausea, vomiting, diarrhea, loss of appetite, headache, dizziness	Stomach upset	Stomach bleeding, liver damage, kidney damage	History of stomach ulcers, liver or kidney disease
Nabumetone (Relafen)	Arthritis pain	Nausea, vomiting, diarrhea, loss of appetite, headache, dizziness	Stomach upset	Stomach bleeding, liver damage, kidney damage	History of stomach ulcers, liver or kidney disease
Naproxen (Aleve, Naprosyn, Naprelan, Anaprox)	Arthritis pain	Nausea, vomiting, diarrhea, loss of appetite, headache, dizziness	Stomach upset	Stomach bleeding, liver damage, kidney damage	History of stomach ulcers, liver or kidney disease

Drug	Use	Common, Benign Side Effects	Serious Side Effects	Life-threatening Side Effects	Reasons Not to Take
COX-2 Inhibitors					
High Risk					
Celecoxib (Celebrex)	Arthritis pain	Constipation, reflux, flushes, nausea, vomiting, diarrhea, loss of appetite, headache, dizziness	High blood pressure, migraine, stomach upset	Heart attacks, strokes, stomach bleeding, heart failure, heart arrhythmias	History of heart disease
Lumiracoxib (Prexige)	Arthritis pain	Constipation, reflux, flushes, nausea, vomiting, diarrhea, loss of appetite, headache, dizziness	High blood pressure, migraine, stomach upset	Heart attack, liver damage	History of heart disease
Rheumatoid Arthritis Medications					
Tumor Necrosis Factor (TNF) Inhibitors					
Moderate Risk					
Etanercept (Enbrel)	Rheumatoid arthritis	Headache, nausea, dizziness, cough, rash	Stomach pain	Infections, multiple sclerosis (rare), loss of blood cells	Hyper-sensitivity, active infection, anemia, heart failure
Disease-Modifying Antirheumatic Drugs (DMARDs)					
High Risk					
Methotrexate (Rheumatrex)	Rheumatoid arthritis	Sore throat, stomach pain, nausea, vomiting	Bruising, fever, chills	Bone-marrow suppression, stomach ulcer, hepatic fibrosis, pneumonitis, allergic reaction	Pregnancy, lactation, liver disease, unwilling-ness to undergo repeated blood tests

Drug	Use	Common, Benign Side Effects	Serious Side Effects	Life-threatening Side Effects	Reasons Not to Take
Penicillamine (Cuprimine)	Rheumatoid arthritis	Rash, nausea, vomiting	Skin lesions, stomach pain, diarrhea	Bone-marrow suppression, myasthenia gravis (rare), ulcers, liver dysfunction	Penicillin allergy, pregnancy, breast-feeding, liver or kidney disorder, gold-salt treatment
Leflunomide (Arava)	Rheumatoid arthritis	Rash, nausea	Hair loss, hypertension, stomach upset	Liver dysfunction, respiratory infection	Liver dysfunction, hepatitis, pregnancy
Gold Compounds					
High Risk					
Auranofin (Ridaura)	Rheumatoid arthritis	Nausea, vomiting, rash, skin pigment change	Diarrhea, stomach pain	Fatal bone-marrow suppression, renal damage (rare)	Sjogren's Syndrome, SLE, CHF, HTN, urticaria, colitis, gold sensitivity, pregnancy, breast-feeding; in general use only as last resort
Gold sodium thiomalate (Myocrisin)	Rheumatoid arthritis	Skin redness	Loss of skin	Loss of platelets and blood cells, kidney damage	History of kidney or blood disorder, gold sensitivity, pregnancy, breast-feeding; in general use only as last resort

Drug	Use	Common, Benign Side Effects	Serious Side Effects	Life-threatening Side Effects	Reasons Not to Take
Low-Back Pain Muscle Relaxers					
Moderate Risk					
Carisoprodol (Soma)	Low-back pain	Drowsiness, dizziness, loss of appetite, vomiting, diarrhea	Memory loss, blurred vision	Confusion, coma (overdose)	Not recommended
Chlorzoxazone (Parafon)	Low-back pain	Drowsiness, dizziness, loss of appetite, vomiting, diarrhea	Memory loss, blurred vision	Confusion, coma (overdose)	Not recommended
Cyclobenzaprine (Flexeril)	Low-back pain	Drowsiness, dizziness, loss of appetite, vomiting, diarrhea	Memory loss, blurred vision	Confusion, coma (overdose)	Not recommended
Methocarbamol (Robaxin)	Low-back pain	Drowsiness, dizziness, loss of appetite, vomiting, diarrhea	Memory loss, blurred vision	Confusion, coma (overdose)	Not recommended
Orphenadrine (Norflex)	Low-back pain	Drowsiness, dizziness, loss of appetite, vomiting, diarrhea	Memory loss, blurred vision	Confusion, coma (overdose)	Not recommended

3.

Acne Treatments

Acne is a troubling disorder that at its worst is associated with considerable facial disfigurement and scarring and at its best with embarrassing and annoying outbreaks and inflammation. It's also the most common skin condition in the U.S., affecting 17 million people. Eighty-five percent of the population gets acne in young adulthood. For most, the condition clears up by the age of thirty. Acne is caused by blockage of the pores leading from the sebaceous glands, which secret an oily substance called sebum. When these glands become blocked, they can become infected, leading to comedones (pimples) and, in more extreme cases, nodules (inflamed bumps that are often tender) or cysts (pus-filled lesions). When the acne heals it can often leave the skin scarred.

For teens and adults alike, even mild acne can be a social disaster—reason enough to pursue all sorts of remedies, including pharmaceutical ones. You need only think back to your high school prom or even a recent job interview that was marred by an outbreak of red bumps to know how inconvenient bad skin can be.

First-Line Treatments

Antibiotics and topical creams are usually the first defense dermatologists recommend in fighting acne. Antibiotics (all of which must be obtained by prescription) include drugs in the tetracycline class of antibiotics, including tetracycline (Achromycin), doxycycline (Vibra tabs), demeclocycline (Declomycin), and minocycline (Minocin). They were developed from a common mold and share a four-ring chemical structure. They work by inhibiting protein synthesis in bacteria, thereby inhibiting growth of the bacteria in the sebaceous glands that lead to acne. They also reduce the normal bacterial flora in your intestines that you need for digestion. Common side effects are nausea, vomiting, diarrhea, and abdominal pain. These drugs can worsen kidney damage in patients with kidney dysfunction and so should not be taken by those who have kidney problems. Women who are pregnant should consult with their doctor about whether to take antibiotics; some are safer than others.

Antibiotics can also cause liver damage and sun sensitivity. (See Chapter 10 for more about the general uses and risks of antibiotics.) These side effects, however, are not common. In general, these drugs are fairly safe for healthy people, but they aren't as effective in the treatment of acne as medications like Accutane (isotretinoin). Several prescription and nonprescription topical ointments can work in tandem with antibiotic treatment. In general, ointments are safer than ingested pills because very little of the active ingredients gets into your bloodstream.

Benzoyl peroxide cream (NeoBenz Micro, Basiron, Brevoxyl, Stioxyl, Panoxyl, Proactiv) is an effective and safe first-line treatment that can be purchased over the counter or obtained by prescription. Benzoyl peroxide increases skin turnover, which helps clean pores, as well as directly inhibiting bacteria. Side effects can include skin dryness and irritation. Benzoyl peroxide can cause sun sensitivity, so sunscreen should be used in conjunction with this treatment. Other topical compounds include azelaic acid, salicylic acid, and topical antibiotics. Azelaic acid has anti-inflammatory and antibiotic properties as well as direct effects on the skin to break up whiteheads. Sulfur has similar anti-inflammatory and antibiotic effects and is available in a variety of prescription and nonprescription topical applications. Some studies have shown that zinc oxide is effective in the treatment of acne.[1] Side effects with zinc oxide are minimal.

Other topical treatments, like tazarotene, tretinoin, or adapalene gels, are in the retinoid class of compounds and must be obtained by prescription. They are safer than orally taken retinoids, however, because they don't get into the bloodstream in very high concentrations. Nevertheless, they shouldn't be taken during pregnancy. Side effects include skin dryness, skin peeling, and sun sensitivity.

The Accutane Paradox

The most commonly used medication for acne that is resistant to first-line therapies is isotretinoin (Accutane, 13-Cis-retinoic acid). Accutane belongs to the class of compounds called retinoids, which includes the active form of vitamin A. Originally approved as a second-line treatment for cystic and nodular acne, Accutane inhibits sebaceous-gland secretions. Since its approval for the indication of cystic acne by the FDA in 1982, Accutane, manufactured by the Swiss-based company Roche, has been prescribed for 2 million patients in the U.S. and more than 8 million patients worldwide.

Extremely effective in treating severe acne, Accutane quickly became very successful, bringing in more than a billion dollars a year in sales, the result, in part, of doctors who also started prescribing it for patients suffering from "treatment-resistant" acne or the "psychological consequences of acne." Within a short time, fewer than 20% of patients taking Accutane met the original criteria for the treatment of acne; today most patients are using isotretinoin for treatment-resistant or nodular acne or for acne that has caused emotional pain. That's because orally administered Accutane is the single most effective way to clear up acne. It's very important, however, to be aware of the possible devastating risks associated with the medication.

Soon after the introduction of Accutane as a treatment for cystic acne, troubling reports of depression and suicide associated with its use started to surface. Dozens of cases in the U.S., France, Germany, England, Ireland, and other countries popped up in the medical literature, all within just a few years of its introduction to the market. The cases of Accutane-related depression and suicide reported to the World Health Organization (WHO) and the Food and Drug Administration were much higher than those of similar events related to other treatments for acne, such as antibiotics. By 2000 Accutane had earned the distinction of having the largest number of reports of side effects to agencies like the WHO of any drug in the world.[2]

As I said earlier, Accutane is only a minor modification of the active form of vitamin A. Vitamin A is found naturally in foods like liver, carrots, and other orange vegetables in the form of beta-carotene. When vitamin A is digested, the beta-carotene is converted to retinoic acid, which has biological effects. For example, Arctic explorers in the ninteenth century who lived almost exclusively on polar bear liver, an extremely rich source of vitamin A, developed symptoms of confusion and psychosis. Large doses of vitamin A can have a number of other neurological and mental effects, including fatigue, decreased interest, headache, double vision, aggression, personality changes, depression, psychosis, and a swelling of the brain, called pseudotumor cerebri, that can be fatal. Side effects are eliminated when dosage of vitamin A is discontinued.

Many patients who recovered from depression after they stopped taking Accutane became depressed again after restarting it, and some patients exhibited bizarre, even psychotic behavior. There are verifiable accounts of young men and women lighting themselves on fire and jumping off bridges. Questions about the relationship between Accutane and depression and suicide have been swirling around for the past fifteen years. Internal memos in 1984 (just two years after Accutane hit the market) between the FDA and Roche stated that there "probably" was a relationship in some patients. In 1986 Roche changed the package insert to include information that some patients had reported becoming depressed on Accutane. As reported in *USA Today* on December 7, 2004 (Kevin McCoy, "Drug Maker Rebuffed Call to

Monitor Users"), however, as of 2004 the company's spokespersons still publicly denied that there was a "causal relationship" between Accutane and depression, meaning that depression spontaneously developed, unrelated to Accutane, but secondary to other causes.

French regulatory authorities required that Roche place a warning about suicide on the label in 1997; however, the FDA did not even learn about this for another year, when it required the company to put a similar label on Accutane sold in the U.S. In 1997 Dr. Peter Schifferdecker, a doctor working for Roche in Switzerland, wrote in a report for the FDA that Accutane "probably caused" depression, that doctors and patients should be warned, and that patients should be monitored for the development of the condition. As reported in *USA Today*, the company's U.S. marketing team "rewrote" his report because of concerns about its "impact on marketing strategy and product liability," removing the language about how Accutane could cause depression in some patients.

The FDA received an edited report that did not include these concerns about depression. In 1988, based on the FDA's request, Roche included a warning regarding depression, psychosis, and rare suicidal ideation, suicide attempts, and suicide.

In 1999 Liam Grant, the father of an adolescent boy from Ireland who had killed himself after taking Accutane, contacted me after hearing about some of my research on brain imaging of patients with depression. Several years before, the French division of Hoffman-LaRoche placed a warning on the drug's packaging that stated it could cause depression and suicide. However, this did not help the son of the man who contacted me, because the doctor and the drug company did not tell him about the risk of depression and suicide. He donated money to Emory to fund research to determine whether the drug affected the brain and led to changes that could cause depression or suicide.

In 2000 Roche changed the package warning to include depression, psychosis, and suicide as possible side effects. It took the suicide in 2000, of a boy being treated with Accutane who was the son of U.S. Congressman Bart Stupak (D-Michigan), to get the attention of the FDA, which convened an advisory committee to discuss the relationship between Accutane and depression that same year. The committee concluded that "more research" was needed on the topic. In 2002 Accutane's label was changed yet again to warn of "depression, psychosis and, rarely, suicidal ideation, suicide attempts, suicide, and aggressive and/or violent behaviors." However, after planning a study with Roche, the acting head of FDA Drug Surveillance concluded in 2002 that such a study could not be blinded because patients would know from the side effects (like skin dryness) what they were on and that therefore the study should not be performed. At that time the FDA knew of 173 cases of suicide from its MedWatch Program. Assuming that 1% of cases get reported, that would mean 17,300 cases of suicide.

My study of the effects of Accutane on brain function using brain imaging was first presented in November 2004. My theory was that if Accutane affected the brain and caused depression in that way, we should be able to detect it with brain imaging. My colleagues and I did in fact find that Accutane caused a decrease in function in the orbitofrontal cortex. That was identical to what we found in patients who developed depression. This showed that Accutane was affecting brain areas that were known to underlie depression.[3] It also countered the argument that Accutane couldn't be causing depression because it doesn't go into the brain; it's an acne drug.

Other work funded by Mr. Grant showed that Accutane inhibited the growth of neurons in an area of the brain called the hippocampus, which is involved in memory and emotion. This area is smaller in patients with depression, suggesting atrophy. In fact, antidepressants promote the growth of neurons in the hippocampus, which is thought to explain how antidepressants work to treat depression. Other studies showed that Accutane caused behavioral abnormalities in animals.

Following the release of my study and the animal studies, the FDA changed the warning on its Web site to read, as a direct result of this research:

- Preclinical and neuroimaging data suggest that isotretinoin produces behavioral effects (i.e. activation) in rats, impairment of neuronal division in the murine hippocampus, and reductions in orbitofrontal brain metabolic rates in humans. This preclinical and neuroimaging data may suggest biological plausibility for the suspected psychiatric adverse events associated with isotretinoin.

- From isotretinoin's initial marketing in 1982 through August 2004, 4,992 spontaneous reports of psychiatric disturbances associated with using isotretinoin in patients in the United States have been submitted to the FDA.

Once studies were published and word of the results reached the popular press, I was contacted by a number of people who had developed psychiatric side effects after taking Accutane. One family from Missouri was particularly desperate to talk to me. They drove all the way from their home state to Georgia to meet with me. The entire family, including the parents, two sisters, and the young boy who had taken the Accutane, filed into my office. The father related a most incredible story: Soon after starting Accutane, his son told the family that the deceased rocker Jim Morrison was talking to him through monkeys and telling him to commit suicide on April 15, 2004. When the boy finished relating the story, his parents checked him into a locked psychiatric facility on April 14, 2004, a sound decision in my professional opinion. After he stopped taking Accutane his psychosis and suicidal thinking stopped, and he continues to be free of symptoms to this day.

As I mentioned earlier, *USA Today* reported that Roche was still committed to its position that there was no "causal relationship" between Accutane and depression. At the same time Martin Huber, Roche's global head of drug safety, testified under oath in a deposition that Roche's internal assessments showed that Accutane "probably caused" depression and other psychiatric ailments in some users and that the rate of depression among Accutane users was 1.5 times higher than that among nonusers. Roche pointed out that depression is so common in the general population that you can't pick out an increased signal over background noise. On the other hand, what is the probability of developing depression solely by chance during a four-month course of treatment? Although the prevalence of depression (meaning that it has occurred at some time in your life) is

16%, the actual *incidence* (developing new-onset depression) during any given year is only 1.6%.

Therefore, in the four-month period of an isotretinoin trial, about 0.5% of patients would spontaneously develop depression. Estimates of the incidence of depression following treatment with isotretinoin range from 1% to 4% to 6%. More than 6 million patients have been treated with Accutane. If 3% of patients treated with Accutane were to develop depression while taking isotretinoin who otherwise would not have, 180,000 people could have developed depression from Accutane since its introduction. This is higher than the estimated numbers of patients who have suffered a heart attack from taking Vioxx.

BEYOND DEPRESSION

Another devastating side effect was also discovered *after* the drug reached the market: Taken during pregnancy, Accutane causes disfiguring birth defects, including thymus gland abnormalities, parathyroid hormone deficiency, cerebral abnormalities, hydrocephalus, cranial nerve defects, cardiovascular abnormalities, ear defects, absent external auditory canals, eye abnormalities, facial dysmorphia, cleft palate, and skull abnormalities. Birth defects come with a single dose and affect a quarter of babies. Half of all "Accutane babies" have a reduction in IQ.

On November 18, 2004, FDA scientist David Graham created a firestorm of controversy by telling a Senate committee that Accutane should be studied for possible withdrawal. On November 23 the FDA announced it would require prescribers, patients, and pharmacies to register for Accutane and women to test negative for pregnancy and demonstrate a one-month history of being on two forms of birth control before getting a prescription. Now you, your doctor, and your pharmacist have to be registered on a computer (www.ipledgeprogram.com) with evidence of a negative pregnancy test and one month of being on two forms of birth control before your pharmacist can fill your Accutane prescription.

Although the effects of Accutane on the developing brain of the fetus might well have prompted the drug company, the FDA, or the National Institutes of Health to posit that the drug might also affect the brains of teenagers and adults taking the drug, no research has been initiated to test this hypothesis. The fact is that drug companies usually don't support research that might reveal their drug to have a damaging or deadly side effect.

Less serious than suicidal depression and birth defects, Accutane can cause severe headaches in about 20% of patients and, more rarely, pseudotumor cerebri (a swelling of the brain that can be fatal). Other serious side effects include ulcerative colitis, irritable bowel syndrome, severe joint pain, cholesterol elevation, and liver damage. Cholesterol and liver-enzyme levels need to be monitored during treatment, and treatment should be stopped if they are elevated.

Other Systemic Treatments for Acne

A few other systemic treatments for acne have unpleasant side effects but so far have not been linked to severe depression or suicide, making them safer alternatives for teens with acne.

DAPSONE

Dapsone is an anti-inflammatory medication used in the treatment of leprosy whose mechanism of action is poorly understood. It can be used as a second line of treatment for acne. Side effects include upset stomach, vomiting, sore throat, fever, and sun sensitivity. It should not be taken by pregnant or breastfeeding women or by patients with anemia or liver disease.

SPIRONOLACTONE

An aldosterone receptor antagonist that works by altering hormones, spironolactone is sometimes used as a second-line treatment for acne. Side effects include vomiting, dizziness, headache, irregular periods, hair growth, deepening of the voice, and, more rarely, confusion, movement problems, and blurred vision. It too should never be taken by women who are pregnant or breast-feeding or by patients with liver or kidney disease.

Alternative Treatments

So are there alternatives? Stress and diet may be related to the development of acne. Reducing stress with relaxation techniques or other methods may be helpful. Non-Westernized cultures have lower rates of acne, suggesting that diet may be a factor. There is some evidence that diets high in sugar increase insulin levels and reduce inherent retinoid levels, increasing the risk of acne. Data from the Nurses' Health Study of more than 47,335 women showed a 22% increase in severe acne in women who frequently drank milk as teenagers. There was no association with increased acne for those who frequently ate chocolate or drank soda.

Oral contraceptives help women with acne by decreasing testosterone levels and thereby affecting sebaceous-gland production. Laser therapies also work, but they are costly and painful.

The Bottom Line

Prevention is the first-line treatment for acne, and diet plays a big part in it. First, drink less milk and stay away from high-sugar and processed foods, all of which have been shown to cause breakouts. Exercise regularly and make other shifts in behavior to reduce stress, another reason people get pimples. If you want to try a medication, start with over-the-counter topical benzoyl peroxide cream. If that doesn't work, you may need to see a doctor for a combination benzoyl peroxide and/or antibiotic cream, or a course of oral antibiotics. The next step would be a retinoid cream like retinal. The last-resort course of treatment would be isotretinoin or a similar medication.

Drug	Use	Common, Benign Side Effects	Serious Side Effects	Life-threatening Side Effects	Reasons Not to Take
Antibiotics					
Moderate Risk					
Tetracycline (Achromycin)	Acne	Nausea, vomiting	Diarrhea, tooth damage, skin sensitivity	Liver or kidney toxicity (rare), hypersensitivity, sun sensitivity	Allergy, kidney or liver disease, pregnancy, lactation
Doxycycline (Vibra)	Acne	Nausea, vomiting	Diarrhea, tooth damage, skin sensitivity	Liver or kidney toxicity (rare), hypersensitivity, sun sensitivity	Allergy, kidney or liver disease, pregnancy, lactation
Demeclocycline (Declomycin)	Acne	Nausea, vomiting	Diarrhea, tooth damage, skin sensitivity, sunburn	Liver or kidney toxicity (rare), hypersensitivity, sun sensitivity	Allergy, kidney or liver disease, pregnancy, lactation
Minocycline (Minocin)	Acne	Nausea, vomiting	Diarrhea, tooth damage, skin sensitivity, dizziness, vertigo	Liver or kidney toxicity (rare), hypersensitivity, sun sensitivity	Allergy, kidney or liver disease, pregnancy, lactation
Topical Ointments					
Low Risk					
Benzoyl peroxide	Acne	Dry skin, skin irritation	Sun sensitivity, rash, blistering	None	None
Azelaic acid	Acne	Itching, burning, stinging, tingling	Rash	None	None
Sulfur	Acne	Skin irritation, itching	Sun sensitivity, bruising	Allergic reaction, jaundice	Kidney disease, allergies to sulfa
Zinc oxide	Acne	Dry skin, skin irritation	Sun sensitivity	None	None

Drug	Use	Common, Benign Side Effects	Serious Side Effects	Life-threatening Side Effects	Reasons Not to Take
Salicylic acid	Acne	Skin irritation	Dizziness	Confusion, drowsiness, vomiting	None
Tretinoin (Retin-A)	Acne	Dry skin, skin irritation	Sun sensitivity	Allergic reaction	Allergy to medication
Adapalene	Acne	Dry skin, skin irritation	Sun sensitivity	Allergic reaction	Allergy to medication
Tazarotene	Acne	Dry skin, skin irritation	Sun sensitivity	Allergic reaction	Allergy to medication

Oral Retinoids

High Risk

Drug	Use	Common, Benign Side Effects	Serious Side Effects	Life-threatening Side Effects	Reasons Not to Take
Isotretinoin (Accutane)	Acne	Headache, dry skin, dry eyes, skin peeling	Elevated lipids, osteoporosis	Depression, psychosis, aggression, suicide, irritable bowel disease, birth defects, bone and joint pain, brain swelling, liver damage	Current depression, pregnancy

Anti-inflammatory Medications

Moderate Risk

Drug	Use	Common, Benign Side Effects	Serious Side Effects	Life-threatening Side Effects	Reasons Not to Take
Dapsone (Avlosulfun)	Acne	Stomach upset, sore throat, fever	Sun sensitivity, rash, pale skin	Mental changes, bleeding, vomiting	Pregnancy, lactation, anemia, liver disease

Aldosterone Receptor Antagonists

Moderate Risk

Drug	Use	Common, Benign Side Effects	Serious Side Effects	Life-threatening Side Effects	Reasons Not to Take
Spironolactone (Aldactone)	Acne	Headache, diarrhea	Hair growth, deepening of the voice, breast enlargement, impotence	Confusion, blurred vision, dizziness, vomiting	Pregnancy, lactation, liver or kidney disease, taking antihypertensives

4.

LDL Cholesterol–Lowering Medications (Statins)

I've studied the human heart my whole life. I trust Lipitor to help keep my heart healthy. —Dr. Robert Jarvik, inventor of the Jarvik artificial heart

This quote is featured prominently on the official Web site of Lipitor, and yes, you've seen his earnest face on TV, in magazines, and popping up on the Internet. The truth is that most people who received Jarvik's artificial heart didn't live for more than a year. Should we trust him now to be recommending statins?

Based on the studies I review below, the answer is no. And I am afraid there are a lot of people who are getting more harm than good from Lipitor and other LDL cholesterol–lowering statin drugs like it.

Remember when Tom Cruise had a meltdown and started jumping on Oprah's couch and when he shouted at Matt Lauer that he didn't know anything about psychiatric drugs? In the aftermath of those episodes, an anchorwoman from the television show *Dateline* asked me to provide a psychiatric perspective on Cruise's comments. The show never aired (it got bumped by the Iraq War), but the conversation I had with the anchorwoman as I sat perched on a high stool waiting for the cameraman to get set up was memorable.

"It's ironic that I am acting as a spokesman for taking drugs, since I am writing a book that says that many people are taking drugs they don't need," I said.

"What drugs are you writing about?" she asked.

"Everything: antidepressants, statins, meds for hypertension."

"My husband is a tennis pro," she said. "He went to his doctor, who checked his cholesterol and put him on Lipitor. He developed muscle pain, and now he can't play tennis anymore."

"That's called myalgia," I responded. "It's a possible side effect of statins. If he was a tennis pro he probably didn't have any risk factors for heart disease, like obesity, smoking, diabetes, or high blood pressure, right?"

"Right. He's only forty years old and in perfect health."

"And he went to the doctor because you nagged him because he hadn't had a checkup in years?"

"Right."

Poor woman. Should I tell her that the American Medical Association does not recommend regular checkups for healthy people not on medications? And for exactly this reason? Her husband would have been better off not going to the doctor. And this wasn't the first time I had heard about a wife who was sorry that she pushed her husband to go in for a checkup.

The term *cholesterol* is tossed around very casually today. Everyone seems to be aware that it can be "good" or "bad," and "high" or "low." Many of you have probably had your cholesterol tested, and I'm betting a good percentage of you are taking an LDL cholesterol–lowering medication. In this chapter I will try to help you answer the question of whether you are really a candidate for these medicines by reviewing the risks and benefits associated with the most commonly prescribed cholesterol-lowering meds.

I'll begin by explaining that cholesterol is a soft, waxy substance found in the bloodstream and cells and that it is not inherently bad. Rather, it is an essential part of a healthy body that is used for producing cell membranes and some hormones, among other functions. It occurs in two ways: The body manufactures some, and the remainder comes from the cholesterol found in the fat in the animal products we consume, such as meat (including poultry), fish, eggs, butter, cheese, and whole milk. Fruits, vegetables, and whole grains do not contain cholesterol. Processed foods, such as doughnuts, that contain trans fats (a type of unsaturated fat associated with increased risk for heart disease), and even whole or unprocessed foods with saturated fats, such as beef, cause your body to make more cholesterol.

Cholesterol can't dissolve in the blood; it must be transported to and from the cells by carriers called lipoproteins. High-density lipoprotein (HDL), known as "good" cholesterol, carries cholesterol away from your arteries. Your body makes HDL cholesterol for your protection. Studies suggest that high levels of HDL cholesterol reduce your risk of heart attack.

Low-density lipoprotein (LDL) is known as "bad" cholesterol. Too much LDL cholesterol, a condition known as hypercholesterolemia, can clog arteries and increase the risk of heart attack and stroke. Cholesterol collects in a damaged section of the artery wall in something called a plaque, which is a collection of calcium, cholesterol, and inflammatory scar tissue. The plaque can either build up to the point that it clogs the artery, or it can rupture and clog the artery that way. The disease also increases the risk of stroke, which is caused by the clogging of an artery in the brain.

Because cholesterol is found in arteries of the heart that have become clogged, it is assumed that lowering cholesterol will solve the problem. However, the association between elevated cholesterol and heart disease is not as direct as it sounds. Nevertheless, the connection has prompted drugmakers to come up with pharmaceutical solutions to lower bad cholesterol.

Your doctor decides you need cholesterol-lowering medication based on his or her calculation of risk factors that have been quantified by a study called the Framingham Study. These factors include obesity, family history of heart disease, smoking, diabetes, and high blood pressure. Your specific data (i.e., weight, blood pressure, etc.) are fed into a computer, and out comes a risk score that tells the doctor whether you need medication. The relevance of this score, however, is limited. For instance, increasing age increases the score. Just because old age is a risk factor for heart disease, however, doesn't mean you are automatically a good candidate for a statin. One study that hasn't received much media attention (the PROSPER study, which I discuss later) showed that men over age seventy without heart disease had no heart disease–prevention benefit from statins. But the point system adds on a point for every five years over age forty-five up to age eighty. In other words, since an eighty-year-old is more likely to have a cardiac event just because his aged heart is more likely to give out, our medical system is going to give him a statin, even if it causes more harm than good. This isn't the only limitation of the score. For instance, it is assumed that men and women are the same. However, as I will show you below, they are not.

Early Treatments

Introduced in the late 1960s, the first generation of the lipid-lowering drugs came in the form of resins and fibrates, which included gemfibrozil (Lopid) and fenofibrate (Tricor). Fibrates were found to lower LDL cholesterol and prevent heart disease, but they were also found to actually *increase* overall mortality by as much as *47%*.[1] Animal studies showed that these drugs caused cancer; in some cases the cancer risk was seen at blood levels only three- to fourfold higher than those seen in the normal treatment of high cholesterol. These medications also cause nausea, bloating, fatty stools, and potential nutritional deficiency. As a result of all this, they are no longer prescribed very often. Since the fibrates (e.g., gemfibrozil) can cause cancer and may actually increase mortality, I recommend that these medications should not be taken.

Another class of older drugs, called bile acid sequestrants [e.g., cholestyramine (Locholest, Questran)], binds cholesterol in the gut and decreases its absorption. It lowers cholesterol, including "good" HDL levels. This drug can cause nutritional deficiencies through interference with absorption, as well as bloating and constipation, and should be avoided.

Ezetimibe (Zetia) is a drug that blocks absorption of LDL cholesterol by the small intestine, thus lowering LDL cholesterol levels in the blood. Zetia acts on cells lining the small intestine to interfere with their uptake of cholesterol by a mechanism that is not completely understood. Side effects of Zetia include fever, headache, muscle pain, runny nose, and sore throat. More rarely it can cause hives and liver damage. Zetia is sometimes used on its own by people who cannot tolerate the side effects of statins, which are reviewed in the following section. Generally, however, they are used in combination with statins.

Vitamin B$_3$, or niacin (Niaspan), yet another cholesterol-lowering option, is found in a number of plants. A deficiency of this vitamin causes pellagra, which is associated with diarrhea, skin inflammation, and dementia. Niacin does lower cholesterol. However, it is associated with a number of side effects, including flushing (a sudden rushing of blood to the face accompanied by a feeling of heat in the face that can be very uncomfortable), which limit its use. But if you can cope with the side effects, there is no reason not to take niacin, since it is not associated with any lasting conditions.

The Status of Statins

The search for better cholesterol-lowering drugs led to the development of statins, a class of drugs that lower LDL cholesterol by blocking an enzyme that churns out LDL cholesterol in the liver, called HMG CoEnzymeA reductase. The enthusiasm among doctors for statins has resulted in the writing of prescriptions for 13 million people each year, many of whom don't derive any health benefits, as I'll explain in detail here. Generic and brand names include rosuvastatin (Crestor), fluvastatin (Lescol), atorvastatin (Lipitor), lovastatin (Mevacor), pravastatin (Pravachol), and simvastatin (Zocor). Lipitor rings up $6 billion a year in sales; Zocor, $5 billion; and the others are close behind.

Indeed, in their enthusiasm for statins and other drugs, some cardiologists advocate the development of a "polypill" that would include a statin, a beta-blocker, aspirin, and maybe an angiotensin-converting enzyme (ACE) inhibitor. The idea is that everyone, even those considered normal, would take a polypill to prevent heart disease.

Pfizer is one of the biggest pharmaceutical companies in the world largely because of the success of Lipitor, its best-selling drug. The fact that Lipitor is scheduled to go off patent in 2010 led the company to look for new cholesterol-lowering drugs with unique mechanisms of action. Torcetrapib, slated to be Pfizer's next drug, works by raising HDL, the "good cholesterol," and thus has a mechanism of action that is complementary to that of Lipitor, which lowers LDL, the "bad cholesterol." Pfizer expected Torcetrapib to be its next best-selling medication.

Unfortunately, after reviewing the data from a clinical trial of Torcetrapib, the independent monitors found that the drug appeared to be causing more subjects to die of heart attacks and other complications of high blood pressure than seen with placebo. Based on this finding the trial was immediately halted, and Pfizer withdrew its application to the FDA for approval of Torcetrapib. The lesson from Torcetrapib is that just because medications have actions that we think should be helpful (like raising HDL cholesterol), that doesn't mean they necessarily will be. In the case of statins, lowering LDL cholesterol is not always associated with lowering mortality or even in some cases heart attack risk.

Again, 13 million Americans take statins each year. However, if we were to follow the recommendations of the Expert Panel on Detection, Evaluation, and Treatment of High Blood Cholesterol in Adults, endorsed by the American College of Cardiology and the American Heart Association, *every* American over age forty-five with an LDL greater than 130 mg/dL would be taking statins. Since half of Americans over age thirty-five have an LDL greater than 130, that would mean that almost half of all Americans, or 100 million people, should, theoretically, be taking statins. Since a year of statins costs up to $3,000, that would come to $300 billion a year. We might get there yet; there has been a recent push to prescribe statins even for people with normal LDL cholesterol, which would push LDL to extremely low levels.

In my opinion this push to give statins to people with normal cholesterol concentrations is a cause for concern. For one thing, we are introducing people who do not have a disease to medications with potentially dangerous side effects. Second, the body requires cholesterol for a number of vital processes, like the construction of cell membranes. Very low cholesterol concentrations have been linked to depression and suicide, possibly because of the impairment in the ability to maintain neurons in the brain.

For those of you who may be taking statins right now, you have probably seen an amazing reduction in your bad cholesterol levels, perhaps as much as 20%. "What a great drug!" It's a popular refrain, one I have heard from friends and colleagues who take the drugs. However, there is convincing evidence that statins aren't a miracle solution.

First, taking a statin won't prevent you from having a heart attack or dying if you have heart disease. It only slightly lowers your risk and, again, only if you are known to have heart disease. I have heard my American physician colleagues say things about statins like "They ought to put that stuff in the drinking water." It therefore shouldn't be a surprise that American guidelines for who should take statins (which are written by American doctors), if followed by everyone, would have more of us on statins than any other country in the world. In fact, U.S. guidelines would have one out of four Americans on a statin. If this was helpful you would expect that we would have fewer deaths from heart attacks than other countries. However, our heart attack death rates are no different from those in countries such as New Zealand, where the criteria for who should take a statin are stricter, and where the percentage of the population that would be recommended to take a statin is half what it is in the U.S.

And statins are not without their risks. A paper published in the *Journal of the American College of Cardiology* in 2007 found that when cholesterol levels were pushed to very low concentrations (LDL < 100 mg/dL) using the high doses of statins currently in vogue with many U.S. doctors, there was a statistically significant increase in cancer rates. If you are over age seventy, evidence from the PROSPER study I review on page 67 suggests that statins given even at normal doses increase cancer rates by 25%

with no benefit for heart-disease prevention if you don't have a prior history of heart disease.

For every hundred people known to have heart disease who take a statin for five years, three will die of a heart attack even though their cholesterol was lowered with a statin. Only one will be saved from dying of a heart attack. That translates into the much-vaunted 25% reduction in risk, based on "relative risk." This means that the number of patients who died from a heart attack by the end of five years when the study ended was 25% smaller in the statin group than in the placebo group. But that number is misleading. Since the number of people who died from a heart attack was small to begin with, what it actually means is that your own personal risk of dying from a heart attack was reduced by only 0.2% per year, the figure for what is known as "absolute risk." Obviously a 25% reduction sounds a lot better than a 0.2% reduction, and not surprisingly the makers of statins use the 25% "relative risk" figure because it makes their drug look better. The second number (0.2%) doesn't look so great, and that doesn't take into account the risks from statins themselves, which I will get to shortly.

What about the evidence for heart-attack prevention if you *don't* have a prior history of heart disease? Of the five major studies purportedly involving patients at high risk for heart disease because of their risk factors (high cholesterol, diabetes, smoking, hypertension, family history) but who don't currently have known heart disease, all of which I describe in more detail on pages 63–68, one of them, the ALLHAT study,[2] showed no effect on heart attacks, and two (CARDS[3] and AFCAPS/TexCAPS[4]) showed some effect. The remaining two involved patients who were represented as being free of heart disease, but probably were not, either because they had anginal chest pain (Pravastatin Prevention)[5] or an abnormal angiogram (ASCOT-LLA),[6] even if they hadn't had an actual heart attack.

In all of these studies, the risk of adverse events, which include, in addition to heart attacks and strokes, liver damage, development of cancer, or another major health problem, was identical for patients treated with statin or placebo.

THE STUDIES

Over the past twenty years, there have been numerous studies done on statins that have involved at least eighty thousand people. The large number of subjects studied may sound reassuring, but you should understand that if there are small differences between an active drug and a placebo, researchers *need* large numbers of subjects to be able to show an effect. Some of the studies have involved patients with a history of heart disease (i.e., they had a heart attack, or had heart disease diagnosed with a nuclear perfusion scan or similar test), and so-called secondary prevention to prevent recurrence of a heart attack; others involved patients without a history of heart disease, and were primary-prevention studies. There were no primary-prevention studies that looked only at patients with no risk factors other than elevated cholesterol. As I will demonstrate in this chapter, there are several points that can be taken away from these studies:

- Men without a history of heart disease, multiple risk factors, or familial hypercholesterolemia should not take statins.
- Men over age seventy without heart disease should not take statins.
- Women of any age without heart disease should not take statins.
- For men with multiple risk factors and women with heart disease, statins may prevent a heart attack, but they won't save your life.
- Although some studies have shown a reduction in mortality with statins in men under age sixty-five with established heart disease a larger number have not.
- Diet and exercise are always better than statins.

The fine print in these studies reveals some crucial information about the safety and efficacy of statins in patients with high cholesterol but no family history or risk of heart disease. Stay with me here as I review the research literature and show you why taking statins is most likely an unnecessary expense and risk if you are otherwise healthy.

In order to assess the ability of a variety of medications to prevent heart attack, the National Institutes of Health (NIH) sponsored the Antihypertensive and Lipid Lowering Treatment to Prevent Heart Attack Trial (ALLHAT). This study assessed, in addition to antihypertensive treatments, the ability of the statin drug pravastatin (Pravachol) as opposed to usual care to reduce mortality in 10,355 high-risk men and women over the age of fifty-five with LDL cholesterol over 120 mg/dL and triglycerides less than 350 mg/dL who were not already being treated for high cholesterol. In addition to high cholesterol, participants had high blood pressure as well as one other risk factor for heart disease (e.g., diabetes, smoking, obesity) and therefore represented the typical patient who would normally be put on a statin. Fourteen percent had a known history of heart disease, and 35% had diabetes.

The study found identical mortality rates between the two groups at five years, and no significant difference in heart attacks and similar heart disease–related events: 9.3% of the pravastatin group compared to 10.4% of the nonpravastatin group experienced cardiac events. The study was criticized by a number of doctors in the field because patients and doctors knew what they were taking, and many of the usual-care group started taking statins because of the education they received while being in the study. Though cardiac events and mortality remained basically the same between the two groups, LDL cholesterol was reduced more in the pravastatin group (28%) than in the usual-care group (11%), showing that there was a greater effect on cholesterol in the treatment group.

The Heart Protection Study (HPS) randomized 20,536 patients from the U.K. with high cholesterol and a history of heart disease, vascular disease, high blood pressure, and/or diabetes, giving them either simvastatin or a placebo.[7] Sixty-five percent of the participants had a known history of heart disease. The study found a statistically significant reduction in heart attacks, cardiac deaths, and related vascular events. However, again, the results showed a modest reduction of 3.1% (8.7% vs. 11.8%). There was also a statistically significant 1.8% reduction in absolute risk of death from all causes. Reductions were seen for both women (most of whom were postmenopausal) and diabetics. Simvastatin had some negative non–heart-related outcomes, however. There were 243 cases of cancer in the simvastatin group vs. 202 in the placebo group, an increase of about 22% that was of borderline statistical significance.

The Long-Term Intervention with Pravastatin in Ischaemic Disease (LIPID) study examined 9,014 patients with high cholesterol and a history of heart disease randomized to pravastatin (Pravachol) or placebo.[8] This study showed a 1.9% reduction in heart-disease–related death and a 3.1% reduction in overall mortality that was statistically significant. However, there were no differences in heart attacks and/or cardiac deaths in the women on pravastatin (12%) when compared with those on placebo (14%).

The Cholesterol and Recurrent Events (CARE) study randomized 4,159 patients (men and postmenopausal women) with a history of heart attack, giving them either pravastatin (Pravachol) or a placebo.[9] Subjects on pravastatin had heart attacks and/or cardiac-related death in 10.2% of cases as opposed to 13.2% of those taking a placebo. One hundred nineteen (6%) patients taking the placebo died from heart disease as opposed to ninety-six (5%) taking pravastatin. However, only seventy-five (3.6%) taking the placebo died from noncardiac causes as opposed to eighty-four (4%) taking pravastatin. There were twice as many violent deaths (e.g., suicide, accidents) in the pravastatin group, but there were no differences in overall mortality between the groups. There were significant reductions in heart attacks and related events in women when looked at separately.

The Myocardial Ischemia Reduction with Aggressive Cholesterol Lowering (MIRACL) Study compared atorvastatin (Lipitor) treatment to placebo in 3,086 male and female patients with a recent heart attack or unstable angina.[10] Although the study did show a 2.6% reduction in a combined measure of death and/or heart attack or related events (14.8% vs. 17.4%), it was of marginal statistical significance. There were no differences in mortality or nonfatal heart attack between the groups. Most of the benefits were from reduction of recurrent anginal chest pain. An elevation in liver enzymes of three times over normal occurred in thirty-eight atorvastatin patients (2.5%) vs. nine (0.6%) on placebo, an increase of four-fold. Results for women were not reported separately.

In the Lescol Intervention Prevention Study (LIPS), 1,677 patients with heart disease who had been treated with angioplasty were randomized to fluvastatin (Lescol) or placebo.[11] (Combined) risk of heart attack, death, or repeat angioplasty was 21.4% in the fluvastatin group vs. 26.7% in the placebo group. There were no differences in mortality between the groups. Although only 16% of the subjects were women, there was not a statistically significant reduction in women when looked at alone. Ten patients in the fluvastatin group (1.2%) vs. three (.4%) in the placebo group had a significant increase in liver enzymes, a threefold increased risk.

The West of Scotland Coronary Prevention Study Group (WOSCOPS) study assessed 6,595 men at high risk of heart attack due to elevated cholesterol levels and risk factors for heart disease. There was a 2.4% reduction in heart attack or cardiac death, although overall mortality was not affected.[12] One hundred sixteen in the pravastatin group vs. 106 on placebo developed cancer.

In the Scandinavian Simvastatin Survival Study (4S)[13] 4,444 men and postmenopausal women with a history of anginal pain or heart attack were randomized and given either a placebo or simvastatin. There were significantly more deaths in the placebo group (12%) than in the simvastatin group (8%) and a 9% increase in heart attacks and other heart-related events with placebo. Women showed no reduction in mortality, although there was a reduction in heart attacks and related events.

In the Stroke Prevention by Aggressive Reduction in Cholesterol Levels (SPARCL) study 4,731 patients with a history of stroke or transient ischemic attack (TIA) (see page 74) within the past six months and LDL cholesterol of 100–190 mg per deciliter were randomly assigned to receive atorvastatin or placebo for five years. A 2.2% reduction in strokes was at the borderline of statistical significance. There were no reductions in total mortality or cardiovascular mortality in patients treated with atorvastatin vs. placebo.[14]

These studies show that statins do reduce recurrent heart attacks in patients with a history of heart disease, although whether they save lives is not as clear. The problem with all of these studies is that the participants had heart disease; you can't draw any conclusions about statin use for people who don't have a history of heart disease from this research, even though it is often cited and used for this purpose.

One of the studies of patients with risk factors but with no known heart disease, The Air Force/Texas Coronary Atherosclerosis Prevention Study (AFCAPS/TexCAPS), included 5,608 men and 997 postmenopausal women who were randomized to take either lovastatin (Mevacor) or a placebo. This study did find a statistically significant reduction in a combined outcome of heart attacks, unstable angina (worsening and/or uncontrollable chest pain), and/or heart-related death. However, the absolute reduction was only 2% (5.5% rate in the placebo group vs. 3.5% in the treated group). There was no difference in deaths between the lovastatin (eighty) and placebo (seventy-seven) groups. There were seventeen deaths from cardiovascular-related causes in the lovastatin group and twenty-five in the placebo group; however, there were sixty-three deaths from noncardiovascular causes in the lovastatin group and fifty-two in the placebo group, suggesting that the benefits of survival from heart disease–related causes might be outweighed by other drug-induced health risks, echoing earlier concerns. Consistent with these findings, lovastatin caused a significant doubling in cases of liver damage as measured by significant increases in liver enzymes.

The Anglo-Scandinavian Cardiac Outcomes Trial–Lipid Lowering Arm (ASCOT-LLA) Study examined 10,305 patients with hypertension and at least three other cardiac risk factors randomized to take either atorvastatin (Lipitor) or a placebo. One hundred fifty-four placebo patients had a fatal or nonfatal heart attack as opposed to one hundred in the atorvastatin group. There were no significant differences in death between atorvastatin (185) and placebo (212). There was no reduction in heart attacks for women on atorvastatin (19, or 1.9%) vs. placebo (17, or 1.8%).

In the Pravastatin in Elderly Individuals at Risk of Vascular Disease (PROSPER) Study 8,804 male and female patients over age seventy with a history of heart or vascular disease and/or risk factors for heart disease were treated with pravastatin (Pravachol) or placebo. Four hundred eight on pravastatin had a stroke or heart attack compared to 473 on placebo, with no differences in mortality. There were no significant reductions in heart disease and/or stroke in women, diabetics, or patients without a prior history of heart disease.

There was, however, a 25% *increase* in cancer with statin treatment, which was statistically significant, with as many as one new case of cancer per year for every one hundred patients treated with pravastatin in the last years of the trial.[15] And we don't know how many patients developed cancer after the five-year trial was over. The authors of the study wrote that these results were due to the "play of chance" or to preexisting occult cancer, which gives the impression that they were trying to explain away something that didn't fit with their expected outcome.

WOMEN AND STATINS

You may have read that heart disease is underdiagnosed in women and that they are missing treatments with lifesaving potential. For instance, in the May 10, 2004, edition of *Newsweek,* it was reported that heart disease is a "grave threat to women's health, but no one needs to take it lying down. Statin drugs (Zocor, Lipitor, Pravachol and others) can slash a woman's heart-attack risk by more than a third—just as they do in men . . . should you be taking one of these medications?"

The answer is probably not. In a study that combined all of the available information on women from the different clinical trials, the authors found *no reduction in heart attacks or mortality in women with high cholesterol who did not have a history of heart disease.*[16] That means that if you are a woman with high cholesterol and no history of heart disease, you should not take a statin.

But what if my cholesterol is elevated? you might ask. Just because your cholesterol is high and statins reduce it doesn't mean that statins prevent heart attacks or death. As with the ALLHAT study, LDL cholesterol came down with statins but there was no reduction in mortality.

At this time there is no evidence that statins save the lives of women even if they do have a history of heart disease. Although the Heart Protection Study (HPS) did show a reduction in heart attacks (with no reduction in mortality) for postmenopausal women with heart disease, more of the studies I have reviewed above, including ASCOT, LIPID, and PROSPER, did not show any benefit. The 4S study showed a 12% *increase* in overall mortality, even though there was a 24% reduction in heart-disease–related mortality. The CARE study showed a twelvefold increase in breast cancer, which may explain the increased overall mortality with statins in spite of the reduced cardiac mortality for women in that study. *For women without heart disease or premenopausal women (even with risk factors for heart disease) there is no proven benefit to taking statins.* However, this has not stopped a consortium of experts from advocating statins for women without heart disease.[17]

DIABETES AND STATINS

A couple of studies showing a reduction of heart attacks in diabetics without heart disease have received so much attention that the National Cholesterol Education Panel of the National Institutes of Health has been spurred to call diabetics "heart-disease equivalents." However, more recent studies like ASCOT, PROSPER, and ALLHAT, show no benefit for diabetics without heart disease.

Other studies show that patients with heart disease and diabetes had no more benefit than patients without diabetes; in fact, when looked at alone, the diabetic group did not have a reduction in major cardiovascular outcomes (heart attack, cardiac death, strokes).[18] In other words, the research doesn't support the idea that diabetes is a "cardiac equivalent" beyond its role as another risk factor for heart disease. Also, 90% of diabetics in these trials had type 2 diabetes (non–insulin-dependent), which is caused primarily by obesity. Type 2 diabetics also often have other multiple risk factors. In other words, they probably have undetected heart disease. So rather than take a pill that has dubious potential benefit and definite risk, type 2 diabetics who smoke would benefit more from quitting cigarettes, exercising, and losing weight. Such behavior modifications would help their diabetes as well as dramatically cut their risk of heart disease. I recognize that none of these changes are easy to make, but they are lifesaving and life-extending.

STATINS AND SIDE EFFECTS

Some of the most critical findings on the negative side effects of statins are buried in tables and fine print with little or no discussion in the text of the papers that report the results of the major clinical trials. For example, animal studies show that *all lipid-lowering drugs have been associated with an increased risk for cancer.*[19] Because of this, an FDA advisory panel recommended withholding approval of an earlier-generation lipid-lowering drug. The FDA went ahead and approved it anyway. In some animal studies, the risks of cancer are present at levels similar to those used in the "aggressive lipid-lowering regimens" employed in some research studies today. In nine of the twelve largest statin studies that have reported cancer rates, there was a 3% increase in the development of new cancers overall in patients on statins above and beyond cancers developed by those on placebo.

I added up the cancer rates reported in the major trials I reviewed above and found that patients taking statins have a 7% greater risk of cancer mortality than that of patients taking placebo. In one study of women, for whom evidence of the benefit from statins is not very strong, some particularly alarming results were twelve cases of breast cancer among those on statins vs. one in the placebo group. Some cancers can take up to twenty years to develop, so we don't know how many patients developed cancer after the five-year trial was finished. These drugs have not been on the market that long, so the studies don't show long-term effects. In the Pravastatin in Elderly Individuals at Risk of Vascular Disease (PROSPER) study, there was a 25% *increase* in cancer with statin treatment, which was statistically significant. As many as one new case of cancer per year for every one hundred patients treated with Pravachol developed in the last years of the trial. These patients got more cancer but absolutely no heart-disease prevention (i.e., reduction in heart attacks). Although some analyses combining data from multiple studies have shown no statistically significant increases in cancer with statins,[20] the fact that statins can cause cancer in animals, as well as more recent studies showing an increased risk of cancer with high-dose statins, is cause for concern.

The liver can also be adversely affected by statins. The statin trials that have published the pertinent data show a 32% increase in the number of patients on statins vs. those on placebo who had serious elevations of liver enzymes, indicating significant liver damage. I added up the number of reports of liver disease reported in all of the studies reviewed above and found that for every four people saved from a heart attack, one person developed serious liver disease. There are also problems with a current proposal by the makers of Mevacor to sell it over the counter. Liver monitoring is recommended for anyone taking Mevacor; without a physician, however, how do you monitor your own liver function? By drawing your own blood and sending it to the lab?

Statins also may increase the risk for depression. Cholesterol is the essential building block of neurotransmitters and hormones, changes in which have been associated with the development of depression. This may explain why many patients feel so much worse when their cholesterol is lowered. Statins increase the risk of a recurrence in patients who have previously been treated for depression; if you take a statin after being treated with an antidepressant, your risk of a recurrence is 61% vs. 40% if you don't take a statin.[21]

Another potential problem with statins is the risk of rhabdomyolysis, a severe degenerative muscle disease that can lead to kidney failure and death. Statins commonly cause mild muscle aches and pains, flu-like symptoms, and back pain. Myopathy involves severe muscle pain often associated with the elevation of an enzyme called creatine kinase (CK) that is released from the muscle. Myopathy can proceed to full-blown rhabdomyolysis and possible death. A total of 338 cases of fatal rhabdomyolysis with statin treatment have been reported worldwide; the true number, however, is probably ten to a hundred times that, a formula based on the FDA's own analysis of the true number of actual negative outcomes with drugs vs. the outcomes that are reported. One of the statins, cerivastatin (Baycol), was removed from the market because of at least thirty-one reports of fatal rhabdomyolysis. Crestor (Rosuvastatin) is another statin currently in the spotlight because it is associated with deaths from kidney failure; it has been identified in congressional testimony as a particularly dangerous drug that is still on the market. Crestor is one of the most potent statins.

Because of concerns about Crestor, in 2003 a consumer group urged the FDA to withhold approval of Crestor; however, the FDA still approved it. Since that time there have been 65 cases of rhabdomyolysis with Crestor reported to the FDA, some of them fatal. Although death from statins is rare, given the large number of people who take these drugs, muscle pain (myalgia) in the absence of changes in laboratory values like CK are more common, affecting 2% to 3% of patients. Studies have shown that myalgia can be associated with changes in muscle tissue.

All of the statins can cause problems with memory and joint pains. In fact, on Web sites like askthepatient.com statins are one of the most negatively rated drugs around. Probably because of these side effects, 40% of patients stop taking them in the first six months of treatment. Other side effects include impotence, abdominal pain, dizziness, and constipation.

The use of statins for patients over seventy is not recommended because of the risk of myopathy and rhabdomyolysis. However, these guidelines are not followed by most doctors, due to either lack of knowledge about the guidelines (e.g., 21% of patients prescribed statins were shown to be over seventy) or other reasons. And this is in spite of the fact that statins have been shown to have no effect in preventing heart attacks in patients over seventy in the PROSPER trial I reviewed above.

Recent research shows that there may not be as direct a relationship between "bad" LDL cholesterol and heart-disease risk as we have been led to believe. I recently read about the work of Rodney Hayward, M.D., Timothy Hofer, M.D., and Sandeep Vijan, M.D., who looked at the relationship between LDL cholesterol and heart disease. Normally we are encouraged to keep our LDL cholesterol below 130 mg/dL. These researchers wanted to know what lowering the LDL of very-high-risk patients to less than 70 mg/dL and that of high-risk patients to less than 100 mg/dL would do because they could find no studies showing that reducing LDL cholesterol below the normal level of 130 mg/dL is beneficial in reducing heart-disease risk. The authors concluded that "current clinical evidence does not demonstrate that increasing statin doses to achieve proposed low LDL cholesterol levels is beneficial or safe."[22]

ASPIRIN FOR THE PREVENTION OF HEART DISEASE

We've all heard about the importance of aspirin for the prevention of heart disease. But is it really true?

In a recent analysis of the published literature on people without heart disease, researchers examined a total of 51,342 women and 44,114 men from a range of studies who did not have heart disease but had risk factors for heart disease.[23] Daily aspirin in women reduced cardiovascular disease by 12%, which was statistically significant, with a 17% reduction in stroke and no effect on heart attacks or cardiovascular mortality. However, for any given woman, the *absolute risk reduction,* or how much the risk of heart attack was actually reduced in that individual, was only 0.3% over a six-year period. And aspirin increased the risk of major bleeding by 68%. For men there was a 14% reduction of cardiovascular events that was related primarily to a 32% reduction in heart attacks, with no effect on strokes or cardiovascular mortality. That figure translates into a 0.37% absolute reduction over a six-year period. And men had a 72% increase in major bleeding. Aspirin did not save any lives in men or women. And for every stroke in women or heart attack in men that is prevented by aspirin, there is one major gastrointestinal bleeding event caused by aspirin. Based on these figures, I do not recommend taking aspirin if you don't have heart disease.

For men with a history of heart disease, the Antithrombotic Trialists Collaboration (ATC) Study showed that taking baby aspirin every day can reduce your risk of death from heart disease by about 17%.[24] Translated, this means you are reducing your absolute risk, a concept I explained in my discussion of women and aspirin, by about 1% per year. Although technically the risk of stomach bleeding is outweighed by the heart benefits of aspirin (which can only be shown when large numbers of patients are studied), in terms of what that means to you personally, the differences are not that great. If you don't mind taking it, you can get some advantage, but not as much as you think.

In patients with strokes or transient ischemic attacks (TIAs), small strokes that don't cause permanent damage, aspirin plus dipyridamole (a blood-vessel dilator) has been shown to be associated with a 13% rate of cardiovascular event compared to 16% on aspirin alone, a difference that is statistically significant.[25]

CLOPIDOGREL (PLAVIX)

Since aspirin can be picked up in any drugstore for mere pennies a pill, the drug companies have been looking for something that does the same thing but that requires a prescription, and that can be promoted as being better than aspirin or as being a beneficial addition to aspirin. Clopidogrel (Plavix) is a pill that is promoted as complementing the effects of aspirin based on its ability to inhibit the cyclooxygenase pathway, which is said to work with aspirin by blocking platelets and therefore inhibiting blood clotting, thereby preventing heart attacks. The Clopidogrel vs. Aspirin in Patients at Risk of Ischaemic Events (CAPRIE) trial randomly assigned 19,185 patients with a history of recent stroke or heart attack to receive clopidogrel or aspirin for two years. Patients on clopidogrel had a 5.32% annual rate of a heart attack or stroke, compared with 5.83% for those on aspirin, a difference that was barely statistically significant.[26]

The CHARISMA (Clopidogrel for High Atherothrombotic Risk and Ischemia Stabilization, Management, and Avoidance) trial involved 15,603 patients with heart disease or risk factors for heart disease who were given clopidogrel plus aspirin or aspirin alone. There was no difference between the groups in combined incidence of heart attack, stroke, or death from cardiovascular causes.[27] In the ClOpidogrel and Metoprolol in Myocardial Infarction Trial (COMMIT), 45,852 patients who had suffered a heart attack within the past 24 hours were given clopidogrel or placebo in addition to aspirin. Clopidogrel patients had a 9% reduction in a combined measure of death, heart attack, or stroke, a difference that was statistically significant.[28] An analysis of all of the published studies showed a 10% reduction in heart attacks and strokes in patients with a history of cardiovascular disease when clopidogrel was added to aspirin. These differences, however, translate to a less than 1% reduction in absolute risk.

In the Management of ATherothrombosis with Clopidogrel in High-risk Patients (MATCH)[29] study, 7,599 patients with recent stroke or TIA and one other risk factor for heart disease were randomly assigned to receive clopidogrel or clopidogrel plus aspirin. There was no difference in the rates of combined stroke, heart attack, or hospitalization between the clopidogrel group (17%) and the clopidogrel plus aspirin group (16%); a 1.3% increase in bleeding was not statistically significant. In another study, 320 patients who had developed a bleeding ulcer while taking aspirin to prevent heart disease and whose ulcers had healed were randomized for a year to retreatment with aspirin or clopidogrel. All of them also received esomeprazole. The patients who took clopidogrel had more gastrointestinal bleeding (8.6%) than the aspirin patients (0.7%), a difference that is striking.[30]

Based on these conflicting results and the only marginally greater benefit as well as the higher cost of clopidogrel, I recommend using aspirin over clopidogrel if you have a history of heart attack or stroke. I would not consider it mandatory (or useful) to take either if you don't have a history of heart disease.

Alternative Medicine

There has long been interest in the use of vitamins and other alternative or "natural" remedies to treat heart disease. Yet the value of such treatments is mixed at best.

VITAMINS

There is some connection between oxidative stress and heart disease, and the known role of vitamins C and E as antioxidants. However a large body of research, including large studies of tens of thousands of patients, has shown that vitamins do not prevent heart disease.[31] In fact, they may actually have the opposite effect. In one large study, male physicians given beta-carotene (the precursor of vitamin A) showed no differences in rates of heart disease compared to those given a placebo.[32] In the Beta-Carotene and Retinol Efficacy Trial (CARET), 18,314 smokers randomized to beta-carotene and vitamin A in doses equal to four carrots a day had 17% more heart disease and were 17% more likely to die.[33]

In the Alpha-Tocopherol, Beta-Carotene (ATBC) Cancer Prevention study smokers were treated with beta-carotene and alpha tocopherol (vitamin E) or placebo. There was an 8% increase in total mortality in the beta-carotene–supplemented group.[34] Smokers with a prior history of heart attack in this study had a 75% increase in heart attack with beta-carotene therapy.[35] Subjects getting vitamin E had a 2% increase in mortality. Looking at all these studies together, there is an increased risk of heart disease with vitamin A and beta-carotene associated with a 29% increase in mortality when the two are combined.[36]

Trials for vitamin E have not shown that it prevents heart disease,[37–40] with the exception of one study showing a modest decrease in heart attacks.[41] Other studies like ATBC showed an increase in strokes. When Vivekananthan and colleagues combined data from several previously published studies, no heart-protective effects of vitamin E were shown. In fact, if anything, there was a slight *increase* in mortality, although only about 2%, which is less than that for vitamin A and beta-carotene.

One study by Waters and colleagues of vitamin E combined with vitamin C showed that vitamins actually accelerated the progression of thickening of the coronary arteries and doubled the risk of dying of heart disease.[42] Another study of a combination of antioxidants, including vitamins E, C, beta-carotene, and selenium, showed that vitamins actually blocked the effects of anticholesterol treatment (simvastatin plus niacin) on reducing atherosclerosis and preventing heart attacks and strokes.[43] The vitamins in this study interfered with the ability of the other medications to raise HDL (good) cholesterol. When Bjelakovic and colleagues looked at data from several published studies in which vitamin E was given with beta-carotene, there was a 10% overall increase in mortality that nobody can explain. Based on these studies, there is no role for vitamins in the treatment or prevention of heart disease.

HRT AND HEART DISEASE

Since heart disease increases in women after menopause, researchers have long theorized that estrogen and progesterone (which decline after menopause) protect women from heart disease. However, this theory was never tested in properly controlled trials until tens of thousands of women were unnecessarily exposed to hormone replacement therapy (HRT) for the prevention of heart disease. There was also the purported benefit that HRT would make you look better and improve your sex life.

However, none of these claims held up to the test of time. The original evidence supporting the claim that HRT prevented heart attacks was based on what are called observational studies. Women who chose to take HRT were compared to those who didn't and were found to have fewer heart attacks. It turned out that the women who took HRT also were more health conscious and did other things, like exercise and eat a healthy diet, that protected them from heart attack. The HRT didn't do anything. However, ten years of major marketing to women and billions of dollars in sales went by. The pharmaceutical companies had hit the mother lode of all markets: not just patients with a disease but all women over age fifty.

The observational study, however, is often inherently flawed when applied to medications. It is easy to have other factors creep into the study and affect the results. For example, women who get prescribed HRT might be more likely to be concerned about their health and to exercise, watch their diet, or do other things unrelated to HRT that will promote their health. Observational studies, in other words, are not able to prove anything. They are like circumstantial evidence presented in a courtroom. The only way to answer a question like "Does HRT prevent heart attacks?" is to do a controlled study in which women get either HRT or a sugar pill without their or their doctor's knowledge of which one they are on. At the end of five years, the outcomes (i.e., heart attacks) of the two groups are compared. It took so long to conduct such studies because it was argued by many doctors that it would be unethical to give a sugar pill when HRT had such obvious benefits.

More recently, controlled trials have been performed, and their results are pretty shocking. Not only did HRT (estrogen and progesterone) not prevent heart attacks, it actually increased them. There was a statistically significant 24% increase in risk of heart attack or cardiac death with equine estrogen and medroxy-progesterone (Prempro) in the Women's Health Initiative (WHI) study,[44] while another study, the Heart and Estrogen/Progesterone Replacement Study (HERS), found no protective effect in women with a history of heart disease.[45, 46] HRT also increased the risk of breast cancer by 24%[47] and the risk of stroke by 41%, and doubled the risk of pulmonary embolus (blood clot in the lung).[48] For every one hundred women treated with HRT in the WHI, one woman developed a serious adverse event directly related to HRT. In the HERS study, there was a 10% increase in mortality with HRT, related in part to a doubling of the risk of potentially lethal blood clots.[49] The study by Waters and colleagues mentioned above showed that HRT accelerated the progression of thickening of the coronary arteries and doubled the risk of dying of heart disease. Based on these findings, there is no role for HRT in heart-disease prevention.

SOY

A natural product that has been promoted as a preventative for heart disease, soy is a vegetable protein present in tofu, a food widely consumed in Asia. It is also sold in health-food stores as a supplement for that purpose. Studies have found that replacing animal fat with soy results in a reduction of LDL cholesterol of 13%.[50] If you want to reduce your intake of animal fat, soy and other legumes (beans) are a good alternative source of protein. The effects of soy, however, are probably related to the reduction in animal-fat intake rather than to any specific effects of the soy itself.

COENZYME Q10

Coenzyme Q10, which occurs naturally in the body, is involved in energy transfer in something called the mitochondria, which are like the power station for the cells of the body. Since it decreases normally with age, the connection was made with the increase in heart-disease risk with age. In other words, people thought that coenzyme Q10 might protect against heart disease, and that the loss of it with aging might explain why heart-disease risk goes up with aging. The natural next step was to try to use supplements of coenzyme Q10 to prevent heart disease. Studies of coenzyme Q10 supplementation, however, have shown only modest changes in heart function, with no effect on what we care most about, which is prevention of heart attacks.

CHOLESTIN

Cholestin is an ancient remedy that has been used in Chinese medicine for centuries for the treatment of heart problems. Derived from yeast on red rice, it is called red rice yeast extract. It has eight statin compounds that are HMG coenzymeA reductase inhibitors, just like statins, that have been shown to reduce cholesterol. Because they are chemically identical to statins, they therefore have the same risks as the statins.

FISH OIL

Studies of fish oils and fish-oil extracts in the form of pills and formulas for the prevention of heart disease have not been uniformly promising. Patients with a history of heart attack have had the best results. In the GISSI Prevenzione study, 11,000 Italian post–heart attack patients on standard medication therapy who took 850 mg of omega-3 fatty acids (present in fish oil) each day had a 45% reduction in negative cardiac-health outcomes. In another study, extracts of n-3 polyunsaturated fatty acids also led to a significant reduction in heart attacks in men with heart disease.[51] Contrary to public opinion and to what you read in the papers, however, omega-3 fatty acids will not *prevent* heart disease.

A recent analysis of 41 studies of omega-3 fatty acids with a total of 36,913 participants[52] showed no reduction in cardiovascular events or total mortality with omega-3 supplementation using fish oils and other supplements. There was a 7% increase in cancer, which was not statistically significant.

In the Study on Omega-3 Fatty Acids and Ventricular Arrhythmia (SOFA), 546 patients with implantable fibrillators and ventricular arrhythmias were randomized to receive 2g/day fish oil or placebo. Thirty percent of the fish-oil group had their defibrillator go off or died compared to 33% of the placebo group (not a significant difference).[53]

In addition to not helping prevent heart disease, omega-3 fatty acids in the form of fish-oil supplements may even cause harm in some heart-disease patients. In the DART-2 study 3,114 men with stable angina (chest pain) were randomly assigned to receive omega-3 supplements or placebo. Instead of being protected from heart disease, the omega-3 group had a statistically significant increase in sudden death and cardiac death.[54] The increase in deaths occurred more often in those taking fish-oil capsules than in those eating oily fish. In another study two hundred patients with a history of a potentially lethal heart arrhythmia called ventricular tachy-cardia were given omega-3s or placebo.[55] The number of potentially lethal ventricular tachycardias increased in those given the omega-3s.

Fish-oil supplements or other food products to which omega-3 fatty acids have been added do not prevent heart disease in people without a history of heart disease and it is questionable whether they have beneficial effects in people with a history of heart disease. I do not recommend taking them unless you have had a heart attack, and in that case you should confer with your doctor, since they may exacerbate heart arrhythmias. You can get the same benefits by eating foods, like fish, that contain omega-3, and people who ate those foods in the clinical trials did better than those who took the supplements. In addition, if you take too many fish-oil supplements you might end up smelling like a fish! Better to eat a four- to six-ounce serving of seafood in your diet at least twice a week.

OTHER NATURAL REMEDIES

Fenugreek is a dried seed that contains fiber and steroid saponins that de-crease glucose levels and cholesterol as demonstrated by clinical trials. Gu-gulipid (Guggul gum) a natural product from India, has also been shown to reduce cholesterol. Neither of these products has been assessed for its ability to prevent or treat heart disease.

Green tea has been promoted for its beneficial effects on heart health as well as for other reasons. In the Ohsaki National Health Insurance Cohort Study, an eleven-year study of 40,530 Japanese adults ages forty to seventy-nine, green-tea consumption was associated with a reduced risk of death and death related to cardiovascular disease.[56] I am not ready to accept the results of this study, because people who drink green tea may be more health conscious in general, and this may have led to biased results. A double-blind randomized trial of green tea is needed.

Diet, Exercise, and
Behavioral Approaches

Heart disease is an ailment of modern civilization and behavior—and one, therefore, that can be treated effectively and with dramatic results by making fairly simple lifestyle changes. People in African villages don't need bypass operations. Studies have consistently shown that rates of heart disease are higher in Western cultures, that heart disease rates go up in countries that adopt Western diet and lifestyles, and that modifications of diet reduce heart disease. Some of the differences may not be attributable to diet per se but rather to how food is raised and the industrialization of American agriculture (e.g., the effects of corn-fed vs. pasture-fed animals). However, it is clear that the majority of heart disease is caused by factors associated with Western civilization, such as a fat- and sugar-laden diet and a lack of exercise.

There are also "nonmedical" factors not directly related to lifestyle that increase the risk of heart disease, like low income, lack of social support, depression, marginalization in society, and stress in childhood. I can't fix all of these social ills with this book, but I just want you to understand that it is not as simple as a "one disease/one pill" kind of thing.

Exercising for just thirty minutes a day reduces your risk of developing heart disease by 30%. This can include anything from running, playing tennis, or just vigorous walking. And there is no need to obtain a minimal heart rate. If you are older and don't run or play a sport you should incorporate a daily thirty-minute walk into your routine. That is better for you than statins by any measure. And exercise has no side effects that we don't know about yet.

If you have risk factors and don't yet have heart disease, you should address them. Improving your diet will help you lower your cholesterol and prevent heart disease. In fact, following the low-fat diet advocated by the

National Cholesterol Education Program lowers LDL cholesterol as well as treatment with a statin and without the side effects.[57]

The so-called Mediterranean diet (vegetables, legumes, fruit, cereals, and fish) reduces heart-disease risk and prolongs life.[58] Patients with heart disease who followed the Mediterranean diet had a 50% to 70% reduction in recurrent heart attacks.[59] These results are *twice as good as those of any medication.*

It's a pretty simple diet to follow over the long term. Eat at least one serving of fruit every day, which I define as one apple, one banana, one peach, one cup of blueberries, and so on. Have three or four servings of vegetables every day: a cup of broccoli, two or three cups of leafy greens, a cup of tomatoes, etc. Five to seven one-cup or two-ounce servings of whole grains, beans, and starch, such as cracked wheat, whole-wheat pasta, lentils, and sweet potatoes, should also be consumed on a daily basis. Meat and other animal proteins, like eggs and dairy, should be limited to once or twice a week. The mortality of people who followed this diet was cut in half over a four-year period. In this diet saturated fats (butter, animal fat) are replaced by unsaturated fats (seed oils) and monounsaturated fats (olive oil), and wine and nuts are included. In fact, olive oil has been shown in laboratory studies to improve endothelial function (translation: increases the flexibility of your coronary arteries, which can be beneficial for reducing your risk of heart attacks).

The recent Women's Health Initiative (WHI) study, mentioned on page 78, showed that a low-fat diet did not reduce heart disease.[60] The problem with that study is that it lumped all fats together. We now know that some fats are better than others. For example, there are fats in foods like olive oil and fish that actually promote heart health. As an example, the generic low-fat diet of the WHI reduced LDL cholesterol by only ten points, whereas a diet high in fruits and vegetables, soy, and nuts, and low in animal fat dropped cholesterol by 30%, a figure that equaled the effects of a statin (33%).

A low-carb diet does *not* prevent heart disease. Look at the doctor who developed it: He died of a heart attack. In addition, women subjects from the Nurses' Health Study (82,802) who had low carbohydrate intake did not experience a reduced occurrence of heart disease. Eating a high-sugar diet increased the risk of heart disease by 90%. High vegetable intake was associated with a 30% reduction in heart disease.[61]

Eating fish is good for your heart, but beware of eating a lot of fish high in mercury (a pollutant that gets into fish), like swordfish, tuna, and other large oceangoing fish, during pregnancy, as they can cause birth defects. Foods that are a part of the Mediterranean diet, like fish, olive oil, and nuts, increase "good" HDL cholesterol and reduce "bad" LDL cholesterol. These foods are high in omega-3 fatty acids [like docosahexaenoic acid (DHA) and eicosapentaenoic acid (EPA)] and low in omega-6 fatty acids. Omega-3s are better at increasing good cholesterol and lowering bad cholesterol than are omega-6s. It is often pointed out that ancient diets had a ratio of omega-3 to omega-6 of 1:1, whereas current diets have much higher amounts of omega-6, largely through the substitution of calories in the form of leafy plants with grains and seeds.

When I was a medical student at Duke in 1985, I distinctly remember sitting on the front porch of my house in Durham, North Carolina, and reading an article in *The New England Journal of Medicine* that described how the Inuit people of the Arctic, who had a diet high in fish and low in other meat, had much lower rates of heart disease. That observation led to the idea that the omega-3 fatty acids in fish prevented heart disease, which naturally led aggressive marketers to try to put it in a pill or a bottle and sell it. There is a lot of other stuff in fish, however, and it is not clear if the health benefits can be attributed directly to eating fish or to what you avoid by eating fish instead of other stuff.

The Bottom Line

I argue that if you are healthy; exercise; are not overweight; don't smoke; don't have a family history of heart disease, familial hypercholesterolemia, hypertension, or diabetes but have high cholesterol, you should *not* take a statin or any cholesterol-lowering drug. It's better to change your lifestyle.

Decrease the amount of animal fat you consume. Don't eat processed and junk food that has artificial ingredients like partially hydrogenated oils ("trans" fat). Trans fat is artificially produced oil that is widely used in restaurants and in the production of processed foods. It is present in many potato and corn chips, crackers, doughnuts, french fries, and other processed foods. It has been likened to putting sand into the gears of a watch; it will slowly wear your body out over time. Restaurant fried foods like french fries are a particularly bad culprit, because the oil in restaurants is used over and over and in the process breaks down and becomes even more harmful.

And toast yourself after you make these changes with a glass or two of wine (or beer) a day, if you want to; moderate amounts of wine and beer also reduce heart-disease risk.

If you don't have heart disease or risk factors for heart disease, you don't need to get your cholesterol checked, no matter what anyone tells you. Why do I say this? Because the only reason to get your cholesterol checked is to see if you need treatment. And since statins won't help you, there is no need to get it checked. The only exception is if you have familial hypercholesterolemia, in which case you will have a relative who died young from heart disease. If you are a woman of any age or a man over seventy without heart disease, don't get your cholesterol checked and don't take statins. If you're a man with multiple risk factors (obesity, smoking, hypertension, family history), change the risk factors! If you can't, a statin will decrease heart attacks a little, maybe, but won't save your life. Ditto for women with heart disease. If you don't have heart disease, don't take aspirin or clopidogrel. If you are a man with heart disease, you should take a statin and aspirin. I don't think one statin is better than another. The statins like Crestor that have greater potency are offset by more side effects. I recommend taking a statin that you can buy in generic form, like atorvastatin (generic Lipitor), since it costs much less.

Drug	Use	Common, Benign Side Effects	Serious Side Effects	Life-threatening Side Effects	Reasons Not to Take
Fibrates					
Moderate Risk					
Gemfibrozil (Gemcor, Lopid)	Hypercho-lesterolemia	Bloating, nausea, diarrhea, dyspepsia	Diarrhea, stomach pain, liver damage, gallbladder disease	Increased mortality, possible cancer	Liver or kidney disease, hypersen-sitivity, breast-feeding
Clofibrate (Atromid-S)	Hypercho-lesterolemia	Bloating, nausea, diarrhea, dyspepsia	Diarrhea, stomach pain, liver damage, gallbladder disease	Increased mortality, possible cancer	Liver or kidney disease, hypersen-sitivity, breast-feeding
Fenofibrate (Tricor)	Hypercho-lesterolemia	Bloating, nausea, diarrhea, dyspepsia	Diarrhea, stomach pain, liver damage, gallbladder disease	Increased mortality, possible cancer	Liver or kidney disease, hypersen-sitivity, breast-feeding
Vitamin B$_3$					
Low Risk					
Nicotinic acid (Niacin, Niaspan)	Hypercho-lesterolemia	Nausea, vomiting, stomach pain	Flushing	Activation of stomach ulcer, liver damage (rare)	Liver dysfunction, ulcers, hypo-tension, bleeding

Drug	Use	Common, Benign Side Effects	Serious Side Effects	Life-threatening Side Effects	Reasons Not to Take
Bile Acid Sequestrants					
Low Risk					
Cholestyramine (Locholest, Questran)	Hypercho-lesterolemia	Bloating, nausea, vomiting, heartburn, fatty stools, dizziness, fatigue	Constipation, stomach pain	Nutritional deficiency, interference with absorption of vitamins, bleeding	Nutritional deficiency, intoler-ability
Colestipol (Colestid)	Hypercho-lesterolemia	Bloating, nausea, vomiting, heartburn, fatty stools, dizziness, fatigue	Constipation, stomach pain	Nutritional deficiency, interference with absorption of vitamins, bleeding	Nutritional deficiency, intoler-ability
Cholesterol-Absorption Inhibitors					
Low Risk					
Ezetimibe (Zetia)	Hypercho-lesterolemia	Fever, headache, muscle pain, runny nose, sore throat	Hives	Liver damage	Liver disease, pregnancy, breast-feeding
Statins					
Moderate Risk					
Fluvastatin (Lescol)	Hypercho-lesterolemia	Dizziness, constipation, nausea, vomiting	Myopathy, joint pain, memory impairment, impotence, stomach pain	Liver damage, rhabdomyolysis with kidney damage	Liver disease, pregnancy, breast-feeding, men over seventy, women without heart disease

Drug	Use	Common, Benign Side Effects	Serious Side Effects	Life-threatening Side Effects	Reasons Not to Take
Atorvastatin (Lipitor)	Hypercho-lesterolemia	Dizziness, constipation, nausea, vomiting	Myopathy, joint pain, memory impairment, impotence, stomach pain	Liver damage, rhabdomyolysis with kidney damage	Liver disease, pregnancy, breast-feeding, men over seventy, women without heart disease
Lovastatin (Mevacor)	Hypercho-lesterolemia	Dizziness, constipation, nausea, vomiting	Myopathy, joint pain, memory impairment, impotence, stomach pain	Liver damage, rhabdomyolysis with kidney damage	Liver disease, pregnancy, breast-feeding, men over seventy, women without heart disease
Pravastatin (Pravachol)	Hypercho-lesterolemia	Dizziness, constipation, nausea, vomiting	Myopathy, joint pain, memory impairment, impotence, stomach pain	Liver damage, rhabdomyolysis with kidney damage	Liver disease, pregnancy, breast-feeding, men over seventy, women without heart disease
Simvastatin (Zocor)	Hypercho-lesterolemia	Dizziness, constipation, nausea, vomiting	Myopathy, joint pain, memory impairment, impotence, stomach pain	Liver damage, rhabdomyolysis with kidney damage	Liver disease, pregnancy, breast-feeding, men over seventy, women without heart disease

Drug	Use	Common, Benign Side Effects	Serious Side Effects	Life-threatening Side Effects	Reasons Not to Take
High Risk					
Rosuvastatin (Crestor)	Hypercho-lesterolemia	Dizziness, constipation, nausea, vomiting	Myopathy, joint pain, memory impairment, impotence, stomach pain	Liver damage, rhabdomyolysis with kidney damage	Liver disease, pregnancy, breast-feeding, men over seventy, women without heart disease

5.

Antihypertensives

Summertime and the living is easy, right? Well, it may be for some people, but for me it's a time to dust off my frequent-flyer miles, pack up the kids, and hit the airways for visits to my parents and in-laws. This year it was also a chance to review their medications. First stop Sicily, where a quick check showed that my seventy-something mother-in-law was on Cardura and had been for years. Hadn't her doctors heard about the results of the ALLHAT study, published more than ten years ago, which, as I will review on page 96, showed this alpha-blocker antihypertension medication to have a greater risk of death than treatment with other medications? After winging back across the Atlantic I didn't find the American establishment to be much better: In the States my seventy-something father was being treated for hypertension with the angiotensin-converting enzyme (ACE) inhibitor lisinopril. Didn't his health-care providers know that diuretics like hydrochlorothiazide cost one third as much, are more effective, and don't have the side effects of ACE inhibitors like the dry cough that nearly drove him crazy?

Hypertension, or high blood pressure, often described as a silent killer, affects 50 million Americans. Hypertension usually occurs without symp-toms, but if your blood pressure gets really high you can develop headache, dizziness, blurred vision, ringing in the ears, or nose bleeds. Most people find out that they have high blood pressure by getting a routine blood-pressure check at their doctor's office or more easily and cheaply at many pharmacies. If untreated (about 30% of people with high blood pressure don't know they have it) it can quietly damage your organs and set the course for developing other life-threatening diseases, including stroke, heart disease, and kidney failure.

Hypertension occurs when the body holds on to too much water, which increases the volume of blood in the heart, arteries, and veins and thus in-creases the pressure against the walls of the heart and blood vessels. Some-times the heart beats too hard, which also can increase the pressure. Either situation leads to high blood pressure, which, over time, damages the blood vessels.

Blood pressure is measured in units of millimeters of mercury (mm Hg), which is the amount of atmospheric pressure required to support a column of mercury 1 millimeter high. Blood pressure has a number for systolic and diastolic blood pressure. Your systolic pressure, the pressure in the vessels when the heart beats, should be less than 140 mm Hg. Your diastolic pressure, the pressure between heartbeats, should be less than 90 mm Hg.

Like heart disease, hypertension is a disease of modern civilization. Hypertension is a product of the way our bodies have evolved over the centuries to retain water and avoid dehydration. We tend to retain salt (sodium chloride, or NaCl), because, prior to modern times, salt was rela-tively rare. When salt is retained in our blood vessels, they hold on to water by means of the osmotic effect, thereby preventing water from being excreted as much as it otherwise would be through the kidneys and into the urine.

Granted, not everyone is sensitive to salt to the same degree. However, there is no doubt that the population as a whole eats much more salt than in the past, probably at least two or three times as much, and these habits are having an adverse effect on our health, including raising blood pressure.

Since early man did not have easy access to salt, he didn't have to worry about eating too many salted potato chips and having his blood pressure go through the roof. In fact, for water retention, salt served an important purpose: It was a good thing if you were living on the savannah and wouldn't be eating or drinking for several hours. If you live in twenty-first-century America and eat fast food three times a day, however, it's a bad thing. Ancient man also got more exercise, ate less food in general (not by choice), and didn't smoke, take drugs, or drink alcohol. However, those tough conditions did lead to more infection; and being eaten by tigers and falling off cliffs were occupational hazards. Luckily, those folks didn't have to also worry about their blood pressure zooming up after eating a burger and fries.

Cheeseburgers notwithstanding, our earliest need for salt developed in us a taste for salty foods, which we have never lost. In cooking, salt enhances the flavor of other foods, and many cooks feel it is an essential ingredient in the kitchen. Salting your pasta water with a handful of sea salt is not going to cause high blood pressure. Most of the oversalting in our system comes from the preprepared, packaged, and many frozen foods (with the exception of flash-frozen fruits and vegetables) we eat as well as from restaurant and fast foods. Food makers put huge amounts of salt in their food to enhance flavor, to hide the lack of other natural flavorings, and to act as a preservative. Look at any food label, and you will see astronomical percentages of salt in food, often more than 25% of a serving. The best way to avoid excess sodium in food is to buy fresh, unprocessed whole foods and prepare your own meals. If you buy canned beans and vegetables, low sodium or not, you should rinse them well, as this removes about 40% of the sodium.

Pharmaceutical Solutions

Americans spend $15 billion a year on medications to control high blood pressure. In my opinion much of this money is wasted because many of the medications prescribed cost ten times more than other, older medications that work as well or better.[1] But most important, high blood pressure can be solved for free—by changing your diet, including reducing the amount of salt you eat, and by exercising. Even if you are on high-blood-pressure meds, you should cut back on salt.

The medicines available today—diuretics, beta-blockers, angiotensin-converting enzyme (ACE) inhibitors, alpha-receptor blockers, and calcium channel blockers—work in one of three ways. Diuretics make your kidneys pass more water, so your blood volume is less. Beta-blockers decrease the pumping of the heart, while ACE inhibitors, alpha-receptor blockers, and calcium channel blockers dilate the blood vessels.

DIURETICS

There are two types of diuretics, the first group of antihypertensive medications. Thiazide diuretics increase urine output and decrease the volume of fluid in your circulation by increasing sodium excretion from the kidneys, which drags water along with it. Examples include hydrochlorothiazide (Esidrix, Hydrodiuril, Microzide) and chlorthalidone (Hygroton). They work very well, are safer than other, newer meds used to treat hypertension, and because they are off patent and available in generic versions, cost a fraction of what other drugs cost. They also have some beneficial side effects. Thiazides promote calcium retention and prevent bone loss and fractures. However, they can negatively interact with an extensive list of medications, which are listed in the *Physicians' Desk Reference.*

Their main problem is that they cause frequent urination, which is inconvenient to say the least. They can also be associated with a loss of potassium from the blood. Potassium, a mineral essential for bodily function, is present is many fruits and vegetables, including broccoli, orange juice, potatoes, bananas, soybeans, avocados, apricots, pomegranates, parsnips and turnips. Potassium is essential for muscle action as well as function of the nerves. Low serum potassium, or hypokalemia, is a potentially fatal condition that can be associated with symptoms of muscle weakness, confusion, dizziness that can lead to falls, and heart arrhythmias. For people with a healthy diet, it is not a problem. To avoid the problem of potassium depletion with diuretics you can also take potassium supplements orally every day. One of these drugs, the so-called thiazide-like diuretic indapamide (Lozol), can cause life-threatening drops of sodium in the blood. In 1992 the Australian authorities reported 164 cases of this potentially life-threatening condition, which is associated with confusion, lethargy, nausea, vomiting, dizziness, loss of appetite, fatigue, fainting, sleepiness, and possible convulsions. Since it doesn't work better than hydrochlorothiazide and is potentially dangerous, I don't recommend that you use it.

Loop diuretics are more powerful medications. Brand names include furosemide (Lasix) and bumetidine (Bumex). They block the pump in the kidneys that transports sodium, potassium, and chloride, and cause a stronger output of urine. However, because of their strong action, they can cause life-threatening depletions of potassium, calcium, and magnesium, which can increase the risk of insomnia, falls, confusion, and heat stroke as well as that of blood clots and stroke. Lasix increases the loss of thiamine (vitamin B_1) in the urine, which can lead to memory deficiency and other problems, but this side effect can be corrected with vitamin supplementation. Lasix also increases calcium excretion in the urine, which leads to thinning of the bones and risk of fracture. For these reasons, thiazide diuretics should be used before Lasix or Bumex for the treatment of hypertension, unless there is fluid retention and a failure of kidney function.

Because the risk of potassium deficiency is so great with diuretics, the pharmaceutical companies saw a new market in "potassium-sparing diuretics." Examples of these include eplerenone (Inspra), spironolactone (Aldactone), and amiloride, which is sold as Moduretic in combination with hydrochlorothiazide, and triamterine (Dyrenium), which is currently sold as part of Dyazide or Maxide, a combination of hydrochlorothiazide and triamterene. Because they act to stop the depletion of potassium, they can actually cause toxic increases in potassium in the blood, leading to renal failure. They typically are sold in combination with thiazide. The FDA does not usually approve combination drugs, which tend to be more difficult to manage, because you can't adjust the doses of the two different medications separately. It is not clear why the FDA approved these drugs. Potassium-sparing diuretics also increase risk of heat stroke. For all these reasons they should be avoided.

BETA-BLOCKERS

Again, beta-blockers, the second type of hypertension drug, act by making your heart beat less hard. Common beta-blocker medications are metoprolol (Toprol XL, Lopressor), atenolol (Tenormin), carvedilol (Coreg), bisoprolol (Zebeta), and propanolol (Inderal). Specifically, they work by blocking the noradrenergic beta-1 receptor in the heart, which is responsible for making the heart pump. Because there are also noradrenergic receptors in the brain, in addition to those in the heart, these drugs can also cause side effects related to the nervous system. These include tingling in the hands and feet, nausea, constipation, and, more rarely, dizziness, nightmares, impotence, and depression. These neurological side effects are more common with the older drugs like propanolol, since newer drugs like atenolol were designed to act more selectively on the heart. One drawback of atenolol is that it doesn't seem to lower "central" blood pressure, the blood pressure in your aorta and central arteries (which is what matters most) as much as the blood pressure in your arm, where it is commonly measured.

This may explain why the risk of stroke is 16% higher with atenolol than with hydrochlorothiazide.[2] Since almost all research studies have been on atenolol, we don't know if this applies to other beta-blockers like metoprolol or propanolol. Based on the information we have, however, I recommend using one of the other beta-blockers.

Since beta-blockers inhibit heart function, if your heart isn't working right, they can sometimes cause heart failure, which would be associated with fatigue, chest pain, or a sudden weight gain caused by water retention.

DRUGS THAT ACT ON THE ADRENERGIC RECEPTORS

Alpha-blockers, including doxazosin (Cardura), prazosin (Minipress), and terazosin (Hytrin), block the alpha noradrenergic receptor in the heart and blood vessels. A related drug, called labetalol (Normodyne), blocks both alpha and beta receptors. The Antihypertensive and Lipid Lowering Treatment to Prevent Heart Attack Trial (ALLHAT), a study sponsored by the NIH, compared different types of antihypertensive treatments in 33,357 patients with high blood pressure and one other risk factor for heart disease. Since ALLHAT, which I review in more detail on pages 100–101, was not sponsored by a drug company, it did not have to fit into the marketing agenda of any particular company, enabling the investigators to compare different drugs, both old and cheap (diuretics, alpha-blockers, and beta-blockers), and new and expensive (ACE inhibitors and calcium channel blockers). ALLHAT showed that when compared to diuretics, the alpha-blocker Cardura was twice as likely to cause heart failure and increased the risk of stroke and all cardiovascular disease. In view of this outcome the study was stopped early, and the authors of ALLHAT concluded that alpha-blockers should not be used in the treatment of hypertension.[1] Based on these findings I believe that there is no role for alpha-blockers in the treatment of patients with hypertension.

Another drug that works on adrenergic receptors, clonidine (Catapres), stimulates the alpha-2 norepinephrine receptor, which lowers blood pressure by putting a brake on the norepinephrine (catecholamine) system. Missing a dose or two of clonidine causes sweating, tremor, flushing, and very high blood pressure. It also causes depression and skin reactions. With time, the body adapts to clonidine, and it becomes less effective. Because of these factors and because it doesn't work all that well I do not recommend using clonidine for blood-pressure control.

NITRATES

Nitroglycerin (Nitroquick, Nitrobid, Nitrodur, Nitrol, Minitran, Nitrostat, Deponit) is a vasodilator that is often used for the acute relief of chest pain. Vasodilators work by dilating (i.e., enlarging) blood vessels in the heart, which increases the flow of blood to the parts of the heart that are not getting enough. This condition, called myocardial ischemia, can lead to chest pain and possible heart attack. Since vasodilators change blood flow to the brain as well as to the heart, they can be associated with neurological side effects, including dizziness, headache, blurred vision, nausea, rapid pulse, and light-headedness. Another side effect is postural hypotension with rising: If you sit up too quickly the blood doesn't get pumped to your brain right away and you can end up feeling dizzy and possibly fall or pass out.

The most important side effect to note is that when these drugs are taken with meds for the treatment of sexual dysfunction, such as Viagra, they can be very dangerous and cause heart attack. Most doctors know that they should not prescribe nitroglycerin for someone who is already taking a drug for sexual dysfunction. As I mentioned in Chapter 1, prescription errors can occur in as many as 25% of cases. I can promise you that, unfortunately, somewhere in the U.S. at this moment someone is writing an inappropriate prescription for Viagra. Think about all the junk e-mails about Cialis or similar drugs you get. There are some people getting nitro from their doctors who aren't telling their doctors that they are taking Cialis. Even worse, e-mail sources of prescription drugs are notoriously unreliable, so you really don't know what you might be taking.

ANGIOTENSIN-CONVERTING ENZYME
(ACE) INHIBITORS

ACE inhibitors, one of the newest types of hypertension drugs, act on the reninangiotensin system, which regulates blood pressure and kidney function. Normally, the angiotensin-converting enzyme converts the molecule angiotensin I to angiotensin II, a potent vasoconstrictor that makes the blood vessels close down. Blocking the angiotensin-converting enzyme makes the blood vessels relax, thereby decreasing blood pressure. Examples of this type of drug include lisinopril (Prinivil), enalapril (Vasotec), ramipril (Altace), benazepril (Lotensin), fosinopril (Monopril), and captopril (Capoten). Side effects of ACE inhibitors include headache, flushing, low blood pressure, trouble breathing, diarrhea, rash, and, more rarely, dizziness, heart failure, or stroke. One of the most annoying side effects is a persistent dry cough.

Eleven percent of patients taking ACE inhibitors develop chronic dry cough. For anyone who has experienced this side effect, you know that it is so annoying (to you and those around you) that it is impossible to continue on the drug. In rare cases ACE inhibitors can cause an emergency-level swelling of the face, lips, and tongue, and can be fatal if there is swelling of the larynx. Even more rarely, ACE inhibitors can cause a loss of white blood cells that can be fatal if the drug is not stopped.

Angiotensin-receptor blockers (ARBs), like valsartan (Diovan), irbesartan (Avapro), olmesartan (Benicar), candesartan (Atacand), and losartan (Cozaar, which is Hyzaar when combined with hydrochlorothiazide) act on the angiotensin receptor to block its effects, thereby reducing blood pressure. Side effects include dizziness, diarrhea, rash, and, more rarely, anxiety, muscle pains, upper respiratory tract infection, low blood pressure, or elevations in potassium.

Both the ACE inhibitors and the angiotensin-receptor blockers can have harmful effects on the fetus when taken during pregnancy, including fetal death. They can also cause dangerous elevations of potassium in the blood.

CALCIUM CHANNEL BLOCKERS

Calcium channel blockers act on the lining of the blood vessels. When these channels let calcium in, the blood vessels constrict. By blocking the calcium channels, these drugs cause the vessels to relax, and as a result blood pressure goes down. Examples of this type of drug include amlodipine (Norvasc), verapamil (Calan), nifedipine (Procardia, Adalat), and diltiazem (Tiazac). Side effects include constipation, dizziness, headache, nausea, and, more rarely, low blood pressure, heart failure, or arrhythmias.

Calcium channel blockers can be associated with headache, nausea, or dizziness. They also are associated with an accumulation of bodily fluids that can lead to heart failure. In the International Nifedipine GITS Study: Intervention as a Goal in Hypertension Treatment (IN-SIGHT), there were eight times as many patients who developed a swelling of the legs or arms while on a calcium channel blocker as those on a diuretic.[2] A study of the entire Swedish population showed that if you took calcium channel blockers you were more likely to kill yourself by as much as fivefold. They didn't find that to be the case with any of the other antihypertensive drugs after adjusting for use of other cardiac drugs, including beta-blockers.[3] In general, however, suicide is fairly rare.

Efficacy: Are the New Drugs Really Worth Taking?

As I said earlier, diuretics and beta-blockers have been around longer than ACE inhibitors, ARBs, and calcium channel blockers. Drugmakers have argued that the newer drugs have fewer side effects and are more convenient than these old standbys. Because of the unique way they act in the body (acting on the angiotensin system rather than increasing urine production), they have been promoted as being superior to the older drugs and as having fewer side effects, and for many years doctors and patients have accepted these claims at face value. However, as I point out in this chapter, later research has not always borne out these claims.

By the 1990s, the three newer classes of drugs had taken over the anti-hypertensive market. The most important feature of the antihypertensive drugs is how well they control blood pressure, and studies like the Blood Pressure Lowering Treatment Trials Collaboration (BPLTTC) have shown that the better the blood pressure control the fewer the long-term adverse events like heart attacks and strokes.[4] Recent studies, however, have shown that the newer drugs are probably not worth the extra money.

In a variety of studies, including INSIGHT, the NORdic DILtiazem (NORDIL)[5] study, and Controlled ONset Verapamil INvestigation of Cardiovascular Endpoints (CONVINCE),[6] calcium channel blockers have not been found to prevent heart attacks better than diuretics. In fact, in the A Coronary disease Trial Investigating Outcome with Nifedipine (AC-TION) study, the calcium channel blocker nifedipine did not prevent heart attacks or chest pain (angina) any better than did a placebo, or sugar pill.[7] A meta-analysis of all studies combined showed that treatment with calcium channel blockers did not improve mortality more than a placebo, although ACE inhibitors did.[8] Another meta-analysis found that treatment with calcium channel blockers when compared to other drug treatments for high blood pressure was associated with a relative 26% increase in heart attacks, a 25% increase in heart failure, and a 10% increase in major cardiovascular events.[9] Furthermore, for women, calcium channel blockers increased the risk of heart attack or stroke by 18%. Calcium channel blockers have been found to increase the risk of heart failure relative to other antihypertensive drugs in several studies, overall by about 20% in BPLTTC. In spite of this, one of the calcium channel blockers, amlodipine, continues to be a blockbuster drug, with $2 billion a year in sales reported in 2003, a year after the troubling reports of heart failure with calcium channel blockers was published.

In the abovementioned Antihypertensive and Lipid Lowering Treatment to Prevent Heart Attack Trial (ALLHAT), the largest study of antihypertensive medications ever performed, different types of antihypertensive treatments were compared in 33,357 patients with high blood pressure and one other risk factor for heart disease who were randomly assigned to the "old" drug chlorthalidone (diuretic) or to the "new" drugs amlodipine (calcium channel blocker) or lisinopril (ACE inhibitor). Rates of fatal and nonfatal heart attacks were essentially the same among the three treatments.[10] There was a 38% increase in heart failure with amlodipine compared to that with chlorthalidone. For lisinopril there were increased rates of total cardiovascular disease outcomes (10%), stroke (15%), and heart failure (19%) compared to those with chlorthalidone.

Since the time of ALLHAT other studies have not shown that ACE inhibitors and calcium channel blockers work better than diuretics, even though they cost more. And like ALLHAT, some of these studies show cause for concern.

In a series of studies conducted in a total of 67,658 patients, "old drugs" (the beta-blocker atenolol and diuretics) were compared to "new drugs" (calcium channel blockers and ACE inhibitors). These studies did not show that the more expensive new drugs were better or safer; if anything, diuretics were better than all other drugs, an effect that was probably masked by the fact that patients on diuretics were also treated with atenolol (which, as I will explain later, is not the best beta-blocker, or medication in general, that you can take). The NORDIL study compared diltiazem (calcium channel blocker) to diuretics and/or beta-blockers; the CONVINCE study compared verapamil (calcium channel blocker) and atenolol (beta-blocker) with hydrochlorothiazide (diuretic); the INternational VErapamil trandolapril STudy (INVEST)[11] compared verapamil to atenolol; the Swedish Trial in Old Patients 2 (STOP-2)[12] compared calcium channel blockers and ACE inhibitors to beta-blockers and diuretics; and the CAPtopril Prevention Project (CAPPP) compared captopril (ACE inhibitor) to beta-blockers.[13] None of these studies showed differences in rates of heart attacks between "old" and "new" drugs.

Not only was it difficult to show that the new drugs were better than the old (the marketing goal that drove the design of the studies), it wasn't easy to show that taking the drugs was better than doing nothing. For instance, in the ACTION study (A Coronary disease Trial Investigating Outcome with Nifedipine) that I mentioned earlier, 7,665 patients with stable angina received the calcium channel blocker nifedipine or a placebo in a randomized trial. There was no difference in a combined measure of fatal and nonfatal heart attack or stroke, revascularization, or heart failure. Death from heart disease was equal in the groups, and there was a 16% increase in noncardiac deaths with nifedipine that was not statistically significant. Women on nifedipine had an 18% increase in this measure of cardiac events, although the difference was not statistically significant. In the Heart Outcomes Prevention Evaluation (HOPE) study, 9,297 patients at high risk for heart disease were randomized to the ACE inhibitor ramipril or placebo in addition to their usual treatment.[14] A fatal or non-fatal heart attack or stroke occurred in 14.0% of the ramipril patients compared to 17.8% of those on placebo, a difference that was statistically significant. In the Prevention of Events with Angiotensin-Converting Enzyme Inhibition (PEACE) trial, a study of 8,290 patients with heart disease, the addition of the ACE inhibitor trandolapril had no effect on reducing heart attacks and coronary revascularization procedures compared to treatment with a placebo.[15] These results led to the editorial "ACE Inhibitors in Patients with Stable Heart Disease—May They Rest in Peace?"

The Valsartan Antihypertensive Long-term Use Evaluation (VALUE) study compared the ARB valsartan to the calcium channel blocker amlodipine in 15,245 patients over age fifty with high blood pressure and a high risk of heart disease.[16] The study found no difference between the two drugs in fatal and nonfatal heart attacks and other cardiac events. More nonfatal heart attacks occurred with valsartan, but fewer patients developed diabetes. This study led to the editorial "Is There Value in VALUE?"

When new drugs were compared to diuretics alone, their performance was worse. For instance, the Multicenter Isradipine Diuretic Atherosclerosis Study (MIDAS) compared the calcium channel blocker isradipine to the diuretic chlorthalidone in 883 patients with high blood pressure. Twenty-five patients on isradipine had a major cardiovascular event (heart attack, stroke, heart failure, death, or angina) compared with fourteen on a diuretic, a statistically significant difference.[17] In the International Nifedipine GITS Study: Intervention as a Goal in Hypertension Treatment (INSIGHT), 6,321 patients ages fifty-five to eighty with hypertension and one risk factor for heart disease were randomly assigned to nifedipine or co-amilozide (hydrochlorothiazide + amiloride, both diuretics). In the nifedipine group, 200 patients succumbed to cardiovascular death, heart attack, heart failure, or stroke (combined) vs. 182 in the diuretic group, which was not statistically significant. The nifedipine group did have significantly more fatal heart attacks (sixteen vs. five) and nonfatal heart failure (twenty-four vs. eleven).

As I alluded to above, the fact that more studies didn't show that "old drugs" are better than new drugs is probably related to the fact that beta-blockers and diuretics were lumped together, a policy based more on marketing strategy than on science. The fact that beta-blockers may have dragged down diuretics is supported by studies like the Anglo-Scandinavian Cardiac Outcomes Trial Blood Pressure Lowering Arm (ASCOT-BPLA), in which 19,257 patients with high blood pressure and risk factors for heart disease were randomized to the calcium channel blocker amlodipine vs. the beta-blocker atenolol. In the case of those who needed medication for blood pressure control, the ACE inhibitor perindopril was added to amlodipine, and bendroflumethiazide (diuretic) was added to atenolol. There was no difference in the number of patients who had heart attacks, both fatal and otherwise (429 vs. 474), although there were fewer strokes (327 vs. 422) and fewer deaths from any cause (738 vs. 820), and fewer patients developed diabetes on amlodipine.[18]

When data from 6,825 patients who were treated with the beta-blocker atenolol vs. a placebo were combined from several different studies, atenolol didn't have a very good performance. There was no effect on mortality (+1%), cardiovascular mortality (-1%) or heart attack (-1%). In 17,671 patients treated with atenolol or a comparison antihypertensive treatment, there was a statistically significant increase in mortality of 13% over those receiving other antihypertensive treatments.[19] Patients with a history of heart attack treated with beta-blockers had a 23% reduction in mortality; however, all of this improvement in mortality was a result of treatment with medications other than atenolol.[20] Atenolol confers little benefit. Other beta-blockers (pindolol, metoprolol, propanolol) seem to be more effective than atenolol. However, almost all of the studies of beta-blockers have been conducted with atenolol, so there is not enough information to make a judgment.

Dr. Bruce Psaty and colleagues from the University of Washington in Seattle looked at all the data from the trials that had been published up to 2003. Overall they found that diuretics were superior to all other treatments.[21] Compared to placebo, diuretics reduced the risk of heart disease by 21%, heart failure by 49%, stroke by 29%, and total mortality by 10% (all significant). Compared to calcium channel blockers, diuretics were responsible for 6% fewer cardiovascular-disease events and 26% less heart failure; compared to ACE inhibitors, there was 12% less heart failure, 6% fewer cardiovascular-disease events, and 14% less stroke. Compared to beta-blockers, diuretics had 11% fewer cardiovascular-disease events. All treatments were similar in their ability to lower blood pressure. The authors concluded that diuretics (but not beta-blockers, as was the recommendation at the time) should be the first line of treatment for high blood pressure.

Most of the studies of antihypertensive medications have involved men. In the only study focused on women, 30,219 women with hypertension without heart disease were assessed for the relationship between antihypertensive therapy and outcome. Use of calcium channel blockers vs. diuretic was associated with a 55% increased risk of cardiovascular death, and diuretic plus calcium channel blocker was associated with an 85%

increased risk of cardiovascular death compared to diuretic plus beta-blocker. The risk increased to 116% when women with diabetes were excluded.[22]

ACE inhibitors and ARB drugs have been shown to be helpful if you have what is called left ventricular dysfunction (when your heart is not pumping correctly), or if you have had a heart attack.[23-25] The Losartan Intervention For Endpoint Reduction in Hypertension study (LIFE) was conducted in 1,195 patients with high blood pressure, diabetes, and left ventricular failure (heart-pump failure). Patients were given the ARB losartan or the beta-blocker atenolol. This study showed a 26% reduction in fatal and nonfatal strokes and heart attacks with losartan compared to atenolol.[25] Another study of 5,010 patients with heart failure showed that addition of the ARB valsartan to the usual treatment regimen caused a 13% reduction in fatal and nonfatal cardiac events and interventions compared to placebo. For those patients on an ACE inhibitor and a beta-blocker, however, there was an increase in cardiac events and mortality when valsartan was added.[26] The Evaluation of Losartan In The Elderly (ELITE II) study randomized 3,152 elderly patients over age sixty with heart failure and left ventricular dysfunction to the ARB losartan or the ACE inhibitor captopril.[27] There were no differences in mortality (11.7% vs. 10.4%), although fewer patients stopped medication in the ARB group (9.7% vs. 14.7%), primarily because of dry cough with the ACE inhibitors. These drugs do not help African Americans with left ventricular dysfunction, however.

A recent study in the U.K. followed patients prospectively using a database of 1.18 million patients. Heart-disease patients who were treated with a statin, aspirin, and beta-blockers had a better rate of survival than those who were not treated with these medications; the addition of an ACE inhibitor, however, yielded no additional benefit in terms of survival.[28]

Lifestyle Changes

As in the treatment or prevention of heart disease, you have a lot more control over your blood pressure than you may realize. High blood pressure is not inevitable. The cavemen didn't have it. If you exercise thirty minutes a day, lose weight, and cut out processed foods that are high in salt, your hypertension will likely disappear.

To this end, if you have high blood pressure, I have to emphasize again that you should stop consumption of all frozen, processed, and fast foods. This means no more trips to McDonald's or the like, potato chip binges, or frozen-food entrees. All of these foods contain extremely high amounts of sodium. Canned vegetables should be avoided, but if you have to eat them, rinse them off. Look for low-sodium versions of chicken stock and broth, prepared soups, crackers, and other foods.

If these measures don't lower your blood pressure, it may be stress that is driving your blood pressure up. A change in your circumstances might help, but that could be unrealistic. Extraordinary circumstances require extraordinary means. We may need to go beyond our usual repertoire to find techniques to cope with these increased stressors, including muscle relaxation, deep breathing, and yoga. Transcendental meditation—a mental technique requiring deep concentration and focus to promote relaxation, reduce stress, and improve overall quality of life—has been shown to not only promote relaxation but actually lower blood pressure. Other methods like mindfulness-based stress reduction reduce anxiety and stress and probably are effective in reducing high blood pressure.

Exercise can also go a long way toward reducing blood pressure.[29] Research studies show that regular exercise lowers blood pressure in 75% of people with hypertension, with reductions of 11 mm Hg in systolic pressure and 8 mm Hg in diastolic pressure. These figures are clinically significant, as demonstrated by a 25% reduction in heart attacks because of reductions in blood pressure. Aerobic exercise is better for blood pressure than resistance exercise. The beneficial effects of exercise on blood pressure are evident in the first twenty-four hours after exercise, and one to two weeks after the last period of exercise. Furthermore, modest exercise (e.g., moderate walking for thirty minutes three times a week) is as effective as more vigorous exercise and may be safer for sedentary individuals starting out on a new exercise program (for whom vigorous exercise before getting in decent shape may trigger a heart attack).

The Bottom Line

First things first. Cut down on the sodium from your diet. That means making your own dinner whenever possible, since processed (including canned and frozen) foods are full of sodium. Exercise by moderate walking for thirty minutes three times a week. Try stress reduction or meditation. Stop smoking. Do not drink alcohol in excessive amounts.

If these changes fail to lower your blood pressure, you may need medication. Start out with the standard and least-expensive treatment: diuretics. Based on the research I outlined earlier, they work better than the newer drugs, and they have fewer side effects overall than the newer medications. This is especially true if you are African American. You should definitely not take an ACE inhibitor or calcium channel blocker if you are not taking a diuretic.

Alpha-blockers should not be taken under any circumstances; these drugs cause more heart problems than do conventional diuretic treatments. Potassium-sparing diuretics are dangerous and should be avoided.

If you can't control your blood pressure with a diuretic, you may need to add another medication. This means going to a beta-blocker, ACE inhibitor, or calcium channel blocker. I do not recommend atenolol; use another beta-blocker like metoprolol. Women should not take a calcium channel blocker. ACE inhibitors or ARB drugs can help Caucasians with left ventricular (heart pump) failure.

Drug	Use	Common, Benign Side Effects	Serious Side Effects	Life-threatening Side Effects	Reasons Not to Take
Thiazide Diuretics					
Low Risk					
Hydrochloro-thiazide (Esidrex, Hydrodiuril, Microzide)	Hyper-tension	Increased urination, dizziness, nausea, vomiting	Hypotension, numbness, headache	Low potassium levels with seizure and death (rare if on potassium supplement), anemia, Stevens-Johnson Syndrome (SJS)	Kidney dysfunction, hyper-sensitivity
Chlorthalidone (Hygroton)	Hyper-tension	Increased urination, dizziness, nausea, vomiting	Hypotension, numbness, headache	Low potassium levels with seizure and death (rare if on potassium supplement	Kidney dysfunction, hyper-sensitivity
Thiazidelike Diuretics					
High Risk					
Indapamide (Lozol)	Hyper-tension	Anxiety, dizziness, numbness, weakness	Stomach pain, irregular heart rate, depression	Sudden drops in potassium, allergic reactions	Should not be used
Potassium-Sparing Diuretics					
High Risk					
Eplerenone (Inspra)	Hyper-tension	Weakness, nausea, vomiting, diarrhea	Fatigue, headache	Kidney failure due to toxic increases in potassium, heat stroke, decreased platelets, anemia	Liver or kidney disease, elevated potassium; do not use

Drug	Use	Common, Benign Side Effects	Serious Side Effects	Life-threatening Side Effects	Reasons Not to Take
Spironolactone (Aldactone)	Hyper-tension	Weakness, nausea, vomiting, diarrhea	Fatigue, headache	Kidney failure due to toxic increases in potassium, heat stroke, decreased platelets, anemia	Liver or kidney disease, elevated potassium; do not use
Amiloride + HCTZ (Moduretic)	Hyper-tension	Weakness, nausea, vomiting, diarrhea	Fatigue, headache	Kidney failure due to toxic increases in potassium, heat stroke, decreased platelets, anemia	Liver or kidney disease, elevated potassium; do not use
Triamterine + HCTZ (Dyazide, Maxide)	Hyper-tension	Weakness, nausea, vomiting, diarrhea	Fatigue, headache	Kidney failure due to toxic increases in potassium, heat stroke, decreased platelets, anemia	Liver or kidney disease, elevated potassium; do not use
Amiloride (Midamor)	Hyper-tension	Weakness, nausea, vomiting, diarrhea	Fatigue, headache	Kidney failure due to toxic increases in potassium, heat stroke, decreased platelets, anemia	Liver or kidney disease, elevated potassium; do not use

Drug	Use	Common, Benign Side Effects	Serious Side Effects	Life-threatening Side Effects	Reasons Not to Take
Beta-Blockers					
Low Risk					
Metoprolol (Toprol XL)	Hyper-tension	Dizziness, rash, nausea, constipation	Nightmares, impotence, depression	Heart failure	Heart failure, some heart arrhythmias
Carvedilol (Coreg)	Hyper-tension	Dizziness, rash, nausea, constipation	Nightmares, impotence, depression	Heart failure	Heart failure, some heart arrhythmias
Bisoprolol (Zebeta)	Hyper-tension	Dizziness, rash, nausea, constipation	Nightmares, impotence, depression	Heart failure	Heart failure, some heart arrhythmias
Propanolol (Inderal)	Hyper-tension	Dizziness, rash, nausea, constipation	Nightmares, impotence, depression	Heart failure	Heart failure, some heart arrhythmias
Medium Risk					
Atenolol (Tenormin)	Hyper-tension	Dizziness, rash, nausea, constipation	Nightmares, impotence, depression	Heart failure	Heart failure, some heart arrhythmias
Alpha-Blockers					
High Risk					
Doxazosin (Cardura)	Hyper-tension	Dizziness, headache, palpitations, nausea	Orthostatic hypotension	Heart failure, stroke	Should not use
Prazosin (Minipress) Terazosin (Hytrin)	Hyper-tension	Dizziness, headache, palpitations, nausea	Orthostatic hypotension	Heart failure, stroke	Should not use

Drug	Use	Common, Benign Side Effects	Serious Side Effects	Life-threatening Side Effects	Reasons Not to Take
Combined Alpha- and Beta-Blockers					
High Risk					
Labetalol (Normodyne)	Hypertension	Weakness, fatigue, dizziness	Impotence, diarrhea, bronchospasm, rash, muscle cramps	Orthostatic hypotension	Heart block, asthma; do not recommend
Alpha-2 Agonists					
Moderate Risk					
Clonidine (Catapres)	Hypertension	Sweating, flushing, dry mouth, dizziness, sedation, constipation, nausea, vomiting	Depression, nightmares, skin reactions, orthostatic hypotension	Seizures, low blood pressure with overdose	Hypersensitivity; do not recommend
Loop Diuretics					
Moderate Risk					
Furosemide (Lasix)	Hypertension, heart failure	Dizziness, nausea, vomiting, photosensitivity, muscle cramps	Loss of thiamine (vitamin B$_1$), insomnia, confusion, thinning of bones	Depletion of potassium, calcium, and magnesium; blood clots; stroke; falls; heat stroke; dehydration	Hypersensitivity, low urine output
Bumetidine (Bumex)	Hypertension, heart failure	Dizziness, nausea, vomiting, photosensitivity, muscle cramps	Loss of thiamine (vitamin B$_1$), insomnia, confusion, thinning of bones	Depletion of potassium, calcium, and magnesium; blood clots; stroke; falls; heat stroke; dehydration	Hypersensitivity, low urine output

Drug	Use	Common, Benign Side Effects	Serious Side Effects	Life-threatening Side Effects	Reasons Not to Take
Angiotensin-Converting Enzyme (ACE) Inhibitors					
Moderate Risk					
Lisinopril (Prinivil)	Hyper-tension, heart failure	Headache, flushing, nausea, diarrhea, rash	Dry cough, dizziness, swelling, trouble breathing	Heart failure, stroke, orthostatic hypotension, elevated potassium, angioedema, loss of white cells	Patients without ventricular dysfunction, African Americans, pregnancy
Enalapril (Vasotec)	Hyper-tension, heart failure	Headache, flushing, nausea, diarrhea	Dry cough, dizziness, swelling, trouble breathing	Heart failure, stroke, orthostatic hypotension, elevated potassium, angioedema, loss of white cells	Patients without ventricular dysfunction, African Americans, pregnancy
Ramipril (Altace)	Hyper-tension, heart failure	Headache, flushing, nausea, diarrhea	Dry cough, dizziness, swelling, trouble breathing	Heart failure, stroke, orthostatic hypotension, elevated potassium, angioedema, loss of white cells	Patients without ventricular dysfunction, African Americans, pregnancy
Benazepril (Lotensin)	Hyper-tension, heart failure	Headache, flushing, nausea, diarrhea	Dry cough, dizziness, swelling, trouble breathing	Heart failure, stroke, orthostatic hypotension, elevated potassium, angioedema, loss of white cells	Patients without ventricular dysfunction, African Americans, pregnancy

Drug	Use	Common, Benign Side Effects	Serious Side Effects	Life-threatening Side Effects	Reasons Not to Take
Fosinopril (Monopril)	Hypertension, heart failure	Headache, flushing, nausea, diarrhea	Dry cough, dizziness, swelling, trouble breathing	Heart failure, stroke, orthostatic hypotension, elevated potassium, angioedema, loss of white cells	Patients without ventricular dysfunction, African Americans, pregnancy
Captopril (Capoten)	Hypertension, heart failure	Headache, flushing, nausea, diarrhea	Dry cough, dizziness, swelling, trouble breathing	Heart failure, stroke, orthostatic hypotension, elevated potassium, angioedema, loss of white cells	Patients without ventricular dysfunction, African Americans, pregnancy

Angiotensin-Receptor Blockers

Moderate Risk

Drug	Use	Common, Benign Side Effects	Serious Side Effects	Life-threatening Side Effects	Reasons Not to Take
Valsartan (Diovan)	Hypertension	Dizziness, diarrhea, anxiety, rash	Upper respiratory tract infection, myalgia	Potassium elevations, hypotension with overdose	Pregnancy, patients without ventricular dysfunction
Irbesartan (Avapro)	Hypertension	Dizziness, diarrhea, anxiety, rash	Upper respiratory tract infection, myalgia	Potassium elevations, hypotension with overdose	Pregnancy, patients without ventricular dysfunction
Olmesartan (Benicar)	Hypertension	Dizziness, diarrhea, anxiety, rash	Upper respiratory tract infection, myalgia	Potassium elevations, hypotension with overdose	Pregnancy, patients without ventricular dysfunction

Drug	Use	Common, Benign Side Effects	Serious Side Effects	Life-threatening Side Effects	Reasons Not to Take
Candesartan (Atacand)	Hypertension	Dizziness, diarrhea, anxiety, rash	Upper respiratory tract infection, myalgia	Potassium elevations, hypotension with overdose	Pregnancy, patients without ventricular dysfunction
Losartan (Hyzaar)	Hypertension	Dizziness, diarrhea, anxiety, rash	Upper respiratory tract infection, myalgia	Potassium elevations, hypotension with overdose	Pregnancy, patients without ventricular dysfunction
Calcium Channel Blockers					
Moderate Risk					
Amlodipine (Norvasc)	Hypertension, angina	Constipation, dizziness, headache, nausea	Edema, low blood pressure	Heart failure, suicide, arrhythmias	Beta-blockers and diuretics should be tried first; women should not take these for HTN; heart block; severe CHF
Verapamil (Calan)	Hypertension, arrhythmia, angina	Constipation, dizziness, headache, nausea	Edema, low blood pressure	Heart failure, suicide, arrhythmias	Beta-blockers and diuretics should be tried first; women should not take these for HTN; heart block; severe CHF

Drug	Use	Common, Benign Side Effects	Serious Side Effects	Life-threatening Side Effects	Reasons Not to Take
Nifedipine (Procardia, Adalat)	Hypertension, angina	Constipation, dizziness, headache, nausea	Edema, low blood pressure	Heart failure, suicide, arrhythmias	Beta-blockers and diuretics should be tried first; women should not take these for HTN; heart block; severe CHF
Diltiazem (Tiazac)	Hypertension, arrhythmia, angina	Constipation, dizziness, headache, nausea	Edema, low blood pressure	Heart failure, suicide, arrhythmias	Beta-blockers and diuretics should be tried first; women should not take these for HTN; heart block; severe CHF

6.

Diet Pills

I was sitting in a café in Italy this summer, reading a travel book, drinking cappuccino, and watching the people milling around the piazza, when I noticed that something was missing. Where were all the fat people?

Anyone who has traveled outside the U.S. knows one thing: There are more overweight and obese people here than in other countries.

Everything is big in the U.S.A.: Texas, The Mall of America, The Grand Canyon, . . . and us. We are now officially the fattest people in the world. The number of obese Americans has doubled in the past decade. The percentage of overweight adolescents has increased from 6% to 12% in the past two decades. One in four Americans is obese, as defined by a body mass index, or BMI (calculated as weight in kilograms divided by the square of height in meters), of over thirty. In 1999 and 2000 more than 64% of Americans were overweight or obese, as defined by a BMI of twenty-five.

You may not be surprised that one death out of five each year is caused by cigarette smoking, but did you know that an equal number of deaths are caused by obesity? Indeed, obesity has a number of negative health consequences, including early mortality. Heart disease, diabetes, cancer, hypertension, and an overall reduced quality of life are a few of the major problems overweight people face. The rate of obesity-related ailments like type 2 diabetes has doubled every ten years. Obese people also wear out their joints from carrying around extra pounds, which can cause joint disease and joint failure. The cost of these obesity-related health problems is $70 billion per year.

Access to unlimited amounts of food and the large number of jobs that are almost completely sedentary, relatively recent phenomena in human history, have made it very easy for us to eat more calories than we burn—the magic formula for weight gain. (The reverse—burning more calories than we eat—results in weight loss.) For some of us, that means putting on a few pounds a year; for others it means massive weight gain.

Food makers don't help. The recent rapid increase in obesity parallels the widespread availability of fast-food outlets like McDonald's, Wendy's, Burger King, Subway, and Hardees as well as chain restaurants like Olive Garden and Outback Steakhouse, which serve megaportions of food. Every day one out of four Americans eats at a fast-food restaurant, 43% of the time at McDonald's. Convenience-food makers try to *increase* our desire for the items we crave most (fat, sugar, and salt) in order to sell their products, even if they are killing us. The high fat, sodium, and sugar content in fast and prepackaged food creates a mental and physical dependency that draws the customer back again and again.

Many credible scientists and journalists have chronicled this situation. For example, Marion Nestle, Ph.D., a widely respected food scientist and former member of the committee to construct the food pyramid, argues in *Food Politics: How the Food Industry Influences Nutrition and Health* that lobbyists for the American Restaurant Association promote their agenda without regard to the health consequences of individual people. Eric Schlosser, in *Fast Food Nation: The Dark Side of the American Meal*, discusses how fast-food restaurants have figured out that they can increase sales by promoting "super-size" portions of food. Since most of their costs are not related to the food itself, they can ask you if you want a "large order of french fries for ten cents more" and make you feel like you are getting a better value. After all, you are getting cheaper food per pound. Nobody mentions the fact that the extra food is making you fatter and can kill you.

When Morgan Spurlock of documentary *Supersize Me* fame ate at McDonald's every day for a month, he developed liver toxicity, impotence, depression, and obesity, and he physically craved the junk food he was eating (probably related to the strange effects that high-fat foods can have on your brain). The amount of soda in a 7-Eleven "Double Gulp" drink is sixty-four ounces, and contains forty-eight tablespoons of sugar. A day of McDonald's meals contains one pound of sugar. A pound! No wonder we are swelling like balloons.

No Magic Pills for Weight Loss

People often turn to their physician to help them lose weight because it is so difficult. Americans spend billions of dollars every year attempting to lose weight, but their efforts are largely unsuccessful. Some doctors recommend the most natural and difficult path to weight loss, which is to reduce the number of calories consumed and ramp up exercise, and I talk about this method later on in the chapter. However, many patients have tried diets and failed and now want something a bit more powerful to curb their appetite or something to help them curb cravings and a psychological obsession with food. These people will keep going to doctors until they find one willing to write a prescription for a diet drug, and they usually don't have to search for long. Or, lured by the promise of near-magical weight loss, they pick up some ma huang or another dietary supplement at the drugstore.

It's not surprising that the diet-drug industry is robust; not only is the idea of easy weight loss appealing, but the National Institutes of Health recommend that most obese Americans should undergo drug treatment, which means that 100 million Americans could be on drugs for obesity.

However, diet drugs generally have not been shown to help people reach

or sustain their weight-loss goal. Long-term use of diet drugs is also associated with some dangers, most important among them being the risk of
heart attack or other cardiovascular event (even in young people). Another
worrisome consequence of diet pills is primary pulmonary hypertension
(PPH), a disorder typically of unknown cause that is associated with an
increase in the pressure of the arteries in the lungs. The primary manifestation of PPH is breathing problems with exercise. The end result of PPH in
the absence of a lung transplant is usually death. Heidi Connolly, M.D., of
the Mayo Clinic in Rochester, Minnesota, assessed the risk of getting PPH
following treatment with diet pills. She found that there is a sixfold increase in the risk of PPH with diet pills. Pills that were included in this
assessment of risk were dexfenfluramine, fenfluramine, diethylpropion,
clobenzorek, fenproporek, phemetrazine, and other compounds. Patients
taking diet pills for more than three months face a twenty-threefold increased risk. Although PPH is rare, so that the absolute risk of developing
this disorder remains small, the certain lethality of it when it does occur
should be cause for concern. At this point we can say that *any* diet pill that
actually affects appetite (i.e., those affecting sympathetic function) should
be considered risky.

Dr. Connolly and colleagues also found other life-threatening side effects with diet pills, notably the dangerous effects of "fen-phen" (fenfluramine-
phentermine) on the heart. Although the combination of these pills was
never approved by the FDA, by 1996 more than 18 million prescriptions a
year were being written for this combination of pills as a weight-loss treatment. Dr. Connolly and her colleagues noticed an unusual number of
young women showing up in their practices with heart murmurs. In sharing notes, they discovered that the young women had something in common: They were all being treated with fen-phen for weight loss. The doctors
performed ultrasound examinations of the heart and found abnormalities
of the heart valves in twenty-four women, five of whom required cardiac
surgery for valve repair. This discovery led to the withdrawal of fen-phen
from the market.

MERIDIA

One of the most commonly prescribed medications for obesity, sibutramine (Meridia), acts on receptors in the brain that take the neurotransmitters dopamine, norepinephrine, and serotonin back into the neurons. These neurotransmitters are involved in mood as well as appetite regulation. By blocking the reuptake of these neurotransmitters into the neurons, they increase the amount of neurotransmitter that is available in the space between the neurons (the synapse) and therefore increase the effects of these neurotransmitters. It is by means of this effect that the weight-loss properties of Meridia are believed to accrue, although the exact mechanism is not completely understood.

Meridia is one of the "bad five" identified by Dr. David Graham, an FDA employee who, in his testimony before the U.S. Congress in November 2004, identified the five currently approved drugs with the most potential to cause harm. Before Meridia was approved in 1997, an FDA advisory panel voted five to four that the drug's benefits did not outweigh its risks; however, despite the five-to-four vote, the FDA approved its use. (The FDA isn't required to follow the recommendations of its advisory panel, although it's almost unheard-of for it not to.)

Meridia leads to a 4.45-kg (9-lb) weight loss after twelve months of treatment.[1] Some studies have shown up to a 10-kg (22-lb) weight loss with Meridia.[2] Unfortunately, weight returns to pretreatment levels once Meridia is discontinued. Also, multiple studies have not yielded evidence that Meridia (or any other weight-loss drug for that matter) reduces obesity-related death or disease, like heart disease, stroke, and hypertension.

The most common side effect of the drug is palpitations, but it also causes increased blood pressure and stroke. Forty-nine cardiac deaths related to Meridia have been reported to the FDA. Administration to pregnant women can lead to fetal abnormalities. Reports of these side effects led Sidney Wolfe, M.D., director of Public Citizen, a Washington, D.C.–based organization devoted to drug safety that is an offshoot of Ralph Nader's consumer rights–related organization, to petition for the removal of Meridia from the market. In addition, Lester Crawford, while acting director of the FDA, said in 2004 that the risks of Meridia do not outweigh the benefits.

I do not recommend the use of Meridia—or any weight-loss drug for that matter—since no studies have ever shown that weight loss achieved with these drugs can be sustained after the drug is discontinued. Given the potentially dangerous side effects of the only drugs that have shown any weight-loss effects (albeit transient), the possibility of staying on these drugs for life is not an acceptable risk.

DIETHYLPROPION AND PHENTERMINE

Some of the sympathomimetic (amphetaminelike) weight-loss drugs that have been on the market for many years, like diethylpropion (Tenuate) and phentermine (Ionamin), have appropriately developed a bad reputation for their potentially lethal side effects. These drugs, which are intended only for short-term use, have been shown to result in a six- or seven-pound weight loss, which is of borderline statistical significance. Phentermine, the "phen" of the infamous fen-phen, can cause cardiac and lung toxicity. These drugs activate the sympathetic system but have the usual risks of increased blood pressure and risk of heart attack, stroke, or death. They also cause palpitations and central-nervous-system effects. Like amphetamines, they have the potential for abuse and dependence. These risks have led to their ban in Europe. Other similar amphetamines include benzphetamine (Didrex) and phendimetrazine (Bontril).

ORLISTAT

Orlistat (Xenical), another drug approved for the treatment of obesity, prevents the digestion and absorption of some fats by inhibiting the lipase enzyme. Orlistat treatment results in a six-pound weight loss that persists for as long as treatment continues.[3] Gastrointestinal side effects are experienced by 91% of patients vs. 65% on placebo. Diarrhea is very common;

flatulence, bloating, and dyspepsia are less so. Orlistat inhibits absorption of fat-soluble vitamins (A, D, E, K) and can lead to vitamin deficiency, so you should take a vitamin if you are on this drug. Recently a low-dose version of orlistat called Alli (pronounced *ally*) has been approved for over-the-counter use in conjunction with a diet and exercise program, and is being heavily advertised.

NON–DIET DRUGS USED FOR WEIGHT LOSS

A variety of drugs developed for other problems, such as depression, that have also been shown to be effective weight-loss agents are currently being marketed for that purpose. These drugs act on receptors for brain neurotransmitters that are involved in both depression and appetite regulation. Prozac and Paxil, for instance, primarily used in the treatment of depression, also act on these neurochemical systems. Some of these antidepressant drugs have been shown to induce weight loss and are prescribed specifically for this purpose. However, the effects of these drugs on weight are highly variable from drug to drug and from person to person: A drug that may induce weight loss in one person may cause weight gain in another.

One of the antidepressants that has been most studied for weight loss is the selective serotonin reuptake inhibitor (SSRI) fluoxetine, or Prozac. Prozac blocks the transporter that takes serotonin back up into the neurons, leaving more in the synapse (space between the neurons) so that the brain effectively "sees" more serotonin. Fluoxetine can be associated with a significant reduction in weight that is equivalent to that seen with Meridia. Side effects are jumpiness, sleep loss, insomnia, stomach upset, and sexual dysfunction. The antidepressant buproprion (Wellbutrin), also used for weight loss, has shown an average eight-pound weight reduction. Side effects are dry mouth, constipation, and diarrhea.

The epilepsy drugs zonisamide (Zonegran) and topiramate (Topamax), which are also prescribed for weight loss, have shown statistically significant results. The side effects of zonisamide include dizziness, anxiety, restlessness, constipation, stomach pain, and, infrequently, mental changes, including depression and psychosis. Topiramate can cause tingling, confusion, blurred vision, memory problems, stomach pain, depression, or ringing in the ears.

Alternative Medicines

A variety of products are sold in stores as natural weight-loss aids, most of which have not been scientifically evaluated. Seven percent of Americans, most of whom are young women, are using over-the-counter weight-loss products.

Because of the Dietary Supplement and Health Education Act (DSHEA) passed by Congress in 1994, weight-loss and other supplements are not regulated by the FDA, are not required to demonstrate efficacy for the conditions for which they are promoted, and are not even required to prove that they contain what they claim to contain.

Many of the supplements currently promoted for weight loss have sympathomimetic effects; in other words, they are compounds from plants, including herbs, or other natural compounds that stimulate the sympathetic nervous system, and they carry the same risks as prescription drugs that stimulate the sympathetic nervous system.

EPHEDRA

One such supplement is the Chinese plant ma huang, which contains ephedra, a compound similar to ephedrine, which stimulates the sympathetic nervous system. Ephedra increases heart rate, blood pressure, and energy expenditure, stimulating beta-1 and beta-2 adrenergic sympathetic receptors. Ephedra is often combined with caffeine as a weight-loss supplement. Ma huang is also combined with guarana, a Brazilian plant with a high caffeine concentration, and promoted as a weight-loss supplement. A recent meta-analysis by Shekelle and colleagues that pooled the results from several different studies showed that ephedra-containing products result in weight loss of two pounds per month, although no information is available for treatment longer than six months.[4]

Ephedra is one of the most dangerous over-the-counter supplements available today. It accounts for the majority of all reports to the FDA of adverse events for herbs and supplements. In the study of Shekelle and colleagues, it was associated with a two- to threefold increase in psychiatric, autonomic, heart-related, and gastrointestinal side effects. Eighty-seven episodes of heart attack, stroke, seizures, and high blood pressure have been reported to the FDA. It has been associated with several deaths, including that of a pitcher for the Baltimore Orioles, which led to the unusual (for a supplement) step of its ban by the FDA in 1994. The FDA has since revoked the ban.

OTHER OVER-THE-COUNTER REMEDIES

Hydroxycitric acid, sold under the name garcinia, is promoted for weight loss. It has been shown to inhibit the enzymes that convert compounds into coenzyme A, thereby blocking the storage of energy as fat. The evidence related to its ability to promote weight loss is contradictory. Other products, including psyllium, guar gum, chitosan, chromium, and conjugated linoleic acid have shown no effect on weight loss, although they have no major potential toxicities.

Diet and Behavioral Solutions

As I mentioned, Italy doesn't seem to have any obese people, and now I am going to tell you why. It isn't genetics. It isn't exercise (they don't even run for the train). It's this: They don't eat in fast-food restaurants.

Why not? Because they correctly believe that their mothers can cook something for them that's just as good. When they do go to a restaurant, it's one that is not part of a chain and whose cook takes as much care in preparing the food as their mother does. Although they don't know it, they also are helping their health.

Fast- and chain-restaurant food is the worst thing ever to have happened to the American diet. McDonald's, Burger King, and chain restaurants like Applebee's and TGIF pile on the calories in ever-expanding portions, with sodium and fat all far in excess of what we actually need. And since there is a natural tendency to eat everything on your plate, you know the consequence of ordering from their menus.

People who eat fast food three or more times a week have a greater than 90% chance of developing heart disease or diabetes. I don't want to develop heart disease or diabetes, do you? That's why I stopped eating fast food.

I know that I sound like a broken record when I talk about how many diseases are preventable by changing behavior. And I do understand that changing behavior is not easy; the temptation to take a pill to solve a problem is very appealing to many of us. Yet you know what I am going to say: Excess weight is not a "genetic" problem; it is not possible for genes to account for such a dramatic change in obesity in the country in such a short period of time. The only logical explanation is the rapid shift in the amount and kinds of food we eat combined with a lack of exercise. The only lasting, healthy solution for weight loss is to eat less and move more.

These behavioral changes have no side effects, are free (actually save money), and have good long-term outcomes. Unlike drugs, they also have been shown to prolong life and prevent negative health outcomes like stroke, heart attack, diabetes, and hypertension.

Miracle diets come and go, but the bottom line is we gain weight when we eat more calories than we burn, whether they are calories from carbs, protein, or fat. All diets that work, no matter what claims they make, do so because they involve calorie restriction. However, if you are overweight, you can lose excess weight by eating healthfully for your height, age, and activity level. For moderately active women this is between 1,800 and 2,000 calories a day, and for moderately active men it's between 2,000 and 2,400 calories a day. That is certainly not restrictive, but for overeaters, getting back to a normal eating level does take some getting used to. You should derive less than 35% of your total calories from fat and less than 10% from saturated fat. Exercise, at least thirty minutes a day, will speed up weight loss and afford you many cardiovascular and strength benefits besides.

On a practical level, you should eliminate carbonated beverages like (non-"diet") soda, which are high in sugar content. Soda, and in fact almost all processed foods, contains high-fructose corn syrup (HFCS). Fructose goes straight to the liver and increases insulin resistance, which leads to diabetes. So-called "sports drinks" should be eliminated, since they are high in calories. Soda, juice, and energy and sports drinks contain empty calories that will make you fat; they also contain caffeine, which is addictive and makes you consume even more of those useless calories. If you are thirsty, drink water. Replacing sodas and juices with water will help you lose more than five pounds per year, solving the weight problems of most people. I don't advocate drinking any minimal amount of water above what you would drink normally based on your sense of thirst because I don't think there is evidence to support doing so. What I think is most important is replacing calorie-laden drinks with calorie-free water.

You should limit your time at restaurants to once a week. Avoid fast food, which is usually served in excessively large portions: A single meal typically contains twice the fat and saturated fat that you should be eating. Incorporate fresh vegetables into your meals. Eat fruit after every meal. The high fiber decreases the risk of cancer and aids digestion as well as weight loss. Don't eat red meat more than twice a week. Eat three to six ounces of fish or shellfish twice a week or more. Watch out for the mercury in canned tuna. Keep weekly consumption to no more than three six-ounce servings of tuna per week, unless you are pregnant, in which case I recommend avoiding it altogether.

Watch out for fancy diets that promise too much. Treatments that promise you will drop more than a pound a week are too good to be true. You should not follow low-carbohydrate diets or other gimmicks. If you stop eating you won't necessarily lose weight; you will break down protein as quickly as fat. Foods with high fiber include brown bread, brown rice, and fruit. They take longer to pass through the stomach and therefore make you feel fuller, longer.

Several studies have shown sustained weight loss with the Mediterranean diet.[5] This diet is high in vegetables (550 g/day, or 20 oz/day), legumes (9 g/day or 1/3 oz/day), fruits and nuts (360 g/d or 10 oz/day), cereals (180 g/d or 6 oz/day), and fish (24 g/d, or 1 oz/day), and low in other meat, including poultry (120 g/d or 40 oz/day) and dairy products (200 g/d or 70 oz/day). Alcohol consumption was 10 to 50 g (one to four glasses of wine) per day for men and 5 to 25 g (one to two glasses of wine) for women. The diet also involves a high amount of olive oil consumption, and reduces heart disease and cancer risk and prolongs life.[6] People who followed this diet had their mortality cut in half over a four-year period.

This delicious diet substitutes unsaturated fats (seed oils) and monounsaturated fats (olive oil) for saturated fats (butter, animal fat) and also includes wine and nuts. Patients with heart disease who followed the Mediterranean diet had a 50% to 70% reduction in recurrent heart attacks.[7] Overall, this diet had a much more beneficial effect than either statins or weight-loss drugs, and without side effects. You'll lose weight eating this way, and you'll look and feel great.

The Bottom Line

Don't take diet pills, herbs, or supplements. Not for a few weeks, not for a few days, not ever. Not alone and not in combination with a diet program. In my opinion, diet drugs are a bad solution in the long and short term, even for people who have a lot of weight to lose (more than thirty pounds). If you are overweight you need to exercise, stop drinking sugar-added beverages, and cook *all* of your meals at home. If you need to drink soda, make it diet. Water is best. A pill will not solve your problem.

However, if you insist on ignoring my advice and are determined to take a pill, start out with one of the nondiet pills, like Prozac. Although I don't recommend Orlistat and Alli, if you take a multivitamin with either one, the worst thing that will probably happen to you is embarrassing and uncontrollable gas (and other related and more embarrassing events). Do not under any circumstance take Meridia, ephedra, ma huang, phentermine, or any of the other amphetaminelike drugs.

Drug	Use	Common, Benign Side Effects	Serious Side Effects	Life-threatening Side Effects	Reasons Not to Take
Monoamine Reuptake Inhibitors					
High Risk					
Sibutramine (Meridia)	Obesity	Anorexia, constipation, insomnia, headache, dry eyes	Palpitations, dizziness, mood swings, stomach pain	Increased blood pressure and stroke; fetal abnormalities	Do not take
Antidepressants					
Low Risk					
Fluoxetine (Prozac)	Obesity	Nausea, diarrhea, headache, insomnia	Decreased libido, akathisia	Suicidal thoughts, mood swings with dose change	
Buproprion (Wellbutrin)	Obesity	Weight loss, restlessness, dry mouth, constipation, diarrhea		Seizures	Seizure disorder
Anti-epileptics					
Moderate Risk					
Zonisamide (Zonegran)	Obesity	Dizziness, anxiety, restlessness, constipation, stomach pain	Depression	Psychosis	Allergy to sulfa drugs

Drug	Use	Common, Benign Side Effects	Serious Side Effects	Life-threatening Side Effects	Reasons Not to Take
Topiramate (Topamax)	Obesity	Tingling, confusion, blurred vision, memory problems, stomach pain	Ringing in ears	Depression	Allergy to drug

Sympathomimetics

High Risk

Drug	Use	Common, Benign Side Effects	Serious Side Effects	Life-threatening Side Effects	Reasons Not to Take
Diethylproprion (Tenuate)	Obesity	Anxiety	Palpitations, nervous system effects	Increased blood pressure with heart attack	Heart disease
Phentermine (Ionamin)	Obesity	Anxiety	Palpitations, nervous system effects	Increased blood pressure with heart attack	Heart disease
Benzphetamine (Didrex)	Obesity	Anxiety	Palpitations, nervous system effects	Increased blood pressure with heart attack	Heart disease
Phendimetrazine (Bontril)	Obesity	Anxiety	Palpitations, nervous system effects	Increased blood pressure with heart attack	Heart disease

Lipase Enzyme Inhibitors

Moderate Risk

Drug	Use	Common, Benign Side Effects	Serious Side Effects	Life-threatening Side Effects	Reasons Not to Take
Orlistat (Xenical)	Obesity	Flatulence, bloating, dyspepsia, fatty stools	Diarrhea, anxiety, stomach pain	Nutritional malabsorption, vitamin deficiency, kidney stones	Chronic malabsorption, gallbladder disease, pregnancy, breast-feeding, hypersensitivity

7.

Asthma and
Allergy Medications

In March 1988 Dr. Richard Green became the first African-American chancellor of the Board of Education of New York City, an appointment that both the city's parents and children welcomed with enthusiasm. After fourteen months on the job Dr. Green was well on his way to making critical improvements in the city's school system. But all that changed at 1:40 a.m. on May 10, 1989, when Dr. Green suffered a massive asthma attack in his home. At 2:30 a.m. he died at Roosevelt Hospital after attempts to revive him had failed. The fifty-one-year-old left behind a wife and daughter as well as a shocked city. Dr. Green is only one of the 4,000 to 5,000 people who die of an asthma attack each year in the United States. Asthma results in 10 million office visits and 2 million emergency-room visits per year. It affects all races and genders but is slightly more prevalent among African Americans.

Asthma has been on the rise in the U.S. for the past fifty years and is now the most common chronic condition in America, affecting 20 million of us. Asthma occurs when triggers in the environment cause the airways or bronchi in the lungs to contract, making it difficult to breathe and in some cases, like the one above, causing death. There are several reasons that could explain the increase of asthma over the past few decades. It could be because our more limited exposure to infection has made our immune systems more sensitive than those of our ancestors. Unlike our forebears, we also spend more time indoors in controlled environments where we are exposed to dust and mold. The air we breathe, both inside and outside, is more polluted than the air most of our ancestors breathed. Last but not least, we have become more sedentary because of our urban lifestyle, and we have lost the habit of daily exercise.

There is considerable evidence that a lack of outdoor exercise contributes to asthma and that an exercise program helps asthmatics. Our sedentary lifestyle has also led to a surge in obesity (see Chapter 6); there is evidence of an association between obesity and asthma based on the fact that obese people have less room for the lungs to expand, higher levels of the hormone leptin (which is released from fat and is also higher in asthmatics), and higher levels of inflammatory markers (which may contribute to airway reactivity). In fact, as many as 75% of emergency-room asthma admissions are for obese people. Finally, there has been a major change in our diet, including a massive increase in exposure to vitamins and minerals through fortified foods as well as a shift from grain- to corn-based nutrition. There is some evidence that changes in the American diet may have contributed to the increase in asthma, which I review on pages 138–140.

There are two categories of asthma: allergic, also known as extrinsic asthma, and nonallergic, or intrinsic asthma. Allergic asthma, the most common form, which affects 20 million individuals in the U.S., is triggered by an allergic reaction to something that has been inhaled, such as dust mite allergen, pet dander, tree or other plant pollen, mold, or air pollution. Individuals with allergic asthma have high blood levels of a substance called immunoglobulin E (IgE). IgE sitting on the surface of the airways binds allergens and causes mast cells and basophils to release inflammatory factors, which cause the airways to constrict. (IgE in the nose and mouth causes hay fever, and IgE on the skin causes eczema.) Symptoms include coughing, wheezing, shortness of breath or rapid breathing, and chest tightness.

Nonallergic asthma is triggered by factors not related to allergens, such as upper respiratory infections, anxiety, stress, exercise, cold or dry air, hyperventilation, smoke, viruses, medications [aspirin, NSAIDs (see Chapter 2), beta-blockers, and ACE inhibitors (see Chapter 5)], sulfites found in red wine, and gastroesophageal reflux disease (GERD). Like allergic asthma, nonallergic asthma is characterized by airway obstruction and inflammation that can also be treated and partially reversed with medications similar to those used for allergic asthma. Many of the symptoms of nonallergic asthma are the same as those experienced by allergic asthma sufferers. Although blood levels of IgE are normal in the case of nonallergic asthma, a similar type of inflammatory response takes place in the airways for reasons that are not fully understood.

Waiting to Inhale: Medications

Treatment for allergic and nonallergic asthma is similar, with the exceptions that removal of allergens is not part of the therapeutic approach toward nonallergic asthma and that antihistamines do not have therapeutic benefit. In addition, individuals with nonallergic asthma may need to take medications more long term, whereas those with allergic asthma may only need treatment when they are exposed to allergens (such as during springtime, when exposure to pollen is unavoidable).

ALLERGIC ASTHMA TREATMENTS

A number of products that block the histamine receptor (antihistamines) have been developed to treat the allergies that trigger attacks in those suffering from allergic asthma attacks. These include hydroxyzine (Atarax, Vistaril) and its breakdown product cetirizine (Zyrtec). These medications cause sleepiness. Other side effects include dry mouth and urinary retention and, more rarely, confusion, nightmares, nervousness, and irritability. Other older antihistamines, such as chlorpheniramine (Chlor-trimeton), cyproheptadine (Periactin), and diphenhydramine (Benadryl), are associated with the same anticholinergic side effects (dry mouth, confusion, urinary retention).

The so-called second-generation antihistamines, including fexofenadine (Allegra), loratadine (Claratin), and azelastine (Astelin), claim to specifically block the H-1 antihistamine receptor and to cause less drowsiness than the older products, but this is more hype than reality. Side effects are similar to those of the older antihistamines. With all of the antihistamines, drowsiness is dose dependent. It is best to start with a low dose and work up.

One of the best-selling allergy medications on the market is desloratadine (Clarinex), a newer-generation antihistamine medication that is marketed as a magic bullet for allergies. What most people don't know is that Clarinex is merely an old drug, loratadine (Claritin), that is being marketed by the drug company as new and improved. However, Clarinex doesn't add anything to Claritin (other than more money for the coffers of its manufacturer, since Clarinex is still on patent). Clarinex is merely a metabolite (breakdown product) of its precursor, Claritin. That means that twenty minutes after you take Claritin, you will be getting Clarinex, but you'll be paying much less for it than if you had taken Clarinex. For years, folks taking Claritin have been getting Clarinex without knowing it. The company patented the metabolite of its original product and then did a misleading study comparing differing doses of the two medications that came to the erroneous conclusion that Clarinex was less sedating than the older drug. This was misleading because if a drug causes sedation, then higher doses of the drug will cause more sedation, so if you are not comparing the same doses of the drug, you are not making a fair comparison.

This allowed the company to promote Clarinex, which costs much more than the old drug, which went off patent and which in 2004 was bringing in close to a billion dollars a year in sales. Claritin and Clarinex, as far as consumers are concerned, are the same drug; so take Claritin and save some money.

Over-the-counter (OTC) epinephrine inhalers such as Primatene Mist are commonly used for the treatment of mild asthma. More than 115 million Primatene Mist inhalers have been sold over the past twenty years. These inhalers, however, are not as benign as they appear. About 20% of patients using OTC inhalers have severe asthma that needs medical care. Unfortunately, many asthma patients delay professional medical treatment in favor of using their OTC inhalers, often because they lack health insurance, to the point where it may be too late. OTC inhalers can increase heart rate and should not be used by patients with heart or thyroid disease. Over the last twenty years, thirteen deaths, mostly cardiovascular, have been reported to be associated with the use of OTC inhalers. If you have a history of chronic asthma or a history of hospitalization for asthma you should not use OTC inhalers. If asthma symptoms do not resolve in twenty minutes after using an OTC inhaler, you should seek emergency treatment. Delaying medical treatment when you are using OTC inhalers may contribute to the overall severity and chronic nature of the disease over your lifetime.

Prescription short-acting bronchodilators (beta-2 agonists) that are inhaled promote dilation of the airways. The most commonly prescribed inhalers are albuterol (Proventil) and levalbuterol (Xopenex). Side effects include tremors, jitters, and nervousness. There are no known long-term side effects. These medications are designed for temporary relief. Frequent or increasingly frequent use means that the condition is getting worse and further evaluation by a doctor is needed.

Asthma patients can also be treated with steroids in pill form for a short period of time. Corticosteroids can inhibit growth in children and decrease bone-mineral density, although growth inhibition is reversible. Steroids also suppress the immune response, increasing the risk of infection, and decrease bone-mineral density. Other side effects of steroids include low blood sugar, changes in state of consciousness, nausea, seizures, or, in rare cases, death. You can also develop Cushing's disease (an excess production of cortisol in the body), symptoms of which include deposits of fat on the upper back and face, high blood pressure, diabetes, slow wound healing, osteoporosis, cataracts, acne, muscle weakness, ulcers, thinning of the skin, and mood changes. When patients are treated for a long period of time, deaths from adrenal insufficiency have occurred with transfer from oral to inhalation steroids, especially during stressors like surgery. You should not be on steroids for long periods of time.

NONALLERGIC ASTHMA TREATMENTS

Nonallergic asthma is a chronic problem that needs to be treated somewhat differently than allergic asthma, which may come and go with avoidable triggers and seasonal changes. Chronic asthma sufferers are more at risk for fatalities if they are not treated.

Patients with chronic asthma should be treated with inhaled corticosteroids, including fluticasone (Flonase, Flovent), beclomethasone (Qvar, Beconase, Vancenase), flunisolide (Aerobid), budesonide (Rhinocort, Pulmicort), and triamcinolone (Azmacort, Nasacort). Inhaled corticosteroids have the same side effects as systemic steroids but to a much lesser degree. Studies have shown that inhaled corticosteroids (budesonide) can be used intermittently; there is no advantage to regular use of these medications.[1]

Theophylline (theodur, slophyllin) and the related aminophylline drugs are caffeine-related xanthine derivatives that act to dilate the bronchi. Aminophylline can cause rash in some people. They can be given either orally or intravenously for asthma emergencies. Toxicity results in seizures, irregular heartbeats, and pounding heartbeats. They interact with ciprofloxacine and the other fluoroquinolone antibiotics (i.e., those ending with

-xacine) as well as with caffeine. They are not used much anymore because of safety concerns and side effects.

Long-acting beta-2 agonists have been promoted as reducing the need for inhaled quick-relief medication. Drugs on the market include salmeterol (Serevent) and formoterol (Foradil). Serevent, approved in 1994, dilates breathing passages by stimulating the beta-2 adrenergic receptor. At least 300,000 children take this drug.

In November 2004, Dr. David Graham of the FDA isolated Serevent as being one of five dangerous drugs still on the market in testimony before Congress, describing Serevent users as "dying while clutching their inhalers."

In 1996, based on reports of paradoxical bronchospasm (a contraction of the breathing airway or bronchus that impairs breathing and can be fatal) with Serevent, the manufacturer undertook a large multisite randomized placebo-controlled trial, the Salmeterol Multi-center Asthma Research Trial (SMART), a twenty-eight-week safety study comparing salmeterol (Serevent) and placebo in the treatment of asthma.[2] In addition to their usual asthma therapy, patients received either Serevent or a placebo. The study was stopped in 2002 by the study's Data Safety Monitoring Board because of an increase in asthma-related deaths. Analysis of 26,355 patients showed statistically significantly higher rates of asthma-related deaths (thirteen vs. three, relative risk greater than fourfold) in patients on Serevent.

In African Americans, who made up 17% of the study population, the study showed a statistically significantly greater number of respiratory-related deaths and life-threatening events. Many required intubation (a procedure in which a tube is put down the throat to enable a patient to breathe) related to respiratory causes (twenty vs. five for placebo, a fourfold increase). In addition, there was a more than fourfold increase in asthma-related deaths and life-threatening respiratory events in patients taking salmeterol over those taking placebo. Overall the risk of death from any cause or the risk of a life-threatening event was doubled in African Americans, another finding that was statistically significant. The data suggested that the risks of Serevent were greater for African Americans than for Caucasians. About half of the patients were also taking an inhaled corticosteroid. In those patients not taking an inhaled corticosteroid, there were significantly more asthma-related deaths in all patients taking salmeterol than in those taking placebo.

The manufacturers of Serevent initially showed data to the FDA that included the results from the twenty-eight-week trial plus a six-month follow-up period. The results for this period were better than those for the initial twenty-eight weeks alone. However, the initial study protocol was for a twenty-eight-week trial, and the FDA appropriately requested the twenty-eight-week outcomes, which it posted on its Web site in 2005. These results notwithstanding, the potential risks of long-acting beta agonists have long been known. A long-acting beta-agonist drug marketed in New Zealand that was associated with an increase in asthma-related deaths was pulled from the market there in 1976. A recent meta-analysis (for which data from all published studies are combined) of trials from the past twenty years that involved a total of 33,826 asthma patients treated with long-acting beta agonists showed that all drugs in this class are dangerous.[3] Overall there was a statistically significant increase in a number of parameters, including an increase in asthma exacerbations requiring hospitalizations by 2.6-fold, increased life-threatening exacerbations of asthma by 1.8-fold, and increased risk of asthma-related death by 3.5-fold. Based on these findings, I do not recommend use of a long-acting beta-2 agonist.

Advair, which contains Serevent and a steroid, also carries the same black-box warning about increased asthma-related deaths. This hasn't stopped it from running up $2 billion in sales per year. Based on the SMART study we cannot conclude that long-acting beta agonists administered with steroids are safe; in studies where 75% of patients were taking a steroid there was still a twofold increased risk of asthma-related death.

Montelukast (Singulair) and zafirlukast (Accolate) are part of a new generation of asthma medications that are leukotriene antagonists. These medications work by inhibiting the cysteinyl leukotriene (CysLT-1) receptor, which is involved in the inflammatory response. In rare cases they may be associated with Churg-Strauss syndrome, which involves inflammation of the blood vessels. Zileuton (Zyflo) can cause lupus and liver toxicity and requires blood to be checked every six months. These drugs are expensive and have not been shown to be more effective than steroids and antihistamines.

Other new drugs are the mast cell stabilizers like nedocromil (Tilade) and omalizumab (Xolair). Xolair is given by injection every two to four weeks. These meds have only recently been approved by the FDA, and so we have to adopt a wait-and-see attitude.

Diet and Behavior

Although medications often do have a place for asthmatics, in our usual zeal to reach for the pill first, we have neglected other interventions that may play an equal or even greater role in the treatment and prevention of asthma. Inhalers are not as invasive as many oral asthma medications, and steroids, over the short term, can be helpful during a severe attack.

Drugs are often pushed while lifestyle interventions like exercise (which are equally effective based on scientific studies) are ignored and in some cases discouraged. As proof, the Web site of the Asthma and Allergy Foundation of America (www.aafa.org) states, "Exercise—frequently in cold air—is a frequent asthma trigger." Although the site notes that children can exercise with appropriate management, nowhere does it mention the beneficial effects of exercise. All of the treatments listed are medications, and under "Prevention" it lists "take your medication as prescribed" and "identify and minimize contact with your asthma triggers" (one of which is "running, playing, or exercising"!). Why such an emphasis on drugs instead of viable alternatives? The fact that 72% of this particular nonprofit foundation's revenue comes from pharmaceutical companies might have something to do with it.

Sean Lucas, M.D., MPH, and Thomas Platts-Mills, M.D., Ph.D., from the University of Virginia Asthma and Allergic Diseases Center wrote: "[T]he overwhelming majority of studies demonstrated the capacity for asthmatic subjects to exercise safely and significantly improve their cardio-vascular fitness and quality of life . . . the allergy community has placed emphasis on medical therapy and allergen avoidance. . . . It is our belief that an exercise prescription should be part of the treatment for all cases of asthma."[4]

I believe it is important to encourage outdoor play in children as a pre-ventative measure for asthma. As Lucas and Platts-Mills wrote: "The real question is whether prolonged physical activity and, in particular, outdoor play of children plays a role in prophylaxis against persistent wheezing. If so, the decrease in physical activity might have played a major role in recent increases in asthma prevalence and severity."

Allergic asthma can also be treated via avoidance of triggers in the home and environment such as pet dander, mold, dust mites, cockroaches, tree and other plant pollen in spring, secondhand smoke, perfumes, and chemicals, including those found in standard household cleaning products. Wash bedding on a regular basis, decrease humidity, check air-conditioning units for mold, minimize dust, keep pets outside (or don't have one), use an air conditioner (but clean its filter on a regular basis), shower before bed to remove pollen, keep food sealed to decrease insects, and change filters in forced-air cooling and heating systems.

Your doctor can identify your triggers by exposing you to a number of potential allergens and then measuring the inflammatory response. Once the plants, foods, molds, chemicals, or animals you are allergic to have been identified, you can avoid them. In addition, your doctor can perform tests to determine how much of the immunoglobulin IgE you have that is specifically oriented to different potential allergens. These tests are low risk and can provide useful information for deciding on treatment and life-style changes.

A number of studies have shown a relationship between psychological stress and asthma. Using relaxation techniques like deep breathing, progressive muscle relaxation, and meditation can be useful in preventing asthma attacks. Still, for many individuals with chronic asthma, medication is a requirement.

The Bottom Line

Remove things in your environment that can trigger asthma attacks. Develop a good diet and exercise regimen. Use over-the-counter medications for allergies; do not waste money on prescription drugs for these. Do not use OTC medications for chronic asthma. As needed use beta-agonist and steroid inhalers for chronic asthma. If these do not control your asthma use a long-acting beta agonist only as a last resort, and then never in the absence of an inhaled steroid.

Drug	Use	Common, Benign Side Effects	Serious Side Effects	Life-threatening Side Effects	Reasons Not to Take
Histamine Receptor Blockers					
Low Risk					
Hydroxyzine (Atarax, Vistaril)	Allergy	Sleepiness, dry mouth, confusion, urinary retention, nausea, vomiting	Nightmares, nervousness, irritability, viral infection	Agitation	Hypersensitivity, age < 12, pregnancy, breast-feeding
Brompheniramine (Dimetane, Dimetapp)	Allergy	Sleepiness, dry mouth, confusion, urinary retention, nausea, vomiting	Nightmares, nervousness, irritability, viral infection	Agitation	Hypersensitivity, age < 12, pregnancy, breast-feeding

Drug	Use	Common, Benign Side Effects	Serious Side Effects	Life-threatening Side Effects	Reasons Not to Take
Cetirizine (Zyrtec)	Allergy	Sleepiness, dry mouth, confusion, urinary retention, nausea, vomiting	Nightmares, nervousness, irritability, viral infection	Agitation	Hyper-sensitivity, age < 12, pregnancy, breast-feeding
Chlorphen-iramine (Chlor-trimeton)	Allergy	Sleepiness, dry mouth, confusion, urinary retention, nausea, vomiting	Nightmares, nervousness, irritability, viral infection	Agitation	Hyper-sensitivity, age < 12, pregnancy, breast-feeding
Cyproheptadine (Periactin)	Allergy	Sleepiness, dry mouth, confusion, urinary retention, nausea, vomiting	Nightmares, nervousness, irritability, viral infection	Agitation	Hyper-sensitivity, age < 12, pregnancy, breast-feeding
Diphenhydra-mine (Benadryl)	Allergy	Sleepiness, dry mouth, confusion, urinary retention, nausea, vomiting	Nightmares, nervousness, irritability, viral infection	Agitation	Hyper-sensitivity, age < 12, pregnancy, breast-feeding
Fexofenadine (Allegra)	Allergy	Sleepiness, dry mouth, confusion, urinary retention, nausea, vomiting	Nightmares, nervousness, irritability, viral infection	Agitation	Hyper-sensitivity, age < 12, pregnancy, breast-feeding

Drug	Use	Common, Benign Side Effects	Serious Side Effects	Life-threatening Side Effects	Reasons Not to Take
Loratadine (Claritin)	Allergy	Sleepiness, dry mouth, confusion, urinary retention, nausea, vomiting	Nightmares, nervousness, irritability, viral infection	Agitation	Hyper-sensitivity, age < 12, pregnancy, breast-feeding
Azelastine (Astelin)	Allergy	Sleepiness, dry mouth, confusion, urinary retention, nausea, vomiting	Nightmares, nervousness, irritability, viral infection	Agitation	Hyper-sensitivity, age < 12, pregnancy, breast-feeding
Desloratadine (Clarinex)	Allergy	Sleepiness, dry mouth, confusion, urinary retention, nausea, vomiting	Nightmares, nervousness, irritability, viral infection	Agitation	Hyper-sensitivity, age < 12, pregnancy, breast-feeding
Short-Acting Beta-2 Agonist Bronchodilators					
Moderate Risk					
Albuterol (Proventil)	Asthma	Tremors, jitters, nervousness, nausea, vomiting	Palpitations, insomnia	Increased blood pressure, bronchospasm (rare), angioedema (rare)	Hyper-sensitivity
Levalbuterol (Xopenex)	Asthma	Tremors, jitters, nervousness, nausea, vomiting	Palpitations, insomnia	Increased blood pressure, bronchospasm (rare), angioedema (rare)	Hyper-sensitivity

Drug	Use	Common, Benign Side Effects	Serious Side Effects	Life-threatening Side Effects	Reasons Not to Take
Metaproterenol (Alupent)	Asthma	Tremors, jitters, nervousness, nausea, vomiting	Palpitations, insomnia	Increased blood pressure, bronchospasm (rare), angioedema (rare)	Hyper-sensitivity
Pirbuterol (Maxair)	Asthma	Tremors, jitters, nervousness, nausea, vomiting	Palpitations, insomnia	Increased blood pressure, bronchospasm (rare), angioedema (rare)	Hyper-sensitivity
Long-Acting Beta-2 agonists					
High Risk					
Salmeterol (Serevent)	Asthma	Tremors, jitters, nervousness, nausea, vomiting	Palpitations, insomnia	Increased asthma-related deaths in African Americans and those not on inhaled steroids	African Americans; patients not on inhaled steroids
Formoterol (Foradil)	Asthma	Tremors, jitters, nervousness, nausea, vomiting	Palpitations, insomnia	Increased blood pressure, bronchospasm (rare), angioedema (rare)	Hyper-sensitivity
Salmeterol + fluticasone (steroid) (Advair)	Asthma	Tremors, jitters, nervousness, nausea, vomiting	Palpitations, insomnia	Increased blood pressure, bronchospasm (rare), angioedema (rare)	Hyper-sensitivity

Drug	Use	Common, Benign Side Effects	Serious Side Effects	Life-threatening Side Effects	Reasons Not to Take
Terbutaline (Brethine)	Asthma	Tremors, jitters, nervousness, nausea, vomiting	Palpitations, insomnia	Increased blood pressure, bronchospasm (rare), angioedema (rare)	Hyper-sensitivity
Anticholinergics					
Moderate Risk					
Ipratropium bromide (Atrovent)	Asthma	Cough, hoarseness, dry mouth, constipation, urinary retention, blurred vision	Throat irritation	Bronchospasm (rare), anaphylaxis (rare)	Peanut oil or atropine sensitivity
Xanthines					
Moderate Risk					
Theophylline (Theodur, Slophyllin)	Asthma, Chronic Obstructive Pulmonary Disease (COPD)	Rash, nausea, vomiting, diarrhea, restlessness	Confusion, headache, dizziness, insomnia	Seizures, arrhythmias	Patients on Cipro or related antibiotics, hyper-sensitivity to xan-thines, heart or renal disease, ulcers, pregnancy, breast-feeding

Drug	Use	Common, Benign Side Effects	Serious Side Effects	Life-threatening Side Effects	Reasons Not to Take
Aminophylline	Asthma, Chronic Obstructive Pulmonary Disease (COPD)	Rash, nausea, vomiting, diarrhea, restlessness	Confusion, headache, dizziness, insomnia	Seizures, arrhythmias	Patients on Cipro or related antibiotics, hyper-sensitivity to xan-thines, heart or renal disease, ulcers, pregnancy, breast-feeding
Leukotriene Antagonists					
Moderate Risk					
Montelukast (Singulair)	Asthma prophylaxis	Headache, gastritis, runny nose, dizziness, nausea	Stomach pain, joint pain, fever	Churg-Strauss (inflammation of blood vessels—rare), liver failure (rare)	Hyper-sensitivity; do not use for acute wheezing
Zafirlukast (Accolate)	Asthma prophylaxis	Headache, gastritis, runny nose, dizziness, nausea	Stomach pain, joint pain, fever	Churg-Strauss (inflammation of blood vessels—rare), liver failure (rare)	Hyper-sensitivity; do not use for acute wheezing
Zileuton (Zyflo)	Asthma prophylaxis	Headache, gastritis, runny nose, dizziness, nausea	Stomach pain, joint pain, fever	Churg-Strauss (inflammation of blood vessels—rare), lupus (rare), liver failure (rare)	Hyper-sensitivity, pregnancy; do not use for acute wheezing

Drug	Use	Common, Benign Side Effects	Serious Side Effects	Life-threatening Side Effects	Reasons Not to Take
Mast-Cell Stabilizers					
Moderate Risk					
Nedocromil (Tilade)	Asthma prophylaxis	Throat problems (bad taste and irritation), cough, nausea, vomiting	Bronchospasm	Blood cell suppression	Hypersensitivity; do not use for acute wheezing
Omalizumab (Xolair)	Asthma	Throat irritation, cough, nausea, vomiting	Bronchospasm	Allergic reaction, cancer	Hypersensitivity; do not use for acute wheezing
Cromolyn sodium (Intal)	Asthma	Throat problems (bad taste and irritation), cough, nausea, vomiting	Bronchospasm	Allergic reation	Hypersensitivity; do not use for acute wheezing
Corticosteroids					
High Risk					
Fluticasone (Flonase, Flovent)	Asthma	Nausea, sore throat, hoarseness, coughing, dry mouth, fungal infections in mouth	Growth inhibition, decreased bone-mineral density	Seizures, low blood sugar, changes in consciousness, mood changes	Active infection
Beclomethasone (Qvar, Beconase, Vancenase)	Asthma	Nausea, sore throat, hoarseness, coughing, dry mouth, fungal infections in mouth	Growth inhibition, decreased bone-mineral density	Seizures, low blood sugar, changes in consciousness mood changes	Active infection

Drug	Use	Common, Benign Side Effects	Serious Side Effects	Life-threatening Side Effects	Reasons Not to Take
Flunisolide (Aerobid)	Asthma	Nausea, sore throat, hoarseness, coughing, dry mouth, fungal infections in mouth	Growth inhibition, decreased bone-mineral density	Seizures, low blood sugar, changes in consciousness, mood changes	Active infection
Budesonide (Rhinocort, Pulmicort)	Asthma	Nausea, sore throat, hoarseness, coughing, dry mouth, fungal infections in mouth	Growth inhibition, decreased bone-mineral density	Seizures, low blood sugar, changes in consciousness, mood changes	Active infection
Triamcinolone (Azmacort, Nasacort)	Asthma	Nausea, sore throat, hoarseness, coughing, dry mouth, fungal infections in mouth	Growth inhibition, decreased bone-mineral density	Seizures, low blood sugar, changes in consciousness, mood changes	Active infection

8.

Enlarged Prostate

Aging comes with a host of annoyances and problems, both social and medical, as anyone over fifty who has ever tried to understand the appeal of the latest music or fashion or has tried to be as good at a pickup game of basketball as he was in his twenties can attest. Among the medical problems that can impact men is enlarged prostate or benign prostatic hypertrophy, or BPH (also known as enlarging prostate, or EP). Indeed, it happens to almost all men as they age. The thickening of the prostate tissue surrounding the urethra in older men that is associated with urination problems is a part of normal aging and affects some men more than others.

After age fifty most men begin to experience some prostate problems. Fifty percent of men over fifty and 90% of men over eighty have BPH. It sends 6.4 million men to a doctor every year, half of whom consider medication or surgery for treatment. The probability of eventually requiring surgery is 39%. The worst outcomes are a loss of sexual function with surgery, acute urinary retention (the sudden inability to urinate caused by untreated BPH), or damage to the kidneys and bladder. In half of cases

BPH reduces the quality of life for men. Thirty-six percent of spouses of men with BPH surveyed reported that BPH caused a cessation of physical intimacy in their relationships.

The prostate gland, a walnut-size organ in males that is located just below the bladder, helps create semen. Fluid created by the prostate is secreted into the urethra (the tube in the penis that is the conduit for both urine and semen), where it combines with and protects sperm from the testicles. Semen protects sperm and plays an important role in male fertility.

Fertility isn't usually a top priority for most men over fifty, unless they are in a relationship with a woman still in her childbearing years who wants to have children. A more odious condition is BPH. The prostate wraps around the urethra where the urethra exits the bladder. As the prostate enlarges, it squeezes off the urethra, causing urination problems such as the need to urinate frequently day and night, feelings of urgency to urinate, not allowing the bladder to empty completely, and creating weak urine flows that start and stop. BPH is diagnosed by a rectal exam.

BPH is *not* cancer or a precursor to cancer, and it does not increase the risk of prostate cancer. The actual cause of prostate enlargement is unknown. Aside from some link to aging, the testicles may play a role in the growth of the prostate gland. Men who have had their testicles removed at a young age because of testicular cancer or another medical reason do not develop BPH, probably as a result of the ensuing lack of dihydrotestosterone, which has a stimulatory effect on prostate tissue. Similarly, if after developing BPH a man has his testicles removed, the prostate begins to shrink.

Less than half of all men with BPH have symptoms of the disease, which include frequent urination and urgency, urinating at night, weak urine stream, straining to void, dribbling after urination, and incomplete urination. Frequency is caused by mechanical obstruction of the urethra combined with a thickening of the smooth muscle in the bladder wall secondary to the increased resistance from the urethra. This causes the bladder cavity to become smaller, which shortens the times between urination and leads to numerous visits to the restroom.

Treatment is not necessary in the early stages of BPH. Once you *regularly* (several times a week) start urinating less than two hours after the last time you went, feel like your bladder is not empty after urinating, stop and start while urinating, have to push or strain, have a weak stream, can't postpone urinating, and have to get up at night, it is time to do something about it. If you have these problems only once in a while, you won't necessarily benefit from treatment.

Common Medical Treatments

ALPHA ADRENERGIC RECEPTOR BLOCKERS

Alpha adrenergic receptor blocker medications, including doxazosin (Cardura), prazosin (Minipress), alfuzosin (Uroxatral), and terazosin (Hytrin), cause a relaxation of prostate smooth muscle and increase urine flow. The FDA has approved all of these medications for the treatment of BPH, with the exception of Minipress, a medication that has been on the market for the treatment of hypertension for many years. Your doctor has the right to prescribe it for you "off label" for the treatment of BPH if he or she thinks it is indicated. There are no current plans to obtain an indication for Minipress for the treatment of BPH, since it has been off patent for many years. All of the alpha adrenergic receptor blocker medications have similar side effects, including dizziness, postural hypotension (passing out if you stand up too quickly), and fatigue. The potential benefit from relief of BPH symptoms is usually worth the side effects of these medications. However, Uroxatral has cardiac side effects (lengthening of the Q-T interval) and should not be used in patients with liver problems.

TAMSULOSIN

Tamsulosin (Flomax) is a selective blocker of the alpha-1A adrenergic receptor that has fewer side effects than the other alpha-blockers because it is more selective to the alpha-1A adrenergic receptor than the other drugs reviewed above. The other alpha-blockers block adrenergic receptors in both the heart and the brain as well as in the prostate. For this reason they can block the smooth muscles in the blood vessels in these areas and cause the blood vessels to dilate. This changes blood flow to the brain, which is associated with dizziness, fatigue, and the possibility of postural hypotension. Since Flomax is more specific to the adrenergic receptors in the prostate, it has fewer of these side effects.

5-ALPHA-REDUCTASE INHIBITORS

One of the most important factors contributing to BPH is dihydrotestosterone (DHT), a male hormone that normally stimulates prostate tissue in adolescent males, enabling them to produce semen and thus rendering them fertile. Later, however, DHT can stimulate prostate tissue in a counterproductive way. Drugs like finasteride (Proscar), a 5-alpha-reductase inhibitor, inhibit the enzyme responsible for the conversion of testosterone to DHT, 5-alpha-reductase, thereby reducing DHT levels as much as 80%. This reduction is associated with a decrease in prostate volume of 20%, since DHT stimulates prostate tissue growth. Side effects include decreased libido, impotence, and ejaculatory disorder. Dutasteride (Duagen), another 5-alpha-reductase inhibitor, blocks both types 1 and 2 5-alpha-reductase and has a side-effect profile similar to that of finasteride.

In the PROscar Safety Plus Efficacy Canadian Two-Year Study (PROSPECT), 613 men with moderate BPH symptoms were started on a two-year course of treatment with Proscar or placebo.[1] Finasteride resulted in a statistically significant reduction in symptom scores: Compared to placebo, with a baseline score of 15.8, the difference between finasteride and placebo was only 0.4, not a very big difference in symptoms. There was about a 10% increase in the rates of urinary flow. Over twice as many (15.8%) finasteride patients as patients on placebo (6.3%) developed impotence. In a study comparing finasteride to the alpha-blocker terazosin and placebo, 1,229 men were randomized to blinded treatment for one year. Change in symptom scores were 2.6 for placebo, 3.2 for finasteride, 6.1 for terazosin, and 6.2 for terazosin and finasteride.[2] For urine flow finasteride was no better than placebo, while terazosin was statistically significantly better than both finasteride and placebo. Impotence was higher with finasteride (9%) than with placebo (5%) or terazosin (6%). In another study of the long-term effects of these drugs, 3,047 patients who were treated with placebo, doxazosin (alpha-blocker), finasteride, or combination therapy were followed for five years. The outcome was a four-point increase in BPH symptom score, urinary retention, or incontinence. Compared to placebo, doxazosin reduced progression by 39% and finasteride by 34% (both statistically significant).[3] Combination therapy, which was even better (66% reduction), was associated with a reduction in the need for surgery, as was finasteride alone.

Based on these findings I recommend the use of alpha-blockers [doxazosin (Cardura), prazosin (Minipress), alfuzosin (Uroxatral), and terazosin (Hytrin) and Flomax] initially, with the addition of Proscar or Duagen, depending on symptom response and side effects.

Surgical Options

Surgical interventions are the final resort if medications do not help. The decision to opt for surgical interventions should be made when your level of discomfort and impairment are so great that you feel there is just no other choice in terms of your quality of life. Surgical alternatives include open prostatectomy, the removal while under general anesthesia of the inner part of the prostate, which has a 98% success rate. This procedure has caused the most problems with sexual dysfunction and impotence. Transurethral resection of the prostate (TURP) is 88% effective. With TURP the doctor inserts a small device into the penis and removes prostate tissue. Complications are blood clots, bleeding, and infection. Seventy percent develop retrograde ejaculation (ejaculation backward into the bladder), which does not affect sexual performance. One percent of men develop incontinence. The estimates of TURP-induced impotence are difficult to estimate since many men in the older age range of BPH patients already have sexual problems. Estimates vary around 5%, and it is possible that there are no true TURP-induced cases of impotence that do not respond to Viagra.

Other treatments for BPH include thermotherapy, laser surgery, and minor incisions. If medications do not help I recommend starting with a TURP. The long-term financial costs of medical and surgical therapies are the same. Left untreated BPH can lead to acute urinary retention (a medical emergency that requires catheterization), kidney and bladder stones, or damage to the urinary system.

Alternative Medicine

A quick search on the Internet for prostate remedies brings up a picture of a kindly doctor in his white coat with the quotation "Are you or someone you love making too many trips to the bathroom? Try my super prostate formula *free* for thirty days." There must be a lot of desperate men and their wives who don't want to go to the doctor but are being driven nuts by frequent potty stops and dribbling streams of urine. Unfortunately, I am sorry to say that none of this stuff is better than or even equivalent to the prescription medications for BPH or surgical alternatives.

Some of the searches for alternative treatments for BPH have come from observations that rates of BPH are lower in Asia. One idea is that this is related to increased soy consumption. Genistein, an isoflavin ingredient in tofu, has been found to decrease the growth of prostate tissue in animal models. Isoflavin derived from red clover is sold in the U.S. as a supplement for prostate conditions. There are no controlled studies to demonstrate its effectiveness.

Other herbs and supplements promoted for BPH include beta-sitosterol, pygeum extract, pumpkin seeds, garlic rye, grass extract, and magnesium. Controlled studies do not exist for these compounds either.

Saw palmetto is a supplement derived from the fruit of *Serenoa repens* or *Sabal serrulatum* (the American dwarf palm), which is native to the southeastern U.S. Saw palmetto is marketed for the treatment of BPH. Saw palmetto is often mixed with nettle root in a formulation for the prostate. Its action is purported to involve anti-inflammatory activity, blocked conversion of testosterone to dihydrotestosterone, and shrinkage of prostate tissue. The primary side effect is stomach upset, which can be reduced by taking it with food.

In one controlled trial saw palmetto was shown to be efficacious in the treatment of BPH. In a more recent study funded by the NIH, 225 men over age forty-nine with moderate to severe symptoms of BPH were randomly assigned to receive saw palmetto or placebo in a double-blind fashion. There were no differences in urinary symptoms, urine flow rates, prostate size, or quality of life.[4] Based on the studies to date I cannot recommend saw palmetto, but given the lack of adverse effects I will not discourage anyone from taking it, either.

Diet and Behavior

I know I harp on the importance of changing your diet and exercising, but unfortunately there isn't much evidence that either does much for BPH. You can review your medication list for drugs that can exacerbate BPH, including tricyclic antidepressants, anticholinergic agents, diuretics, narcotics, and first-generation antihistamines and decongestants. Medical conditions that can look like BPH include urinary tract infections, heart failure, prostate cancer, and diabetes.

The Bottom Line

Initially use the wait-and-see approach. Saw palmetto is relatively free of side effects but probably doesn't work. In terms of medical therapy, I recommend starting out with the alpha-blockers. If these don't work you can add one of the 5-alpha-reductase inhibitors like Proscar. Eventually, if the problem gets worse, you may need surgery.

Drug	Use	Common, Benign Side Effects	Serious Side Effects	Life-threatening Side Effects	Reasons Not to Take
Alpha Blockers					
Moderate Risk					
Doxazosin (Cardura)	BPH	Dizziness, headache, palpitations, nausea	Orthostatic hypotension, sexual dysfunction	Heart failure, stroke	None
Prazosin (Minipress)	BPH	Dizziness, headache, palpitations, nausea	Orthostatic hypotension, sexual dysfunction	Heart failure, stroke	None
Alfuzosin (Uroxatral)	BPH	Dizziness, headache, palpitations, nausea	Orthostatic hypotension, sexual dysfunction	Heart failure, stroke	None
Terazosin (Hytrin)	BPH	Dizziness, headache, palpitations, nausea	Orthostatic hypotension, sexual dysfunction	Heart failure, stroke	None
Tamsulosin (Flomax)	BPH	Dizziness, headache, palpitations, nausea	Orthostatic hypotension, sexual dysfunction	Heart failure, stroke	None

Drug	Use	Common, Benign Side Effects	Serious Side Effects	Life-threatening Side Effects	Reasons Not to Take
5-Alpha-Reductase Inhibitors					
Low Risk					
Finasteride (Proscar)	BPH	Headache, back pain	Decreased libido, impotence, ejaculatory disorder	Allergic reaction	Allergy to finasteride or dutasteride
Dutasteride (Duagen)	BPH	Headache, back pain	Decreased libido, impotence, ejaculatory disorder	Allergic reaction	Allergy to finasteride or dutasteride

9.

Treatment for Ulcers and Gastric Reflux

Ulcers and gastroesophageal reflux disease (GERD), heartburn, and dyspepsia were traditionally known as businessman's diseases, because they were common among mid-twentieth-century professional males who spent a great deal of time sitting in their offices and regularly consumed steak and sauce-laden three-martini lunches. After all, the risk of getting GERD and ulcers increases with excessive alcohol use, stress, smoking, diet, medications (aspirin, NSAIDs), and some medical conditions. I had an uncle who was the quintessential businessman, president of a family-owned beer company, who was overweight and suffered from GERD for many years until he died recently of esophageal cancer. Well, times have changed. Nowadays everyone from the Wall Street tycoon to the overprogrammed suburban soccer mom can suffer from ulcers and GERD. In fact, 350,000 Americans develop ulcers every year, and 3,000 die from them.

Aside from behavior and stress, ulcers can also be caused by an infection with *H. pylori* bacteria. The good news is that the infection can be detected with a simple test and treated with antibiotics. Ulcers occur when stomach acid burns a hole in the wall of the stomach or intestine. Normal acid secretion in the stomach is an important reason why ulcers don't heal. Symptoms of ulcers include stomach pain, indigestion, and bloody vomit; unless you vomit blood (which doesn't always happen with ulcers) it can be hard to tell if you have ulcers, GERD, or functional dyspepsia (described below). Ulcers are diagnosed by endoscopy, a procedure in which the doctor puts a tube with a camera on the end of it down your throat and looks for ulcers. If you have a negative *H. pylori* test and you don't take aspirin, NSAIDs, or COX 2 inhibitors (see Chapter 2), it is unlikely that you have an ulcer. That's because research studies have shown that the number of people with ulcers without the risk factors of a positive *H. pylori* test or treatment with arthritis medications is very low.

Gastroesophageal reflux disease is caused by reflux of acid from the stomach into the esophagus. It is accompanied by symptoms of heartburn (burning pain in the chest under the breastbone) or acid reflux, especially after eating, is more frequent at night, and is relieved by antacids. Other symptoms include belching, regurgitation of food, nausea, vomiting, hoarseness, sore throat, difficulty swallowing, and cough. Untreated, it can increase the risk of cancer of the esophagus. *Dyspepsia* is a general term for stomach upset that occurs after meals and may or may not be due to GERD.

Although both are stomach-related conditions with overlapping symptoms, GERD and ulcers are different: Ulcers occur when gastric acid burns a hole in the stomach; GERD is the result of gastric acid shooting back up through the valve between the stomach and the esophagus and is very common in obese people.

Pharmaceutical Solutions

The first-line treatment of GERD is with over-the-counter antacids like aluminum hydroxide (Amphojel, Maalox), or magnesium combinations, including Phillips' Milk of Magnesia, Gaviscon, and Riopan. Aluminum can cause constipation, and magnesium can cause diarrhea. These compounds work by coating the stomach and provide protection against the corrosive effects of stomach acid. Ulcers need more aggressive treatment, since bleeding from ulcers can be life threatening.

THE HISTORY OF PRESCRIPTION MEDICATIONS

The original medications for the treatment of both GERD and ulcers were the histamine-2 (H2) blockers, like cimetidine (Tagamet), ranitidine (Zantac), and famotidine (Pepcid). These worked by decreasing the amount of acid in the stomach, thereby promoting the healing of ulcers *and* reducing gastric reflux. Patients with reduced kidney or liver function can experience confusion as a side effect with H2 blockers. Other side effects include diarrhea, dizziness, nausea, and headache. Tagamet can also impair sexual function.

PPIS

In 1998 AstraZenica introduced Prilosec (omeprazole), the first of a new class of medications for GERD called proton pump inhibitors (PPIs). PPIs now on the market include lansoprazole (Prevacid), pantoprazole (Protonix), rabeprozale (Aciphex), esomeprazole (Nexium), and omeprazole (Prilosec). They act by blocking the H+ (hydrogen) K+ (potassium) ATPase pump in the stomach, which decreases acid secretion in the stomach. The PPIs have been shown to be more effective than placebo in promoting the healing of ulcers and decreasing the symptoms of GERD.[1] Compared to the older H2-blocker medication ranitidine, PPIs have shown a 33% improvement in ulcer healing. The PPIs decrease acid secretion to a greater degree than H2 blockers and are more effective in treatment, although most of them cost more than the older drugs because they are only available by prescription.

PPIs have a low side-effect profile, with side effects in less than 5% of patients, the most common of which are headache, diarrhea, stomach pain, fever, sore throat, and nausea. The diarrhea may be related to the suppression of acid formation, which alters the natural bacteria content of the gut. Overall, PPIs are fairly safe.

A review of twenty-one randomized controlled trials of PPIs in patients with proven peptic ulcers showed no effect on mortality, but it did reveal a reduction in rebleeding and repeat surgery of about 50%.[2] There is no evidence that any of the PPIs are superior to one another in efficacy or safety. Since omeprazole (Prilosec) is now available as a generic, it is the cheapest and therefore the recommended PPI.

You have probably seen the man on TV talking about the "purple pill," or Nexium (esomeprazole magnesium). This particular purple pill is a replacement of the original purple pill, Prilosec. Both should probably be called the green pill because of all the money they have made and continue to make for the manufacturer, AstraZenica. They are both widely popular and equally effective medications. After its introduction in 1998, sales of Prilosec continued to rise year after year until they reached $1 billion a year in 1995 and peaked at $4 billion a year in 2000, when it was the most popular drug in the world, as reported by National Public Radio (April 18, 2002).

In 2002 AstraZenica convened a team to assess the impact of their blockbuster Prilosec going off patent. In response to the potential revenue loss that generics would cause, they decided to take a variation of the drug (a metabolite) and put it on patent, and then they marketed the new version as an improvement on the original. You see, all molecules come in one version as well as an identical version that is a "mirror version" (i.e., if you held it up to a mirror it would look the same). Prilosec was a mix of left and right, so the company took the left-hand version, and called it Nexium. Then they tested a higher dose of the "new" drug against the "old" drug to "prove" that it was better, and sent out an army of sales-people to convince doctors that this was the case. Needless to say, if you took higher doses of the older Prilosec you would get a regular dose of Nexium, the "purple pill." It was an effective campaign: By 2002 the company had convinced one in six former Prilosec users to switch to Nexium. At $1,500 a year it is much more expensive than the generic versions of Prilosec ($150 a year). Why not just take higher doses of Prilosec? It will eventually get you your Nexium fix for a lot less money.

Irritable Bowel Syndrome

Irritable bowel syndrome (IBS) is a very disabling disorder that affects as many as 20% of all Americans and accounts for 20% to 50% of visits to gastroenterologists. IBS is characterized by symptoms including abdominal pain, altered bowel function, bloating, distension, and feelings of incomplete evacuation (as in, you didn't get rid of everything when you sat on the toilet). Patients have been subclassified according to whether they have predominant symptoms of diarrhea or constipation.

5HT-3 SEROTONIN ANTAGONISTS

Alosetron (Lotronex) and cilansetron (Calmactin) are 5HT-3 serotonin-receptor antagonists, which act by blocking these particular serotonin receptors in the gut and by an incompletely understood mechanism to reduce pain and retard bowel transit in IBS patients. Although both medications have been shown to be effective for IBS, alosetron is effective only in women with IBS.[3]

The 5HT-3 serotonin-receptor antagonists have been very controversial. Concerns about the potential toxicities of these drugs have been countered by the protests of IBS sufferers that they have no other available remedies. Alosetron was introduced in the U.S. in 2000 and subsequently withdrawn because several patients developed ischemic colitis and severe constipation, and three patients died. Cases of ischemic colitis have also been reported with cilansetron. Other possible side effects include headache, diarrhea, and stomach pain.

5HT-4 SEROTONIN-RECEPTOR PARTIAL AGONISTS

Tegaserod (Zelnorm), a 5HT-4 serotonin-receptor partial agonist that promotes contractions of the colon, is effective in women with constipation-predominant IBS. Common side effects include diarrhea in 5% over placebo and headaches in 3% over placebo. It has also been linked more rarely with ischemic colitis, with 20 cases reported to the FDA between 2002 and 2004.

Cromolyn sodium is a mast-cell stabilizer that has been used in the treatment of IBS. Two controlled studies have shown an improvement in IBS symptoms with cromolyn sodium compared to placebo treatment.[4] Side effects include sore throat, bad taste in the mouth, stomach pain, cough, stuffy nose, sneezing, headache, and (more serious) increased difficulty breathing, and swelling of the tongue or throat.

Functional Dyspepsia

Functional dyspepsia (FD) is a disorder characterized by stomach pain or discomfort, which may be accompanied by belching, nausea, bloating, and early satiety without an identifiable abnormality that causes the symptoms. Functional dyspepsia is one of the most common gastrointestinal disorders, affecting as much as 20% of the population. Symptoms of functional dyspepsia are often provoked by eating fatty foods, which can delay the time it takes for food to leave the stomach, making symptoms even worse. There may be other, specific foods that trigger symptoms that you can learn to avoid. (Contrary to myth, spicy foods do not make dyspepsia worse.) Although alcohol, smoking, and caffeine can exacerbate ulcers or GERD, they don't have a specific relationship to functional dyspepsia. Proton pump inhibitors, or PPIs (see page 159), have not been shown to be effective treatments for functional dyspepsia.

Cisapride (Propulsid), used in the treatment of functional dyspepsia, is a medication that stimulates release of the neurotransmitter acetylcholine.

Side effects of Cisapride include diarrhea, nausea, headache, stuffy nose, constipation, and coughing; more rarely it can cause changes in vision, chest pain, mental/mood changes, stomach pain, dizziness, fainting, irregular heartbeat, or allergic reactions. Unfortunately, it also has troublesome cardiac side effects, which restrict its use. One controlled study showed that itopride, a dopamine D2 agonist, was superior to a placebo in improving symptoms of functional dyspepsia.[5]

Alternative Medicines

Patients suffering from gastrointestinal disorders like IBS, FD, and GERD commonly self-medicate with a number of herbs, supplements, and food products. For example, constipation is often treated with herbal therapies that stimulate secretion of fluids into the bowel and muscular contraction of the intestines, the most common of which include senna, cascara, aloe vera, and rhubarb root. One small study of thirty-five patients showed that aloe vera combined with celandin and psyllium was better than placebo in treating constipation.[6] Although it is unclear whether these herbs and supplements are helpful, there is no evidence of potential harm.

As noted earlier, fatty foods can increase the symptoms of dyspepsia. Patients with IBS commonly can't tolerate a number of foods, including milk, wheat, eggs, and fresh fruits and vegetables. IBS patients do not, however, have a greater lactase deficiency (the enzyme that digests dairy products) or inability to absorb sugars (like fructose) when measured in the laboratory, although they may have more symptoms when exposed to these compounds outside the lab. A variety of herbs, food products, and other supplements have been promoted for the treatment of bowel symptoms, constipation and dyspepsia.

Please note that if you have an ulcer that you suspect could be life threatening, I do not recommend trying herbs and supplements first. Get to a doctor for help.

PEPPERMINT OIL

Peppermint oil has been shown to be the most useful of the food products used to treat dyspepsia and IBS. By virtue of its active ingredient, menthol, which relaxes the smooth muscle of the intestines by blocking calcium influx, it has antispasmodic properties. At least three randomized placebo-controlled trials have shown that peppermint oil improves symptoms of IBS (while two did not show an effect).[7, 8] There was heterogeneity among the trials, meaning that the results were not consistent and therefore inconclusive. One study did show that peppermint oil helped symptoms of dyspepsia. Heartburn is a common side effect of peppermint oil treatment. Based on the studies to date I can say it is safe to try peppermint oil for symptoms of IBS or heartburn, since it has no long-term or dangerous side effects.

ARTICHOKE

Another food product that has been promoted as a treatment for dyspepsia is artichoke *(Cynara scolymus)* leaf extract (ALE), whose active compound is thought to be a bitter compound like cynaropicrin. Animal studies have shown that it improves bile flow. One study of 244 patients randomized to ALE or placebo showed an improvement in dyspepsia symptoms and quality-of-life scores with ALE after six weeks of ALE therapy. The difference between the two at the end of treatment was less than 10%, however, so in my view the effects were not very strong. Of course, this is only one study, and I would like to see another controlled trial showing that ALE works for dyspepsia before I recommend it. In the meantime if you have dyspepsia and you want to eat more artichoke leaves, I say *bon appétit.* They certainly can't hurt.

GINGER

Ginger has been used to treat nausea as well as bowel symptoms. Ginger extract is thought to have anti-inflammatory properties, to strengthen the gastric lining, and to stimulate motility of the intestines. Although it has been promoted for the treatment of nausea, controlled studies have shown that it does not decrease postoperative nausea, although it has been shown to work for seasickness and nausea with pregnancy. It is safe and has no side effects that I know of. So next time you have sushi, don't forget the ginger, although I would like to see another controlled trial to affirm that it really works for nausea. There are no controlled studies I know of using ginger for bowel symptoms.

CHINESE HERBAL MEDICINE

Bowel disorders (and a number of other conditions) are traditionally treated in China with Chinese herbal medicine (CHM), which involves regular meetings with the CHM practitioner, who makes individualized adjustments targeted to the specific symptoms of each patient. It is the combination of the different herbs, rather than the individual herbs, that is believed to work for the specific disorder. In the only controlled trial of CHM for bowel disorders, 116 patients with IBS were randomly assigned to receive traditional CHM with an individualized treatment, a standard formula of twenty herbs used in CHM, or a placebo for fourteen weeks of treatment. Both the herbal treatments were better for IBS symptoms than the placebo, but the individualized CHM was not better than the standard fixed formula.[9] This study was well designed and conducted and offers promising results for CHM treatment of IBS, but I would like to see another replication study. In the meantime I won't discourage you from using CHM, but you don't need to pay for an individual practitioner.

PROBIOTICS

Probiotics are live microbial supplements taken to improve the microbial balance of the colon. Probiotics are more commonly used in Europe than in the U.S. and are most popular in France, where 3% of the population takes probiotics on any given day. The bacteria used most often in probiotic products include *Lactobacillus* and the yeast *Saccharomyces boulardii (S. boulardii)*. Probiotics can be taken orally as a supplement and often are added to yogurts and other food products. The concept behind the use of probiotics is that due to modern-day diets, industrialization of the food-production process, and overuse of antibiotics, many of us have developed an imbalance of the bacterial flora in our colon and intestines. It follows that this imbalance causes constipation, diarrhea, dyspepsia, and disturbances in digestion. The addition of probiotics is designed to reduce pathological bacteria like *Clostridium difficile* and *Escherichia coli (E. coli)*.

Studies of probiotics for the treatment of gastrointestinal disorders have not shown consistent results. In controlled trials, probiotics have not been shown to be an effective treatment for constipation in adults or children. One study of *Lactobacillus plantarum* for the treatment of IBS showed an improvement in abdominal pain and flatulence compared to placebo. Another study of seventy-two patients with IBS who got either the probiotics *Lactobacillus salivarius* or *Bifidobacterium infantis* or a placebo drink for eight weeks showed a greater reduction of IBS symptoms with probiotics. A small study of twenty-three IBS patients who got either *Lactobacillus GG* or placebo showed no difference in pain, urgency, or bloating between the two groups.[10]

The studies offer some hope for probiotics in the treatment of IBS, although the results are not conclusive. There is no evidence that probiotics help constipation. In the meantime, before more and better studies are performed, you can take probiotics for IBS symptoms since they have few side effects. As I mention in Chapter 10, in some trials probiotics also have been shown to reduce antibiotic-induced diarrhea when given in conjunction with antibiotics.[11]

Probiotics are believed to work by binding to the wall of the colon, competing for nutrients with pathogenic bacteria, and secreting substances that inhibit the growth of pathological bacteria. If you do buy probiotics or food with probiotic compounds, make sure that they are the probiotics that have been shown to work: *Lactobacillus, S. Boulardii, B. lactis,* and

Streptococcus thermophilus. Since not all bacteria have been shown to be effective, you shouldn't put up with yogurt and other food companies that refuse to tell you which bacteria are in their products. If they won't tell you, don't buy it.

Diet and Behavior in the Treatment of Ulcers, Reflux, and Functional Bowel Disorders

It's amazing how much control we have over our own health just by changing the way we eat. This is certainly the case as far as limiting our chances of developing ulcers, GERD, or IBS. High-fiber/low-fat diets have been shown to be beneficial in preventing diverticulitis in addition to reducing the risk of heart disease, diabetes, and hypertension. High-fiber diets also reduce the risk of ulcer by slowing the movement of food through the stomach and reducing exposure of the intestines to acid. Foods with high fiber include fruits, vegetables, legumes, and brown bread and rice.

In general fatty-food diets can exacerbate all gastrointestinal disorders, including ulcers, GERD, dyspepsia, and IBS. Chocolate, citrus fruits, tomatoes, peppermint, and caffeine can also worsen gastrointestinal problems, although they don't actually cause ulcers. Smoking, excessive alcohol intake, and NSAIDs, aspirin, and COX-2 inhibitors are also to be avoided for ulcer and GERD prevention.

For IBS, food-elimination diets—with elimination of wheat, eggs, dairy products, and fresh fruits and vegetables, depending on the sensitivity of the individual patient—have been attempted with varying success.

FOOD ALLERGENS

The role of food allergens in IBS and dyspepsia is unclear. In certain people some foods may mediate an immune response, characterized by the release of immune mediators like IgE and IgG4. In a subgroup of IBS patients these types of reactions may contribute to their symptoms. Food allergies have been reported for milk, eggs, peanuts, tree nuts, fish, shellfish, soy, and wheat. An allergist can use blood tests or skin pricks to test you for specific foods.

WEIGHT

Obesity can also play a significant role in gastrointestinal problems. Many people with dyspepsia are overweight. Studies have shown that obese people have more gastric reflux than people of normal weight. Obesity promotes dysfunction of the esophagus (remember my uncle?), which leads to reflux. If you are grossly overweight, you need to find a way to lose weight to help your gastrointestinal problems.

Exercise is beneficial for gastrointestinal problems in two ways. First, it leads to weight loss, which improves GERD and dyspepsia. Moderate exercise also directly reduces symptoms of IBS and dyspepsia apart from its role in weight loss and promotes the movement of food out of the stomach and into the intestine. Thirty minutes of sustained movement such as fast walking, running, or strength training four or five times a week is all it takes to improve or eliminate these conditions.

The Bottom Line

Exercise, cook your own meals, and avoid junk food and dining in restaurants. If you have IBS or you have to take antibiotics for an infection, you can try probiotics. Avoid use of antibiotics for colds and flus; they don't help, but they can mess up your gut flora. For those of you with GERD and ulcers I recommend that you stop taking arthritis medications, cut down on excessive alcohol, quit smoking, and, if needed, take an antacid. If this doesn't help, take H2 blockers, and next PPIs.

Drug	Use	Common, Benign Side Effects	Serious Side Effects	Life-threatening Side Effects	Reasons Not to Take
Antacids					
Low Risk					
Aluminum Hydroxide (Amphojel, Maalox)	GERD	Constipation, chalky taste	Dizziness, headache	None	Low phosphate
Magnesium Combinations (Phillips' Milk of Magnesia, Gaviscon, Riopan)	GERD	Diarrhea	Dizziness, headache	None	High magnesium
Histamine 2 (H2) Blockers					
Moderate Risk					
Cimetidine (Tagamet)	GERD, ulcers	Nausea, dizziness, headache	Diarrhea, sexual impairment	Confusion in patients with kidney or liver dysfunction	Hyper-sensitivity, pregnancy, breast-feeding
Ranitidine (Zantac)	GERD, ulcers	Nausea, dizziness, headache	Diarrhea, sexual impairment	Confusion in patients with kidney or liver dysfunction	Hyper-sensitivity, pregnancy, breast-feeding
Famotidine (Pepcid)	GERD, ulcers	Nausea, dizziness, headache	Diarrhea, sexual impairment	Confusion in patients with kidney or liver dysfunction	Hyper-sensitivity, pregnancy, breast-feeding
Nizatidine (Axid AR)	GERD, ulcers	Nausea, dizziness, headache	Diarrhea, sexual impairment	Confusion in patients with kidney or liver dysfunction	Hyper-sensitivity, pregnancy, breast-feeding

Drug	Use	Common, Benign Side Effects	Serious Side Effects	Life-threatening Side Effects	Reasons Not to Take
Aluminum Salts of Sulfated Sucrose					
Sucralfate (Carafate)	Ulcer prevention	Constipation	Dizziness, stomach pain, vomiting	None	Allergic reaction
Irritable Bowel Syndrome Medications					
High Risk					
Alosetron (Lotronex)	IBS	Headache, stomach pain	Diarrhea	Severe constipation, ischemic colitis	History of bowel obstruction
Cilansetron (Calmactin)	IBS	Headache, stomach pain	Diarrhea	Severe constipation, ischemic colitis	History of bowel obstruction
Tegaserod (Zelnorm)	IBS	Headache, stomach pain	Diarrhea	Ischemic colitis, gall-bladder infection (0.1%)	History of bowel obstruction, gallbladder disease, abdominal adhesions
Proton Pump Inhibitors (PPIs)					
Low Risk					
Lansoprazole (Prevacid)	GERD	Headache, diarrhea, nausea	Stomach pain, fevers, sore throat	Dizziness, blurred vision (rare)	Hyper-sensitivity, pregnancy, breast-feeding
Pantoprazole (Protonix)	GERD	Headache, diarrhea, nausea	Stomach pain, fevers, sore throat	Dizziness, blurred vision (rare)	Hyper-sensitivity, pregnancy, breast-feeding

Drug	Use	Common, Benign Side Effects	Serious Side Effects	Life-threatening Side Effects	Reasons Not to Take
Rabeprazole (Aciphex)	GERD	Headache, diarrhea, nausea	Stomach pain, fevers, sore throat	Dizziness, blurred vision (rare)	Hyper-sensitivity, pregnancy, breast-feeding
Esomeprazole (Nexium)	GERD	Headache, diarrhea, nausea	Stomach pain, fevers, sore throat	Dizziness, blurred vision (rare)	Hyper-sensitivity, pregnancy, breast-feeding
Omeprazole (Prilosec)	GERD	Headache, diarrhea, nausea	Stomach pain, fevers, sore throat	Dizziness, blurred vision (rare)	Hyper-sensitivity, pregnancy, breast-feeding

10.

Antibiotics and Vaccines

Many years ago, when I was a medical student at Duke University School of Medicine in Durham, NC, one of the most popular work rotations was serving as a member of Team Doc, the group of interns and fledgling doctors who took care of the basketball team. If you are from the Carolinas, the most important thing in your life besides putting food on your table is Atlantic Coast Conference (ACC, pronounced *I-say-say*) basketball, so the chance to work with the Blue Devils close up was a dream assignment for some of us. Back then our job was to keep the team in tip-top shape. The majority of the time that meant consulting with one of the players when he had a cold. Every Blue Devil who walked into Team Doc's office with a cold walked out with a prescription, often for an antibiotic that would have no effect on his viral illness. But the little piece of paper gave the impression that Team Doc was taking their complaints seriously. The truth is, as I explain in this chapter, they would have been better off getting into bed for a day or two and eating a big bowl of chicken soup.

The Double-Edged Sword
of Antibiotics

The discovery and development of antibiotics over the last century have led to a dramatic reduction in deaths from infection. They are truly miracle drugs. Penicillin has practically eliminated deaths from infectious diseases. Before 1942, if you got cut deeply, you were pretty much a goner. The *Staphylococcus areus* bacteria that normally live peacefully on the surface of your skin would get into your blood supply, penetrate your bones, set up shop, and start replicating themselves until you were dead. In the Civil War, doctors routinely hacked off the limbs of anyone with a deep-cut injury, and pneumonia was often fatal. Tens of thousands of people died every year from rheumatic heart disease, which was caused by a *Streptococcus* childhood infection. *Gonorrhea* and *syphilis* infections were rampant. All of these problems were eliminated with the discovery of penicillin.

However, not all infections are created equal; they can be caused either by bacteria *or* by viruses. Bacteria and viruses differ in that viruses need a host to replicate (i.e., the cells of your body), whereas bacteria can live independently. Antibiotics work only against bacteria; they are useless against viruses. Viruses cause the common cold, most sore throats, the flu, and many gastrointestinal infections. In spite of this, physicians routinely prescribe antibiotics for the treatment of colds, sore throats, and stomach pain. Because these conditions are typically caused by viruses, antibiotics are useless, and these physicians are actually causing harm by increasing the number of antibiotic-resistant bacteria, with the individual patient deriving absolutely no benefit. In fact, most viral illnesses are little more than an inconvenience that can be treated effectively with bed rest and time. Treatment with an antibiotic has no effect in terms of alleviating the symptoms of these illnesses, yet half of all antibiotics are prescribed for viral illnesses or other disorders on which they have no effect.

Remember too that while some bacteria are harmful and even fatal, hundreds of other types inhabit our bodies for our entire lives and actually are vital to our health. For instance, the bacteria that inhabit the colon and intestines aid in digestion by providing useful substances that assist absorption of food and vitamins, including folate and the B vitamins. Taking too many antibiotics inhibits our natural flora and in the process can lead to malnourishment and vitamin deficiency. These same bacteria also neutralize the bile salts and liver toxins dumped into our intestines and colon. Repeated treatment with antibiotics decreases these helpful bacteria and can lead to digestive and other health problems.

Over the past half century there has been a dramatic increase in the U.S. in the production of antibiotics, from 2 million pounds per year in 1954 to more than 50 million pounds per year in 2006, most of which are being given to farm animals. With the shift in the U.S. of agriculture from pasture grazing of animals to feed lots there has been a need to provide massive amounts of antibiotics to farm animals to prevent epidemics of disease. Another advantage of giving antibiotics to farm animals is that they promote growth. Although no one knows exactly why antibiotics do so, some theorize that they eliminate the bacteria that consume nutrients in the gut, thereby enabling the host (i.e., the farm animals) to take up more nutrients.

There is no reason to believe that these effects are not transferable to humans. Indeed, our massive exposure to antibiotics in the meat that we eat and in the runoff from farms into our drinking water, in addition to the antibiotics we are given for a variety of disorders (which may or may not be responsive to antibiotics) may have contributed to the current epidemic of obesity. Data presented at a conference of the Emory Predictive Health Institute showed that depletion of helpful colonic bacteria by antibiotics caused changes in concentrations of hormones that directly influence appetite, like leptin. These studies suggest that massive overuse of antibiotics may be contributing directly to the obesity epidemic that we are wrestling with today.

The Coming Superbugs

Over the last fifty years an increasing number of bacteria have become resistant to older antibiotics. Bacteria multiply very rapidly, so when large numbers of bacteria are exposed to an antibiotic, the possibility of their changing ever so slightly and becoming resistant to that antibiotic is increased. Naturally the antibiotic-sensitive bacteria die out, while the antibiotic-resistant bacteria flourish. For example, the methicillin-resistant bacteria *Staphylococcus areus* developed a strong outer wall that prevented penicillin from penetrating and exerting its effects. These bacteria flourished while the penicillin-sensitive bacteria died out.

Ironically, the development of drug-resistant bacteria favors pharmaceutical companies, because the rise of new strains of resistant bacteria, like methicillin-resistant *Staphylococcus aureus* (staph infection), often coincides with old drugs going off patent. In the past twenty years, there has been more than a thirteenfold increase in the number of bacteria resistant to methicillin. These events have required the development of newer, more expensive antibiotics that companies can accurately argue are more effective than the old drugs.

You can be sure that resistance to new antibiotics will also occur, and that in response drug companies will develop newer, stronger versions of antibiotics with even greater risks to patients because of their greater power. Better antibiotics weed out the weak bacteria. Because of "survival of the fittest," the bacteria that are left on the playing field at the end of the day are even more resistant to the antibiotics we currently have. One antibiotic-resistant superbug often emerges and multiplies.

One hundred thousand people die in hospitals every year from bacterial infections that are largely related to drug-resistant bacteria that have evolved from careless use of high-powered antibiotics to treat non–life-threatening infections or their misuse. Many scientists and infectious-disease specialists predict that we may get to the point where we can't find any new medications that will treat these new forms of bacteria. For instance, new strains of the bacterium *methicillin-resistant Staphylococcus aureus* or MRSA (which is highly resistant to antibiotics) are becoming more common. What was previously a simple cut on the finger can now grow into something that could kill you in a few days. The number of MRSA cases is growing exponentially.

Another particularly negative outcome of antibiotic overuse is the development of *Clostridium difficile,* which occurs when the normal bacteria of the colon are wiped out. *Clostridium difficile* usually attacks hospital patients who have been on multiple antibiotics that have wiped out their normal colonic bacteria. Clindamycin was the antibiotic most commonly associated with *Clostridium difficile* in the 1970s, on the basis of the facts that it was more commonly used in hospitals in debilitated patients and that it had a greater capacity than other antibiotics to wipe out normal bacterial flora. Now, for similar reasons, the second- and third-generation antibiotics, including cefuroxime, cefotaxime, ceftazidime, and ceftriaxone, are more commonly associated with *Clostridium difficile.* Other antibiotics that commonly cause this infection are ampicillin and amoxicillin. An especially drug-resistant bacterium, it is responsible for 3 million cases of diarrhea and inflammation of the colon and 5,000 to 20,000 deaths each year. The newer strains of this bacteria are becoming more toxic and more deadly, and are now resistant to antibiotics like the fluoroquinolones, to which they were previously susceptible.

Ear Infections

Many parents of young children have experienced firsthand the frustrating ineffectiveness of antibiotics and the growing power of infections when trying to address the ubiquitous childhood ear infection. Ear infections occur when bacteria or viruses get into the small air pocket behind the eardrum (middle ear) and cause an infection, which leads to a buildup of pus accompanied by pain, fever, and possibly drainage of pus from the ear.

There is a small tube called the Eustachian tube that connects the middle ear to the throat and that lets air move in and out of the middle ear. In children less than three the Eustachian tube is very small and less able to keep bacteria out. That is why small children are particularly susceptible to ear infections.

When my fourteen-year-old daughter was still in her single digits, she repeatedly got ear infections that caused enough pain to make her cry. (Who could blame her?) Being responsible parents, we would take her to the pediatrician, who would dutifully write a prescription for an antibiotic like amoxicillin. After treatment, her symptoms would go away, and she'd feel fine for a few weeks. Then, the pain and infection would come back, and the whole cycle would begin again. The repeated doctor visits and treatments were expensive, time-consuming, and inconvenient. The antibiotics also killed the normal bacteria in her ear, and selected for survival the worst bacteria, which were even harder to treat the next time. We repeated this useless cycle for several years, but my daughter actually just grew out of getting ear infections.

For years doctors in Holland have been using the "wait-and-see" approach with much success. It turns out that antibiotics have minimal impact on ear infections and that, unless a child is toxic (very visibly ill and unresponsive), simple ear infections are best treated with ibuprofen, a local painkiller for the ear, and otherwise left alone. If the child does not show improvement after three days, then it is time to go to the doctor. In years of treating children this way there have been no adverse outcomes.[1,2] I wish the doctor had followed the wait-and-see approach when my daughter was a child.

Children treated with antibiotics for ear infections have a threefold increase in reinfection. This is related to the fact that normal bacteria in the ear are killed off by antibiotics, thereby creating an environment in which pathogenic bacteria can grab a foothold. In spite of the fact that guidelines state not to treat some types of ear infections with antibiotics, many doctors do so anyway. The type of ear infection that causes fluid discharge from the ear, without evidence of acute infection (bulging eardrum, extreme pain, high fever), is often treated with antibiotics, although it increases the risk of reinfection.

What is the worst thing that could happen if your child got an ear infection? Well, the infection could possibly spread to his or her brain, causing meningitis (which can be fatal or cause brain damage). It could cause hearing loss or infection of the mastoid sinus. However, none of these outcomes have occurred in cases where treatment was delayed for no more than three days. In other words, if you adopt the wait-and-see approach and wait until three days are up (assuming that your child does not look like he or she is about to die or does not in other respects look really sick, (i.e., have an extremely high fever or repetitive vomiting), you will be fine. Just administer pain medications like Tylenol or, if you have them, local medications to reduce ear pain.

Research studies bear out the advantages of the wait-and-see approach. One study of 240 children ages six months to two years showed that treatment with amoxicillin compared to placebo reduced duration of fever from three to two days and symptoms at day four by 13%, with no difference in pain on ear examination. The authors concluded that "this modest effect does not justify prescription of antibiotics at the first visit, provided close surveillance can be guaranteed."[3]

Another study of 315 children ages six months to ten years showed that unless there was high fever, more than 37.5°C (99.5°F), or vomiting, the antibiotics had no effect on pain. And they did not help the children sleep through the night, even three days after the start of the treatment.[4] A meta-analysis of all studies showed that 60% of children treated with a placebo had no pain after twenty-four hours. Early use of antibiotics reduced pain by 41% compared to placebo at two to seven days. Antibiotics doubled the risk of vomiting, diarrhea, or rash. Based on these studies I recommend waiting two days before treatment unless the child has a high fever, is vomiting, or is in a lot of pain.

The Antibiotics

Given the facts on how antibiotics are changing the way we get sick and recover, how do you decide that an antibiotic is right for you? Next time you come down with a cold or flu, instead of demanding a prescription for an antibiotic, ask your doctor whether he or she thinks your viral condition really requires an antibiotic. In the overwhelming majority of cases, if you have the flu, cough, sniffles, or sore throat, you should not go to the doctor. Overuse of antibiotics can decrease the natural bacterial flora in your intestine and colon, and cause malabsorption of food and vitamins, and even worse problems. If you do have a potentially life-threatening infection, you will have to follow your doctor's prescriptions, but these are in fact rare and certainly don't account for more than 10% of infectious diseases. Opening this dialogue will go a long way toward reducing the use of nonessential prescriptions for antibiotics.

It is also helpful to understand the antibiotics—and there are a lot of them—and what they do, including their side effects. Many antibiotics are now so powerful that caution must be used when taking them. In this section I review all the major classes of antibiotics, so buckle up and be prepared for a lot of crazy-sounding names. It's important to know what's out there, however, so that you and your doctor can make the best decision regarding your treatment, because chances are good that sometime in the next twelve months he or she will be tempted to write you a scrip for one of these drugs.

In general, if you do have an infectious disease that requires antibiotic treatment, you should opt for a first-generation antibiotic, because the later-generation medications, like Cipro, can have major side effects, like destruction of cartilage and other effects, which can be easily avoided by using the less-expensive and less-toxic alternatives in the early-generation classes of antibiotics.

PENICILLIN

The first antibiotic, penicillin, was discovered entirely by accident when some mold got into a lab dish of bacteria and someone noticed that it inhibited the growth of the bacteria. Later it was found that penicillin destroys the walls of bacteria by inactivating an enzyme called transpeptidase that is vital to the cross-linking of bacterial cell walls.

The Gram staining method, named after the Danish bacteriologist who originally devised it in 1882, Hans Christian Gram, is one of the most important staining techniques in microbiology. It is almost always the first test used to identify bacteria. The primary color stain of Gram's method is crystal violet. The microorganisms that retain the crystal violet–iodine complex appear purple-brown under microscopic examination (gram-positive). Those that are not stained by crystal violet are referred to as gram-negative and appear red. Gram-negative and gram-positive bacteria have important differences in terms of their susceptibility to antibiotics and their virulence.

Originally penicillin was very effective against gram-positive bacteria like *Staphylococcus* (i.e., staph infection) and *Streptococcus* (i.e., strep throat), which require oxygen to survive (aerobic bacteria). These are the culprits that cause throat infections, pneumonia, and skin infections as well as sexually transmitted diseases like *Gonoccocus,* which causes gonorrhea. Gram-negative bacteria do not require oxygen to survive (anaerobic bacteria) and are not as sensitive to penicillin.

Penicillin is still useful against many strep and staph infections that cause sore throat, skin infections, and some sexually transmitted diseases like gonorrhea. The most common *Streptococcus* infection is strep throat. In spite of the fact that only 10% of those complaining of a sore throat who visit a doctor actually have a *Streptococcus* infection, 75% walk out the door with a prescription for an antibiotic.

As penicillin became so widely used for gram-positive infections, penicillin-resistant bacteria developed, including some that could break down the beta-lactam chemical structure of penicillin by producing an enzyme called beta lactamase. For instance, some strains of *Staphylococcus aureus* developed an enzyme called *penicillinase* that breaks down the chemical structure of penicillin. Naturally, these bacteria were better able to survive and have gone on to out-compete their more penicillin-sensitive colleagues.

The development of bacteria that could defeat penicillin with the penicillinase enzyme led to the development of the penicillinase-resistant penicillins, which are effective against *Staphylococcus* bacteria that produce the penicillinase enzyme but not against the gram-negative bacteria that produce this enzyme. Drugs in this group that can be given orally include cloxacillin (Tegopen) and dicloxacillin (Dycill). Methicillin (Staphcillin) can be given intravenously.

AMINOPENICILLINS

Other drugs in the penicillin class that also inhibit the formation of the cell wall of bacteria but have a broader spectrum of action, known as aminopenicillins, have a chemical structure slightly different from that of penicillin, which makes them more effective against gram-negative bacteria. These drugs, including amoxicillin (Amoxil), ampicillin (Omnipen), and bicampicillin (Spectrobid), are useful for treating ear infections, lung infections, pneumonia, skin infections, and throat infections. They are, however, susceptible to the penicillinase-producing bacteria.

EXTENDED-SPECTRUM PENICILLINS

The extended-spectrum penicillins (antipseudomonal penicillins), including carbenicillin (Geopen), mezlocillin (Mezlin), piperacillin (Zosyn), and ticarcillin (Ticar), have an even broader spectrum than the aminopenicillins. They are, however, also susceptible to the penicillinase-producing bacteria.

Several penicillinlike drugs that interfere with the bacteria's ability to produce a beta-lactamase enzyme have been developed. These drugs, which include clavulanic acid, tazobactam, and sulbactam, bind to the active site of the beta-lactamase enzyme. They are typically given with a beta-lactam antibiotic like penicillin or amoxicillin to enable the penicillin drug to reach its site of action without being attacked. Some drug combinations include Unasyn (ampicillin + sulbactam), Augmentin (amoxicillin + clavulanic acid), Timentin (ticarcillin + clavulanic acid), and Zosyn (piperacillin + tazobactam).

Penicillin (like all antibiotics) can cause diarrhea, as it interferes with the normal bacteria in the intestines. In some cases this upset can progress to pseudomembranous colitis, a potentially dangerous intestinal condition. Eating active-culture yogurt while taking antibiotics can help prevent this condition.

About 5% to 10% of the population is allergic to penicillin. Allergic reactions can involve itching, swelling, breathing difficulties, and even death. Delayed reactions include joint pain, rash, or fever, which can occur several days later. If you know you have a penicillin allergy, you should not take these medications. Penicillin can also cause nausea, vomiting, and diarrhea that are related to the loss of the normal flora of the gastrointestinal tract. However, compared to the newer generations of antibiotics, penicillin is quite safe.

CEPHALOSPORINS

A group of drugs closely related to penicillin, called cephalosporins, also interfere with the structure of the bacterial cell wall. These drugs, which include cefazolin (Kefzol), cefadroxil (Duricef), cephalexin (Keflex), cephradine (Velosef), and cephapirin (Cefadyl), are used in the treatment of penicillin-resistant bacteria. In spite of the fact that they are not the first-line treatment for infections and the fact that penicillin is a less-expensive and equally effective antibiotic, they are often prescribed. Side effects include stomach cramps and pain, diarrhea, fever, skin reactions, joint pain, and nausea. Skin rashes are rather common. Some patients develop pseudomembranous colitis. The drug should be stopped immediately if there is bloody bowel movement or stomach pain. Some people develop headache, dizziness, or weakness. You can also develop damage to your kidneys.

The second-generation cephalosporins, which include cefamandole (Mandol), cefoxitin (Mefoxin), cefonicid (Monocid), cefotetan (Cefotan), and cefmetazole (Zefazone), are less sensitive to bacteria that produce the beta-lactamase enzyme and are more effective against gram-negative bacteria. Cefotetan and cefmetazole can cause bleeding reactions. If you drink alcohol while taking cefotetan or cefmetazole you may experience flushing, shortness of breath, nausea, vomiting, chest pain, and possibly unconsciousness—so don't drink and take antibiotics!

Third-generation cephalosporins include cefixime (Suprax), cefpodoxime (Vantin), ceftibuten (Cedax), cefoperazone (Cefobid), cefotaxime (Claroran), ceftizoxime (Cefizox), ceftriaxone (Rocephin), and ceftazidime (Fortaz). These medications have side effects and mechanisms of action similar to those of earlier generations of cephalosporins and differ only in being less sensitive to beta-lactamase–producing bacteria.

Cefepime (Maxipime), the only fourth-generation cephalosporin, is effective against both gram-positive and gram-negative bacteria and is resistant to beta-lactamase–producing bacteria.

TETRACYCLINES

The tetracycline drugs, including tetracycline (Achromycin), doxycycline (Vibra tabs), demeclocycline (Declomycin), and minocycline (Minocin), work by inhibiting protein synthesis. Developed from a common mold, they share a four-ring chemical structure. The tetracyclines are used to treat rickettsia and *Chlamydia* infections as well as *Streptococcus.* They also can be used for tick fever and acne. Other infections like walking pneumonia, urinary tract inflammation, and prostate infections are also treatable with tetracyclines. Because of the development of multiple tetracycline-resistant bacteria, however, their effectiveness is limited. Common side effects are nausea, vomiting, diarrhea, and abdominal pain. These drugs can worsen kidney damage in patients with kidney dysfunction. They can also cause liver damage and sun sensitivity. These side effects, however, are not common, and in general these drugs are safer than drugs like clindamycin and streptomycin.

AMINOGLYCOSIDES

Aminoglycosides are useful against both gram-positive and gram-negative bacteria, and are used mainly to treat severe urinary tract infections. When combined with cephalosporins they constitute the first-line treatment of severe, life-threatening infections caused by gram-negative bacteria. Given simultaneously with penicillinase-resistant semisynthetic penicillins or with vancomycin they act synergistically against staph infection (*Staphylococci*) but can be used initially only for a few days because they can cause lasting damage to your hearing or kidneys. They are also combined with penicillin G or ampicillin in the treatment of endocarditis.

Aminoglycosides interfere with the ability of bacteria to produce proteins by blocking the transcription of ribonucleic acid (RNA). If they can't produce proteins, the bacteria can't replicate. Drugs in the aminoglycoside group include gentamycin (Garamycin), tobramycin (Nebcin), kanamycin (Kantrex), amikacin (Amikin), paromomycin (Humatin), and streptomycin.

Gentamycin binds to the ribosomes that are responsible for reading the RNA and producing protein. Because gentamycin and related drugs are concentrated in the ear and in the kidneys, they can be very toxic to the kidneys and cause hearing loss. Gentamycin can cause vestibular problems (problems with balance or visual symptoms) in up to 3% of patients. Gentamycin can also cause confusion and neurological symptoms. For these reasons it should be used as a last resort, usually for life-threatening gram-negative infections. Gentamycin and related drugs should not be used by pregnant women.

LINCOSAMIDES

The lincosamide antibiotics, including clindamycin (Cleocin) and linco-mycin (Lincocin), bind to bacterial ribosomes and inhibit bacterial repro-duction. They are effective for both gram-positive and gram-negative infections, but they are very toxic and therefore should be used only for life-threatening infections, like bone or abdominal infections that don't respond to other antibiotics. The most common side effects are nausea and vomiting. They can have serious adverse effects, including inflammation of the intestines, cramps, and severe diarrhea, sometimes bloody. Rash and suppression of platelet and blood counts as well as allergic reactions can also occur. They should not be used by patients with liver dysfunction. Clindamycin can also cause pseudomembranous colitis, which is associated with diarrhea and stomach pain, and is caused by *Clostridium difficile*.

MACROLIDES

The macrolide antibiotics are another group of antibiotics that inhibit the elongation of the protein chain as it is being transcribed from RNA, thereby inhibiting the reproduction of certain strains of bacteria. Medications in this class, which include erythromycin (Erythrocin), azithromycin (Zithro-max), troleandomycin (Tao), dirithromycin (Dynabac), and chlarithromy-cin (Biaxin), are used for treatment of respiratory tract and skin infections. Side effects include allergic reactions to the medication as well as nausea, vomiting, diarrhea, and stomach pain. These drugs should be used with caution by pregnant women and patients with liver disease.

KETALIDES

The ketalide antibiotics have a mechanism of action similar to that of mac-rolides involving inhibition of bacterial protein synthesis. They are used for the treatment of pneumonia, bronchitis, and sinusitis. Five million prescriptions have been written for Ketek (telithromycin). Most common side effects are gastrointestinal: diarrhea, nausea, abdominal pain, and vomiting. Headache and disturbances in taste also occur. Less common side effects include palpitations, blurred vision, and rashes. According to a review of the FDA's Adverse Event Reporting System, by the staff of the Senate Finance Committee, between July 2005 and September 2005 alone, there were two deaths, thirty-five adverse liver reactions, forty-four cardiac events, and eighty visual events in Ketek patients. Sixty-one cases of abnormal vision were reported to the WHO. In the United States, the FDA's Office of Epidemiology and Surveillance identified twelve cases of acute liver failure, resulting in four deaths, and an additional twenty-three cases of acute, serious liver injury in patients taking telithromycin up to April 2006. Since other antibiotics can be used instead of Ketek, I do not recommend its use.

CHLORAMPHENICOL

Chloramphenicol (Chloromycetin), which inhibits protein synthesis in bacteria, has a mechanism of action and side-effect profile that set it apart from other classes of antibiotics. It can also inhibit protein synthesis in bacterial and human mitochondria (the powerhouse of the cell). This is why chloramphenicol can suppress blood-cell formation and, potentially, cause death; therefore it should be used as a last resort. Although rare, some patients have died from chloramphenicol-induced bone suppression, which can occur sometimes after the drug is stopped. This drug should not be used by pregnant women or by patients with kidney or liver disease or with a history of bone marrow suppression. Because of its toxicity, chloramphenicol should not be used for anything other than the treatment of serious infections. More common side effects include headache, nausea, vomiting, and diarrhea. Because of the risk of bone-marrow suppression, chloramphenicol should not be used unless there is a very good reason to do so.

QUINOLONES

First introduced in the 1980s, the quinolone antibiotics, which include drugs like Cipro, inhibit DNA gyrase, an enzyme needed for bacterial DNA replication and therefore bacterial-cell replication. Quinolones are used for lower-respiratory-tract infections, especially in the treatment of infections caused by methicillin-sensitive or -resistant staphylococci, *Pseudomonas,* and intracellular organisms.

The first generation of quinolones, which include nalidixic acid (Neg-Gram) and cinoxacin (Cinobac), are used for uncomplicated urinary tract infections. Not surprisingly, the second generation of these drugs has a mechanism of action similar to that of the first. This group includes norfloxacin (Noroxin), lomefloxacin (Maxaquin), enoxacin (Penetrex), ofloxacin (Floxin), and its best-known member, ciprofloxacin (Cipro), which achieved fame as a prophylactic for anthrax during the terrorist-based mailing of letters laced with the deadly bacteria anthrax. These drugs are also used for kidney infections, sexually transmitted disease, prostate infections, and skin infections. These drugs can cause headache, abdominal pain, vomiting, and nausea and may cause serious sun-sensitivity reactions. Ofloxacin causes insomnia in 13% of patients.

The third-generation quinolone drugs, which include levofloxacin (Levaquin), sparfloxacin (Zagam), gatifloxicin (Tequin), and moxifloxacin (Avelox), are used for bronchitis and pneumonia. Levofloxacin causes headache and nausea in 7% of patients and rarely may cause seizures. Sparfloxacin is associated with phototoxicity (sensitivity to sunlight) in 8% of patients. Moxifloxacin has been associated with exacerbation of liver impairment. Sparfloxacin, moxifloxacin, and gatifloxicin can interact with cardiac drugs, typical antipsychotics, or tricyclic antidepressants to impair the rhythm of the heart.

The fourth-generation quinolone drugs, which are used for the same purposes as the earlier generations as well as for abdominal and pelvic infections, include trovafloxacin (Trovan) and alatrofloxacin (Trovan IV).

Trovafloxacin, which was associated with fourteen known cases of liver failure, has prompted the FDA to recommend limiting its use to life-threatening situations and for no more than fourteen days.

Quinolones, the most commonly used antibiotics today, are widely overprescribed for problems like urinary tract infection, in spite of the fact that they cost more than ten times as much as drugs like Septra and are not more effective. A recent study showed that 81% of patients for whom fluoroquinolones had been prescribed had not been prescribed these drugs appropriately.

The quinolones are potentially very toxic. For example, among women with a new-onset bladder infection, only 37% were given the preferred treatment, which is Septra, whereas 32% were given Cipro. In addition, most women were treated for a week or more, while the preferred treatment is only three days. Cipro is the medication associated with the most complaints on the Web site www.askthepatient.com, where patients log on with their reactions to different medications.

Most of these drugs have interactions with warfarin (Coumadin), a medication used to decrease blood clotting. They also require dosage adjustment in patients with kidney disease. Animal studies show that quinolones can have effects on cartilage in young animals; these drugs are therefore not recommended for children. Fluoroquinolones also have been associated with the development of joint pain, cartilage damage, and even tendon rupture.

SULFONAMIDES

The sulfonamide (sulfa) drugs, which are used to treat urinary tract infections, include sulfamethoxazole/trimethoprim (Septra, Bactrim), sulfisoxazole (Novosoxazole), and sulfasalazine (Azulfidine). Sulfamethoxazole/trimethoprim acts by inhibiting the synthesis of folate, which is required for DNA replication by the bacteria. This drug is generally well tolerated but can cause nausea, vomiting, and diarrhea. Allergic reactions and rash can also occur. More serious but unusual are suppression of bone marrow, or anemia in people deficient in folate, including the elderly, alcoholics, and people with malnutrition or malabsorption. Rare side effects include Stevens-Johnson syndrome, which involves a total body rash and peeling that could be fatal, and crystal formation in the urine, which can lead to kidney damage. Sulfisoxazole has an action similar to that of sulfamethoxazole/trimethoprim as well as similar side effects.

NITROFURANTOINS

Like the sulfonamides, nitrofurantoins (Macrodantin, Macrobid, Furadantin), which inhibit bacteria locally in the urinary tract by an as-yet-unknown mechanism of action, are also used for urinary infections. Common side effects are anorexia, nausea, and vomiting. It can also induce asthma attacks, cause abdominal pain, and suppress blood-cell levels. It can cause severe side effects, especially in the elderly, including peripheral neuropathy and lung scarring. It can also cause birth defects when given to pregnant women.

VANCOMYCIN

Vancomycin, which inhibits bacterial cell-wall formation as well as synthesis of bacterial ribonucleic acid (RNA), is effective against methicillin-resistant staph areus (MRSA). Vancomycin can cause deafness and kidney damage and therefore should be used with caution. (The exact number of patients affected by these side effects is not known.) It can also cause potentially fatal anaphylactic reactions. For these reasons vancomycin should be taken as a last resort.

Antiviral Agents

THE FLU SHOT

Viruses infect human cells by being absorbed into these cells, having their RNA and proteins replicate, and then bursting out of the cells. The most common viral diseases are herpes simplex, herpes zoster (shingles), *Cytomegalovirus,* human papillomavirus (HPV), respiratory syncytial virus (colds), and influenza (flu).

The belief that vaccinations, like flu shots, have eliminated death from infectious disease in the twentieth century is widespread. In fact, much of the reduction in death from infectious disease is due to public-health measures, including improved nutrition and sanitation. And vaccinations are not without potential danger. We still don't know the potential long-term effects of vaccination.

An oft-repeated fact is that 36,000 people die each year from the flu. The government urges citizens to get vaccinated, presumably to prevent these deaths. As a result, every year children under age seven, everyone over sixty-five, all health-care workers, and patients with chronic obstructive pulmonary disease (COPD) and asthma specifically are urged to get the influenza vaccine. *And yet there is no evidence that the flu vaccine does anything at all.* There are no controlled trials that show that a flu shot prevents deaths in children or the elderly. The only positive studies are of patients with COPD, probably because COPD patients have marginal lung function and preventing any flu infections will have a greater impact.

Dr. Tom Jefferson, an epidemiologist working for the Cochrane Collaboration in Rome, Italy, a nonprofit organization that conducts analyses of published clinical trials, led a group that performed a comprehensive review of the published data on flu vaccines. He concluded,[5] "The optimistic and confident tone of some predictions of viral circulation and of the impact of inactivated vaccines, which are at odds with the evidence, is striking. The reasons are probably complex and may involve a 'messy blend of truth conflicts and conflicts of interest making it difficult to separate factual disputes from value disputes' or a manifestation of optimism bias (an unwarranted belief in the efficacy of interventions." In other words, the overuse of the flu vaccine is related to: (1) overzealous policy makers with good intentions but a lack of knowledge of the evidence; (2) the attitude that "it can't hurt"; and (3) the influence of the profit motive in selling millions of flu vaccines.

Most cases of the so-called flu are actually "influenzalike diseases," that is, infections caused by viruses other than the flu that are not prevented by the flu vaccine. In addition, the influenza vaccine does not prevent the most virulent forms of influenza, the ones that can actually cause death. At most there are less than 2,000 cases of influenza-related deaths per year; the remainder are cases of pneumonia that were "associated" with the flu or a flulike illness (in other words, they died from pneumonia but happened to have a flulike illness that probably wouldn't have been prevented by the vaccine) or, less likely, the "true" flu.

If we assume that there are 2,000 flu-related deaths per year and that all of these occur among the elderly, and we follow the guidelines by immunizing everyone over age sixty-five, 0.00004% of those immunized would be saved from an influenza-related death. And even that estimate is optimistic because a substantial number of the elderly who die from influenza are immunocompromised and won't benefit from a flu vaccine anyway.

Pending legislation in the form of the Flu Protection Act will revamp U.S. flu-vaccine policy by requiring the CDC to pay makers for vaccines unsold "through routine market mechanisms." The bill will also require the CDC to conduct a "public awareness campaign" emphasizing "the safety and benefit of recommended vaccines for the public good."

And let me remind you that flu vaccinations are not innocuous. There is conjecture that the mercury and aluminum (metals that are known to have neurotoxic effects) in vaccine shots are associated with long-term adverse consequences. These vaccines can also overstimulate the immune system in ways that are not fully understood. For that reason, I recommend that *only* people with COPD get flu shots.

OSELTAMIVIR AND ZELE

In the past few years there has been mounting concern over bird flu. Are we all about to succumb to a global bird flu pandemic? Not likely. Bird flu is transmitted from birds to birds, not birds to people. Only in extremely rare instances have humans become infected with the bird flu, and there is no reason to believe that that will change.

Should we take drugs to prevent getting the bird flu? No. If bird flu does change and become infectious to humans, the current treatments probably won't work, because the virus will have mutated and changed by that time. At last check there were no cases of bird flu in the U.S. or Europe.

Oseltamivir (Tamiflu) and Zele (Zanamivir) are used in the treatment of the influenza virus and are promoted as potentially useful agents for the prevention of bird flu. Tamiflu is taken as a pill twice a day for five days; Zanamivir is inhaled through a device, called a diskhaler, that delivers the medicine to the lungs. These medications are neuraminidase inhibitors that prevent replication of influenza A and B viruses by interfering with the production and release of the virus from cells that line the respiratory tract. To be useful, they both need to be taken within 48 hours of the onset of flu symptoms.

Tamiflu has been approved for treatment of the flu in children over the age of one and for prevention of the flu in patients over age thirteen. Side effects of both medications include swelling of the sinuses, diarrhea, nausea, and vomiting. Patients with asthma or COPD may experience breathing problems. In November 2006 the FDA approved a labeling supplement precaution about neuropsychiatric events based on postmarketing reports (mostly in children from Japan) of self-injury and delirium with the use of Tamiflu in patients with influenza.

GARDASIL

The human papillomavirus (HPV), a virus that is spread by unprotected sexual intercourse, affects more than half of the world's population. HPV can cause genital warts and in rare cases cervical cancer. Of those who are infected, however, 95% are asymptomatic and never know they have HPV. Although almost all cases of cervical cancer are caused by HPV, HPV is ubiquitous and it is uncommon for HPV to progress to cervical cancer. Cervical cancer kills four thousand women per year, only one tenth the death rate of breast cancer, for example. That means that about 0.002% of women infected with HPV die each year from HPV-induced cervical cancer—not a very impressive number.

In 2006 support for the human papilloma virus (HPV) vaccine Gardasil led Texas to mandate vaccination for all young girls in the state, an action that was followed by similar proposals in a number of other states. But is the HPV vaccine safe and effective? Since the vaccine is new, its long-term consequences are unknown. The known side effects of Gardasil include pain and swelling at the site of injection. Fever occurs in about 1% of cases.

Although it may not be realistic to expect young people to practice safe sex, it is another way to prevent HPV until the vaccine can be investigated further. It should be emphasized, however, that condoms don't always stop infection, since HPV can be spread by parts of the genitals that are not covered by the latex.

ACYCLOVIR

Herpes simplex includes HSV-1 and HSV-2. HSV-1 involves herpes labialis, or cold sores on the lips. HSV-2 can cause both herpes labialis and herpes genitalis, or genital herpes. Genital herpes is more of a concern because it can be spread by sexual contact and is potentially transmittable at childbirth. Genital herpes resides in a dormant state in nerve endings and periodically reactivates, forming lesions that are infectious. When the virus is dormant it is not infectious. A tingling sensation signifies that the virus is about to be expressed; this sensation can be used to predict upcoming periods of infectivity.

Herpes simplex is treated with acyclovir (Zovirax). Other drugs with the *-cyclovir* ending are used for similar purposes. Acyclovir is phosphorylated (a phosphate group is added to the molecule) by the viral enzyme thymidine kinase and then incorporated into the DNA chain of the herpes virus, where it blocks DNA synthesis and therefore replication of the virus. Acyclovir is generally well tolerated but can cause headache, nausea, vomiting, or abdominal pain. More serious side effects include confusion and hallucinations, but these are rare. It also can rarely cause kidney damage.

Antifungals

Fungal infections include Tinea (ringworm), candidiasis, aspergillosis, cryptococcosis, blastomycosis, histoplasmosis, and coccidioidomycosis. Tinea (ringworm) is not actually a worm but a fungus that causes itching, redness, and a spreading circular patch. Different disorders all caused by tinea include athlete's foot, jock itch, ringworm of the scalp, ringworm of the body, and ringworm of the nails. *Candida* is usually present in the mouth, intestines, and vagina. Immunocompromise or overuse of antibiotics can cause an outbreak of *Candida*. Aspergillosis, cryptococcosis, and the other fungal infections occur in immunocompromised individuals, like patients with HIV, in whom they may be life threatening, and therefore are beyond the scope of this book.

Antifungals used to treat aspergillosis, blastomycosis, candidiasis, cryptococcosis, and histoplasmosis are polyene drugs, like amphotericin B, griseofulvin, and nystatin, which bind themselves to membrane sterols in fungal cell membranes, causing cell death. Side effects include anemia, low blood potassium and magnesium, diarrhea, nausea, vomiting, and head-ache. More than 80% of patients given amphotericin develop some level of kidney damage, which has led to the nickname "amphoterrible" among doctors.

AZOLE

The azole drugs ketoconazole (Nizoral), miconazole (Monistat), clotrima-zole (Mycelex, Lotrimin), and fluconazole (Diflucan) inhibit the develop-ment of the fungus membrane. Side effects include diarrhea, nausea, vomiting, and headache. These drugs can also cause liver damage, exfolia-tive skin reactions, kidney damage, and allergic reactions, but these effects are rare. Clotrimazole, which is commonly used for jock itch, ringworm, and athlete's foot, should not be used for diaper rash. In general it is less toxic than other antifungals since it is given topically and thus not highly absorbed into the bloodstream.

Antiprotozoans

Malaria, giardiasis, amoebiasis, trichomoniasis, and toxoplasmosis are protozoans, organisms that can cause infection in humans. Malaria is caused by the parasite *Plasmodium* and is spread by mosquitoes. *Plasmo-dium falciparum* infects red blood cells and is fatal in 1% of cases. Symp-toms include recurrent fever and an anemia that is associated with a drop in energy. If you are traveling abroad, you have to decide whether to use prophylactic medications to prevent malaria. With the increase in world-wide travel and the involvement of the U.S. armed forces overseas, there is a need to ensure that travelers not be exposed to infectious diseases like malaria that are not endemic in the U.S. It is also important, however, to consider the potential detrimental side effects of the medications used to prevent such diseases.

CHLOROQUINE

The first-line treatment for malaria was chloroquine (Aralen), a drug that suppresses malaria but does not prevent relapse. This drug can affect eye function, blood pressure, liver function, and gastrointestinal function. Possible side effects include nausea, vomiting, stomach upset, cramps, loss of appetite, diarrhea, tiredness, weakness, and headache. These effects are most severe in the first few days and usually clear as the body adjusts to the medication. More serious but more rare side effects include blurred vision, ringing in the ears, difficulty hearing, seizures, mood changes, bruising, and allergic reactions.

MEFLOQUINE

Mefloquine (Lariam), a drug commonly used for malaria prophylaxis, has a number of neurological side effects, including dizziness (96%), nausea (82%), and headache (73%). This drug has also been associated with an increase in psychiatric symptoms in 11% to 35% of patients.[6] Possible psychiatric symptoms include paranoia, depression, psychosis, anxiety, and fatigue, and a loss of vigor as well as impairment of motor control.

Rates of depression, anger, fatigue, and loss of vigor were higher with mefloquine than with other prophylactic malaria medications, like atovaquone plus chloroguanine. Mefloquine users have a number of other symptoms, including vertigo in 96%, nausea in 82%, and headache in 73%. In general, symptoms seem to be more prevalent in females. These studies show that caution should be employed before using mefloquine in future overseas travelers.

ATOVAQUONE AND CHLOROGUANINE

The antimalarial drugs atovaquone and chloroguanine were not associated with neuropsychiatric effects and were as effective as mefloquine for malarial prophylaxis. Dihydroartemisinin-piperaquine (Artekin) was shown to be as effective as artesunate-mefloquine in the treatment of malaria-infected children. Since alternative medications like atovaquone and chloroguanine are as effective as mefloquine for malarial prophylaxis and treatment, the latter drug should not be used, especially by patients with neuropsychiatric histories.

METRONIDAZOLE

Metronidazole (Flagyl) is used to treat serious protozoan infections, including giardiasis, trichomonlasis, and amoebiasis. Amoebiasis is caused by a protozoan parasite transmitted by fecally contaminated food or water. Symptoms include diarrhea, fatigue, and abdominal pain. Hikers or travelers who drink infected water can contract giardiasis, which causes diarrhea and malabsorption. Trichomoniasis is a vaginal infection that may cause a discharge but is usually asymptomatic. Toxoplasmosis, which comes from contact with the feces of cats and birds as well as other sources, may cause fever, headache, and sore throat. It works by inhibiting DNA synthesis of fungal organisms. Side effects include tingling, confusion, mood changes, nausea, vomiting, and problems with urination. Other possible side effects include liver dysfunction.

Lice Medications

Scabes is a small skin infection from a mite that usually comes from infected bedding. It can cause excoriated vesicles and pustules in the skin. *Pediculosis* is the medical term for lice, which can affect the head hair or the genital hair. It is transmitted through bedclothes, touch, and genital contact. Over-the-counter topical treatments (Nix, Rid), which use pyrethrin-based ingredients, are generally safe.

LINDANE

The most commonly used prescribed medication for these problems is lindane (Kwell). Doctors apparently have not yet figured out that it doesn't work and has generated some safety concerns. Over the past few decades the effectiveness of lindane has been decreasing because of the emergence of treatment-resistant lice. Lindane kills only 17% of lice after a three-hour period, and none after ten minutes, the recommended time of exposure. Lindane is less effective than prescription malathion and over-the-counter pyrethrin and permethrin. Lindane acts on lice by stimulating their central nervous system similar to DDT. Those with lesions on their head can develop central-nervous-system toxicity if they apply the lotion on the head. This is an obvious concern for the many children who are applying this lotion on top of their head for the elimination of head lice, which they may have to do twice. Side effects include dizziness, headache, tingling, and seizures. There have been three confirmed Lindane-related deaths. Lindane is contraindicated in children with uncontrolled seizure disorders and alcoholics. Only one application is recommended.

MALATHION

Malathion (Ovide) is an organophosphate that kills lice by inhibiting the cholinesterase enzyme. Malathion is the most highly effective pediculicide, killing 88% of lice in ten minutes and 100% in twenty minutes. Malathion also binds to sulfur in the hair shaft and kills lice eggs. Malathion is highly flammable, so children treated for lice should stay away from fires to keep their heads from catching on fire. Side effects are rare and include scalp irritation and eye inflammation (conjunctivitis). Malathion is not absorbed into the body in significant quantities. Although the product label instructs the user to leave it on for eight hours, this is overkill, and can eventually lead to lice resistance, so these recommendations should not be followed. It should not be used by women who are pregnant or breast-feeding.

Alternative Medicines and Recommendations

There are many people who believe that vitamins boost immunity and prevent infections. For many years, the famous scientist Linus Pauling promoted vitamin C in high doses for the prevention and treatment of the common cold; however no one has ever been able to show that prophylactic vitamin C prevents colds. At best, it might reduce the duration of the cold by one day. A 2004 review of placebo-controlled studies in which 200 mg or more of vitamin C was given as a preventative measure showed only a 4% reduction in colds when vitamin C was taken as a treatment before the cold had started. Duration was reduced by 8% in adults and 14% in children, a difference that was statistically significant. Treatment *after* the onset of the cold had no effect on cold duration or symptoms.

One study, however, that showed that prophylaxis reduced cold duration found that subjects who figured out what they were on reported significant reductions in cold duration and severity compared to those who didn't know what they were on. It turned out that subjects could taste the difference between vitamin C and placebo and correctly guess what they were on. When this was accounted for, there was no difference between vitamin C and placebo.[7] This raises questions about the validity of the meager results that purportedly show that prophylaxis reduces the length of a cold. In fact, this is an issue that applies to all studies of herbs and vitamins, since many herbs have a pungent aroma that was probably not adequately concealed in many clinical trials.

ALTERNATIVES AND THE ELDERLY

A review of trials of multivitamin and mineral supplements in the elderly addressed the question of whether vitamins and supplements prevent infections in this population. No reduction in infection rates was reported, though there was a reduction of about seventeen days per year spent with colds in three of the studies reviewed.[8] These three studies, however, were either authored by Ranjit Chandra, M.D. (one of them in *The Lancet*) or published in his journal by a mysterious "Dr. A. L. Jain." As reported by Chris O'Neill-Yates in *The National* (Jan. 30, 2006, "The Secret Life of Dr. Chandra"), there is speculation that the studies probably had never taken place and that "Dr Jain" was probably a fictitious person invented by Dr. Chandra in an attempt to "replicate" his results.

The authors of the review published a correction, excluding the three studies, and stating that ". . . the originally published beneficial difference of 17.5 days is now completely discounted . . . incidence rate ratio for the difference in infection rates [with] exclusion of the one questionable trial that was relevant to this outcome means that the pooled incidence rate is now 1.00 (0.85 to 1.17), not 0.89 (0.78 to 1.03) as published." In other words, whether you were on multivitamin or placebo, the rates of catching a cold were identical. They went on to conclude that if the allegations that these three studies were not reliable were true, then the remaining evidence base suggested no benefit for the use of multivitamins for preventing infections in elderly people. This conclusion was confirmed in 2005 by the Mineral and Vitamin Intervention Study (MAVIS), which randomly assigned 910 men and women over age sixty-five to multivitamin and multimineral treatment or placebo for one year. Those who were taking vitamins experienced a 4% decrease in visits to the doctor's office and a 7% increase in days of infection, neither of which was statistically significant. In summary, if you are elderly, unless you have a vitamin or mineral deficiency, taking a multivitamin confers no benefit.

ECHINACEA

Among other natural remedies said to lesson the risk or severity of colds and infections is echinacea, probably the most popular. Echinacea is a plant native to North America that has been used by Native Americans for centuries to treat infections. At $300 million in annual U.S. sales, echinacea is the most popular herbal remedy for the treatment of colds and other upper respiratory tract infections. In animal studies it has been shown to increase immunologic activity; yet, despite all the promotion of its preventative properties, echinacea has not been shown to be useful in the prevention of colds. Based on some small earlier trials of questionable methodology that were performed primarily in Germany, echinacea was initially claimed to reduce the length of colds. Results of more recent randomized, double-blind trials conducted in the U.S. using appropriate methods, however, have not been consistent with those of the German studies.

For instance, in one study 148 students with new-onset common colds were given either echinacea or a placebo for ten days. The duration of colds for those who took the plant was 6.27 days, and it was 5.75 days for those on placebo.[9] In another study 408 children ages two to eleven were given either echinacea or placebo immediately after the development of cold symptoms.[10] There were no differences in the number of days of symptoms (9 vs. 9) or severity of symptoms. Echinacea-treated patients had statistically significantly more rash (7.1%) than those treated with placebo (2.7%).

In another study 399 volunteers were given either echinacea or placebo and then were exposed to the cold virus. There were no differences in the percentage of volunteers who became infected in the echinacea group (81%) vs. the placebo group (85%) or in other laboratory measures of infection. Based on these studies echinacea treatment of the common cold is not justified.

PROBIOTICS

Probiotics are live microbial supplements taken to improve the microbial balance of the colon. Probiotics are used more commonly in Europe than in the U.S., with the highest usage in France (thirty-two doses per day per 1,000 people). Probiotics for which there is some evidence of efficacy include the bacteria *Lactobacillus* GG and the yeast *Saccharomyces boulardii (S. boulardii)*. Strains of *Lactobacillus* include *L. rhamnosus* GG, *L. acidophilus* NCFM, *L. casei* Shirota, *L. reuteri* MM53, *L. casei* CRL431, *L. rhamnosus* GR-1, and *L. fermentum* RC-14. They can be taken as an oral supplement or consumed as an additive in various yogurts and other food products. Probiotics compete in the gut with pathological bacteria like *Clostridium difficile* and *Escherichia coli (E. coli)*, which can become more prominent after antibiotic treatment and thereby lead to antibiotic-associated diarrhea (AAD). Probiotics, including *Lactobacillus* and *S. boulardii*, have been shown to prevent diarrhea when given in conjunction with antibiotic treatments in children[11] and adults.[12] Probiotics have also been advocated for recurrent urinary tract infections and yeast infections in women. In uncontrolled studies intravaginal application of *Lactobacillus casei* has been shown to restore normal urogenital flora in women and prevent UTIs and yeast infections.

Studies consistently show that probiotics cut the risk of antibiotic-associated diarrhea by more than one half. Children admitted to the hospital who are given probiotics showed a decrease in hospital-based infections.[13] The effects of probiotics on the treatment of AAD has been less studied. Probiotics have also not been shown in controlled trials to be effective for constipation in adults[14] or children.[15] Probiotics are felt to work by binding to the wall of the colon, competing for nutrients with pathogenic bacteria, and secreting substances with antibiotic properties.

Based on these studies I would recommend the use of probiotics to prevent diarrhea if you are prescribed antibiotics. Probiotics have few side effects so if you want to take them daily that is fine; however, there are no studies that show they are beneficial for anything but prevention of diarrhea with antibiotics so you might want to save your money. If you do buy probiotics or food with probiotic compounds make sure that they contain the probiotics that have been shown to work, including *Lactobacillus, S. boulardii, B. lactis,* and *Streptococcus thermophilus.* Studies of *L. acidophilus/Bifidobacterium infantis* or *L. acidophilus/L. bulgaricus* did not show that they were effective treatments for antibiotic-associated diarrhea.[16]

The Bottom Line

I urge you to recognize the harm to yourself and the potential harm to society from taking antibiotics for viral illnesses that do not respond to antibiotics and that may be associated with potentially very harmful side effects. If you don't go to a doctor you don't run the risk of getting an antibiotic prescription. In other words, *never* go to the doctor if you have a cold, flu, sniffles, or cough. Bed rest, drinking fluids like water and herbal tea, and consuming chicken soup is still the best cure for common colds and flu. Washing your hands after contact with the world (going to work, riding the train, etc.) can do more to stop colds than almost anything else I know. Keeping surfaces (counters, doorknobs) in your home clean does the same.

Most of us can figure out when an infectious illness has become serious and potentially life threatening, in which case it could be due to a bacterial infection that needs antibiotic treatment, but understand that this represents probably less than 10% of cases.

If your kids get an ear infection, wait three days before taking them to the doctor, and treat them with pain medications. If they get very high fever, have recurrent vomiting, or look toxic, take them to the doctor.

If you have to take antibiotics, I recommend taking probiotics with them. When you wipe out your normal colonic "flora," or bacteria, with a course of antibiotics, you can be affected by the colonization of more harmful bacteria like *Clostridium difficile* and *Escherichia coli (E. coli),* which can cause antibiotic-associated diarrhea.

As for other uses of probiotics, they seem to help those with irritable bowel syndrome (IBS). I don't see a lot of evidence for helping constipation or diarrhea, and the controlled trials for intravaginal use of probiotics to prevent yeast and urinary tract infections in women simply haven't been done. I think the best way to get those healthy bacteria working for you is to eat a well-balanced diet with cheese and yogurt, which are full of natural bacteria that can work for you, in addition to nuts, fruits, and vegetables.

Drug	Use	Common, Benign Side Effects	Serious Side Effects	Life-threatening Side Effects	Reasons Not to Take
Penicillins					
Low Risk					
Penicillin	Staph and Strep (lung, skin, throat infections), *Gonococcus* (STD) (IM/IV)	Nausea, vomiting	Diarrhea, lethargy, hallucinations, anemia	Allergic reaction	Allergy, renal disease, pregnancy, breast-feeding
Aminopenicillins					
Low Risk					
Amoxicillin (Amoxil)	Respiratory infections, UTIs	Nausea, vomiting	Diarrhea, lethargy, hallucinations, anemia	Allergic reaction	Allergy, renal disease, pregnancy, breast-feeding
Ampicillin (Omnipen)	Meningitis, lung and tissue infections	Nausea, vomiting	Diarrhea, lethargy, hallucinations, anemia	Allergic reaction	Allergy, renal disease, pregnancy, breast-feeding

Drug	Use	Common, Benign Side Effects	Serious Side Effects	Life-threatening Side Effects	Reasons Not to Take
Bicampicillin (Spectrobid)	Pneumonia	Nausea, vomiting	Diarrhea, lethargy, hallucinations, anemia	Allergic reaction	Allergy, renal disease, pregnancy, breast-feeding
Extended-Spectrum Penicillins					
Low Risk					
Carbenicillin (Geopen)	UTIs	Nausea, vomiting	Diarrhea, lethargy, hallucinations, anemia	Allergic reaction	Allergy, renal disease, pregnancy, breast-feeding
Mezlocillin (Mezlin)	Pneumonia, skin infection, joint infection, bone infection, gyn (IM/IV)	Nausea, vomiting	Diarrhea, lethargy, hallucinations, anemia	Allergic reaction	Allergy, renal disease, pregnancy, breast-feeding
Piperacillin (Zosyn)	Pneumonia, skin infection, joint infection, bone infection, gyn (IM/IV)	Nausea, vomiting	Diarrhea, lethargy, hallucinations, anemia	Allergic reaction	Allergy, renal disease, pregnancy, breast-feeding
Ticarcillin (Ticar)	Pneumonia, skin infection, joint infection, bone infection, gyn, abdominal (IM/IV)	Nausea, vomiting	Diarrhea, lethargy, hallucinations, anemia	Allergic reaction	Allergy, renal disease, pregnancy, breast-feeding

Drug	Use	Common, Benign Side Effects	Serious Side Effects	Life-threatening Side Effects	Reasons Not to Take
Penicillinase-Resistant Penicillins					
Low Risk					
Cloxacillin (Tegopen)	Infections resistant to penicillin	Nausea, vomiting	Diarrhea, lethargy, hallucinations, anemia	Allergic reaction	Allergy, renal disease, pregnancy, breast-feeding
Dicloxacillin (Dycill)	Infections resistant to penicillin	Nausea, vomiting	Diarrhea, lethargy, hallucinations, anemia	Allergic reaction	Allergy, renal disease, pregnancy, breast-feeding
Methicillin (Staphcillin)	Infections resistant to penicillin (IM/IV)	Nausea, vomiting	Diarrhea, lethargy, hallucinations, anemia	Allergic reaction	Allergy, renal disease, pregnancy, breast-feeding
Cephalosporins					
Moderate Risk					
Cefazolin (Kefzol)	Severe infections (IM/IV)	Stomach cramps, headache, dizziness, weakness, rash	Diarrhea, fever	Renal damage, allergic reaction, pseudomembranous colitis	Allergy
Cefadroxil (Duricef)	UTIs	Stomach cramps, headache, dizziness, weakness, rash	Diarrhea, fever	Renal damage, allergic reaction, pseudomembranous colitis	Allergy
Cephalexin (Keflex)	Skin, ear infection	Stomach cramps, headache, dizziness, weakness, rash	Diarrhea, fever	Renal damage, allergic reaction, pseudomembranous colitis	Allergy

Drug	Use	Common, Benign Side Effects	Serious Side Effects	Life-threatening Side Effects	Reasons Not to Take
Cephradine (Velosef)	Pneumonia, UTIs, ear infections	Stomach cramps, headache, dizziness, weakness, rash	Diarrhea, fever	Renal damage, allergic reaction, pseudomem-branous colitis	Allergy
Cefixime (Suprax)	UTIs, ear infections	Stomach cramps, headache, dizziness, weakness, rash	Diarrhea, fever	Renal damage, allergic reaction, pseudomem-branous colitis	Allergy
Cefpodoxime (Vantin)	Respiratory infections	Stomach cramps, headache, dizziness, weakness, rash	Diarrhea, fever	Renal damage, allergic reaction, pseudomem-branous colitis	Allergy
Cefaclor (Ceclor)	Ear infections, bronchitis	Stomach cramps, headache, dizziness, weakness, rash	Diarrhea, fever	Renal damage, allergic reaction, pseudomem-branous colitis	Allergy
Cefditoren (Spectracef)	Ear infections, bronchitis	Stomach cramps, headache, dizziness, weakness, rash	Diarrhea, fever	Renal damage, allergic reaction, pseudomem-branous colitis	Allergy
Cefprozil (Cefzil)	Ear infections, bronchitis	Stomach cramps, headache, dizziness, weakness, rash	Diarrhea, fever	Renal damage, allergic reaction, pseudomem-branous colitis	Allergy
Loracarbef (Lorabid)	Respiratory, urinary tract, skin infections	Stomach cramps, headache, dizziness, weakness, rash	Diarrhea, fever	Renal damage, allergic reaction, pseudomem-branous colitis	Allergy

Drug	Use	Common, Benign Side Effects	Serious Side Effects	Life-threatening Side Effects	Reasons Not to Take
Vancomycin					
Moderate Risk					
Vancomycin	Sepsis, heart infections, bone infection, joint infection, *C. difficile*		Hearing loss	Renal toxicity, decreased blood cells, anaphylaxis	Hyper-sensitivity, renal disease, pregnancy, inflamma-tory bowel disease
Aminoglycosides					
Moderate Risk					
Gentamycin (Garamycin)	Broad spectrum	Nausea, vomiting, weight loss	Hearing loss, confusion, numbness, fever, joint pain, blood pressure changes, diarrhea	Renal damage, liver damage, hypersensitivity reactions	Pregnancy, breast-feeding, renal or liver disease
Tobramycin (Nebcin)	Burns, skin wounds	Nausea, vomiting, weight loss	Hearing loss, confusion, numbness, fever, joint pain, blood pressure changes, diarrhea	Renal damage, liver damage, hypersensitivity reactions	Pregnancy, breast-feeding, renal or liver disease
Kanamycin (Kantrex)	*E. coli*	Nausea, vomiting, weight loss	Hearing loss, confusion, numbness, fever, joint pain, blood pressure changes, diarrhea	Renal damage, liver damage, hypersensitivity reactions	Pregnancy, breast-feeding, renal or liver disease

Drug	Use	Common, Benign Side Effects	Serious Side Effects	Life-threatening Side Effects	Reasons Not to Take
Amikacin (Amikin)	Broad spectrum	Nausea, vomiting, weight loss	Hearing loss, confusion, numbness, fever, joint pain, blood pressure changes, diarrhea	Renal damage, liver damage, hypersensitivity reactions	Pregnancy, breast-feeding, renal or liver disease
Paromomycin (Humatin)	Intestinal amoebiasis	Nausea, vomiting, weight loss	Hearing loss, confusion, numbness, fever, joint pain, blood pressure changes, diarrhea	Renal damage, liver damage, hypersensitivity reactions	Pregnancy, breast-feeding, renal or liver disease, intestinal obstruction
Streptomycin	TB	Nausea, vomiting, weight loss	Hearing loss, confusion, numbness, fever, joint pain, blood pressure changes, diarrhea	Renal damage, liver damage, hypersensitivity reactions, neural toxicity	Pregnancy, breast-feeding, renal or liver disease

Lincosamides

High Risk

Drug	Use	Common, Benign Side Effects	Serious Side Effects	Life-threatening Side Effects	Reasons Not to Take
Clindamycin (Cleocin)	Serious staph, strep infections	Nausea, vomiting, abdominal pain	Diarrhea, rash, dry skin	Pseudomem-branous colitis, blood-cell suppression, hypersensitivity reaction	Pregnancy, lactation, asthma, liver or renal disease
Lincomycin (Lincocin)	Serious staph, strep infections	Nausea, vomiting, abdominal pain	Diarrhea, rash, dry skin	Pseudomem-branous colitis, blood-cell suppression, hypersensitivity reaction	Pregnancy, lactation, asthma, liver or renal disease

Drug	Use	Common, Benign Side Effects	Serious Side Effects	Life-threatening Side Effects	Reasons Not to Take
Macrolides					
Moderate Risk					
Erythromycin (Erythrocin)	Respiratory infection, skin infection	Nausea, vomiting	Diarrhea, stomach pain	Liver damage (rare), pseudo-membranous colitis (rare)	
Azithromycin (Zithromax)	Respiratory infection, skin infection	Nausea, vomiting	Diarrhea, stomach pain	Liver damage (rare), pseudo-membranous colitis (rare)	
Troleandomycin (Tao)	Respiratory infection, skin infection	Nausea, vomiting	Diarrhea, stomach pain	Liver damage (rare), pseudo-membranous colitis (rare)	
Dirithromycin (Dynabac)	Respiratory infection, skin infection	Nausea, vomiting	Diarrhea, stomach pain	Liver damage (rare), pseudo-membranous colitis (rare)	
Chlarithromycin (Biaxin)	Respiratory infection, skin infection	Nausea, vomiting	Diarrhea, stomach pain	Liver damage (rare), pseudo-membranous colitis (rare)	
Tetracyclines					
Low Risk					
Tetracycline (Achromycin)	Acne, chlamydia, rickettsia	Nausea, vomiting	Diarrhea, tooth damage, skin sensitivity	Liver toxicity (rare), hyper-sensitivity	Allergy, pregnancy, lactation
Doxycycline (Vibra)	Acne, chlamydia, rickettsia, lyme disease	Nausea, vomiting	Diarrhea, tooth damage, skin sensitivity	Liver toxicity (rare), hyper-sensitivity	Allergy, pregnancy, lactation
Demeclocycline (Declomycin)	Acne, chlamydia, rickettsia	Nausea, vomiting	Diarrhea, tooth damage, skin sensitivity, sunburn	Liver toxicity (rare), hyper-sensitivity	Allergy, pregnancy, lactation

Drug	Use	Common, Benign Side Effects	Serious Side Effects	Life-threatening Side Effects	Reasons Not to Take
Minocycline (Minocin)	Acne, chlamydia, rickettsia, meningitis	Nausea, vomiting	Diarrhea, tooth damage, skin sensitivity, dizziness, vertigo	Liver toxicity (rare), hyper-sensitivity	Allergy, pregnancy, lactation

Chloramphenicol

High Risk

Chloram-phenicol	Broad spectrum	Headache, depression, confusion, nausea, rash, vomiting	Blindness, nerve damage	Bone marrow toxicity with aplastic anemia	Breast-feeding, toxic reaction, minor infection, porphyria, renal or liver disease, G6PD deficiency

Fluoroquinolones

High Risk

Nalidixic acid (NegGram)	Skin infection, STD, ear infections	Nausea, vomiting	Joint pain, tendon rupture, headache, restlessness, depression, sun sensitivity	Heart attack (rare)	Pregnancy, breast-feeding, allergy; should not be taken by children
Cinoxacin (Cinobac)	UTIs	Nausea, vomiting	Joint pain, tendon rupture, headache, restlessness, depression, sun sensitivity	Heart attack (rare)	Pregnancy, breast-feeding, allergy; should not be taken by children

Drug	Use	Common, Benign Side Effects	Serious Side Effects	Life-threatening Side Effects	Reasons Not to Take
Norfloxacin (Noroxin)	UTIs, prostatitis	Nausea, vomiting	Joint pain, tendon rupture, headache, restlessness, depression, sun sensitivity	Heart attack (rare)	Pregnancy, breast-feeding, allergy; should not be taken by children
Lomefloxacin (Maxaquin)	Respiratory infection, UTIs	Nausea, vomiting	Joint pain, tendon rupture, headache, restlessness, depression, sun sensitivity	Heart attack (rare)	Pregnancy, breast-feeding, allergy; should not be taken by children
Ciprofloxacin (Cipro, Ciloxan)	UTIs, respiratory infection, bone infection, joint infection	Nausea, vomiting	Joint pain, tendon rupture, headache, restlessness, depression, sun sensitivity	Heart attack (rare)	Pregnancy, breast-feeding, allergy; should not be taken by children
Enoxacin (Penetrex)	UTIs, STDs	Nausea, vomiting	Joint pain, tendon rupture, headache, restlessness, depression, sun sensitivity	Heart attack (rare)	Pregnancy, breast-feeding, allergy; should not be taken by children
Gatifloxacin (Tequin)	UTIs, pneumonia	Nausea, vomiting	Joint pain, tendon rupture, headache, restlessness, depression, sun sensitivity	Heart attack (rare)	Pregnancy, breast-feeding, allergy; should not be taken by children

Drug	Use	Common, Benign Side Effects	Serious Side Effects	Life-threatening Side Effects	Reasons Not to Take
Gemifloxacin (Factive)	Pneumonia, bronchitis	Nausea, vomiting, rash	Joint pain, tendon rupture, headache, restlessness, depression, sun sensitivity	Heart attack (rare), heart arrhythmia, liver failure	Pregnancy, breast-feeding, allergy; should not be taken by children
Levofloxacin (Levaquin)	Pneumonia, skin infection, UTIs	Nausea, vomiting	Joint pain, tendon rupture, headache, restlessness, depression, sun sensitivity	Heart attack (rare), seizures	Pregnancy, breast-feeding, allergy; should not be taken by children
Lomefloxacin (Maxaquin)	Respiratory infection, UTIs	Nausea, vomiting	Joint pain, tendon rupture, headache, restlessness, depression, sun sensitivity	Heart attack (rare)	Pregnancy, breast-feeding, allergy; should not be taken by children
Norfloxacin (Noroxin)	UTIs, STDs, prostatitis	Nausea, vomiting	Joint pain, tendon rupture, headache, restlessness, depression, sun sensitivity	Heart attack (rare)	Pregnancy, breast-feeding, allergy; should not be taken by children
Ofloxacin (Floxin)	UTIs, prostatitis, gonorrhea	Nausea, vomiting	Joint pain, tendon rupture, headache, restlessness, depression, sun sensitivity	Heart attack (rare)	Pregnancy, breast-feeding, allergy; should not be taken by children

Drug	Use	Common, Benign Side Effects	Serious Side Effects	Life-threatening Side Effects	Reasons Not to Take
Sparfloxacin (Zagam)	Respiratory problems, skin infections	Nausea, vomiting	Joint pain, tendon rupture, headache, restlessness, depression, sun sensitivity	Heart attack (rare), heart arrhythmia	Pregnancy, breast-feeding, allergy, prolonged QT interval; should not be taken by children
Trovafloxacin (Trovan)	Pneumonia (life threatening only)	Nausea, vomiting	Joint pain, tendon rupture, headache, restlessness, depression, sun sensitivity	Heart attack (rare), liver failure, heart arrhythmia	Pregnancy, breast-feeding, allergy, liver disease, prolonged QT interval; should not be taken by children
Moxifloxacin (Avelox)	Pneumonia, sinusitis	Nausea, vomiting	Joint pain, tendon rupture, headache, restlessness, depression, sun sensitivity	Heart attack (rare), liver failure, heart arrhythmia	Pregnancy, breast-feeding, allergy, prolonged QT interval; should not be taken by children
Sulfonamides					
Moderate Risk					
Sulfamethox-azole-trimethoprim (SMZ-TMP, Septra, Bactrim)	UTIs	Nausea, vomiting	Diarrhea, sun sensitivity	Anemia, allergic reaction, crystals in urine	G6PD deficiency, folate deficiency, porphyria, breast-feeding, pregnancy

Drug	Use	Common, Benign Side Effects	Serious Side Effects	Life-threatening Side Effects	Reasons Not to Take
Sulfisoxazole (Novosoxazole)	UTIs	Nausea, vomiting	Diarrhea, sun sensitivity	Anemia, allergic reaction, crystals in urine	G6PD deficiency, folate deficiency, porphyria, breast-feeding, pregnancy
Sulfasalazine (Azulfidine)	UTIs	Nausea, vomiting	Diarrhea, sun sensitivity	Anemia, allergic reaction, crystals in urine	G6PD deficiency, folate deficiency, porphyria, breast-feeding, pregnancy
Nitrofurantoin					
Nitrofurantoin (Furadantin, Macrodantin, Macrobid)	UTIs	Anorexia, nausea, vomiting	Asthma, abdominal pain	Anemia, neuropathy, lung scarring	Renal impairment, pregnancy

11.

Osteoporosis Drugs

When I was a kid there was an older woman who lived by herself in a house near my family's. I remember her as a sweet, outgoing, diminutive person who had a slight hump on her back. Back then I had no idea that she had *osteoporosis,* but given her physical appearance, which was similar to that of many of her contemporaries, she was the iconic image of the "little old lady." It does not have to be that way, of course; not all elderly people develop a bowed back, although we all shrink. The important thing to keep in mind when considering the causes of and treatments for osteoporosis is that it is *not* necessarily a disease; it is a natural fact of life for all of us. Osteoporosis is a thinning of the bones that naturally occurs with aging and that sometimes leads to fracture or a bowed back.

The most disabling fractures in the elderly occur in the hip bone, specifically the femoral neck, which is associated with a considerable loss of mobility. More common are fractures in the vertebral body (the bones of the spine), which usually are not associated with pain but may cause a bowing of the back. In the elderly, 25% of hip fractures lead to a permanent loss of independent function. No wonder many seniors, especially frail ones, live in mortal fear of fractures that may send them to oft-dreaded nursing homes for the rest of their few remaining days (although my neighbor lived out her long life at home).

Bone Density

Bone density, that is, the thickness of your bones, is determined by a bone-mineral density (BMD) test. To determine what constitutes abnormal bone-mineral density, the World Health Organization (WHO) has established specific guidelines based on how much a patient's results deviate from those of the average healthy young woman, or the *t* score. Osteoporosis is defined as a *t* score of less than –2.5, which corresponds to a marked degree of bone thinning. If you have a *t* score of less than –2.5, you are in the bottom 1% in terms of bone density. Osteopenia, bone thinning that is not as severe as osteoporosis, is defined by *t* scores between –1.0 and –2.5. If you have a *t* score in this range, your bone density is so low that only 16% of women would have such a result. As bone thinning progresses you could go from having osteopenia to osteoporosis. The National Osteoporosis Foundation (NOF) recommends BMD testing for postmenopausal women who have a risk factor for osteoporosis (smoking, drinking, lack of exercise, body weight of less than 127 pounds, family history of osteoporotic fracture, or prior vertebral fracture), and all women over the age of sixty-five.

I believe the logic of this measure is deeply flawed; judging older women by standards for young women doesn't make any sense. The *t* scores are calculated by comparing how much a woman deviates from the bone density of a healthy young woman. That's like having a seventy-year-old and a twenty-year-old run a one-hundred-yard dash, and then if the seventy-year-old loses, saying that the older person has a disease. Bone density normally declines with age, and therefore there is no reason to think that this is necessarily a cause for concern. Yet today if you have an abnormal

BMD test, defined as a *t* score of less than –2.5, the NOF guidelines advise you to "talk to your doctor" and provide a description of medications that are used to prevent fractures.

For example, if you are a woman who gets a BMD test and follows the WHO criteria, there is a 50% chance you will be diagnosed with osteoporosis at the age of seventy-two (*t* score < –2.5) and a good chance your doctor will recommend medication. Your risk of having osteopenia (*t* score < –1.0), for which your doctor may recommend medication to "prevent" osteoporosis, is 50% by age fifty-two. In other words, according to the guidelines, half of postmenopausal women should be taking medication for osteoporosis. However, as I show in the next section, recommendations for so many women to take bone medications don't make any sense.

Also, even though BMD predicts fracture and medications increase BMD, that doesn't mean they necessarily prevent fracture (at least not the ones that cause loss of function or pain). This is the old *A* equals *B* and *B* equals *C*, therefore *A* equals *C* rule. Osteopenia causes fracture, and medication reduces osteopenia, therefore medication reduces fracture. Right? Not exactly.

Normally there are two kinds of cells that regulate bone turnover, osteoblasts and osteoclasts. The osteoblasts actively increase bone by laying down calcium and phosphate. Osteoclasts, in turn, chew up bone. In young people there is a balance of the two. When you get older, however, osteoblast activity declines, so your bones get thinner. Popular osteoporosis medications get between the bone and the osteoclast to prevent the osteoclast from breaking down bone and thus increase bone mineral density.

But what doctors and drug makers often don't tell you is that the medications used to treat osteoporosis (see pages 219–226) increase the laying down of calcium on the outer, cortical bone, which is more densely packed. The inner bone, called the trabecular bone, is less dense but forms a latticelike network that is actually more important for the strength of the bone. With aging there is a loss of trabecular bone; therefore there is less area on which calcium can be laid down. Therefore calcium is preferentially laid down on the outer, cortical bone. This may increase your BMD score, but it won't necessarily reduce your risk of fracture. And there are some particularly nasty side effects to deal with, which I will discuss below.

A Brittle Pill: Common Osteoporosis Treatments

One of the drug industry's most charming commercials features a healthy and glamorous-looking sixty-something actress who confides to viewers that she has gotten shorter and that her doctor told her she might have bone fractures. Then she smiles and cheerfully advises women to see their doctors if they have gotten shorter. She also says that osteoporosis may be making women's bones brittle. The words Actonel (risedronate) float across the screen, and a male voice fires off the typical list of possible side effects, caveats, and contraindications.

What she neglects to mention (it's not in her script, obviously) is that Actonel can actually make your bones brittle and that, unfortunately, due to a normal settling of the spine we *all* get shorter with age. The implication that a healthy and active sixty-year-old needs to measure her height and then take drugs if she is shorter than she was when she was in her forties is absurd.

BISPHOSPHONATES

Osteoporosis is commonly treated with bisphosphonates, estrogenlike medications, and supplementation with calcium and vitamin D, with the goal of treatment being the prevention of fractures. The bisphosphonates include risedronate (Actonel), alendronate sodium (Fosamax), etidronate (Didronel), tiludronate (Skelid), pamidronate (Aredia), and zoledronate (Zomeda). Again, they act by getting between the bone cells (osteocytes) and the cells that break down bone (osteoclasts). Doctors prescribe bisphosphonates, often with calcium and vitamin D, to prevent recurrence of fracture and to prevent the first fracture in women with osteopenia or osteoporosis (thinning of the bones). Pamidronate and zoledronate are used intravenously for the treatment of cancers, primarily breast cancer with bone metastases and myeloma.

So are bisphosphonates helpful? Several studies performed in a total of 12,831 postmenopausal women with *t* scores of less than –2.5 (i.e., with osteoporosis) or less than –2.0 (close to the osteoporosis cutoff) looked at the ability of these drugs when compared with placebos to prevent fractures over the course of one to five years. Studies of alendronate (Fosamax) include the Alendronate Phase III Osteoporosis Study,[1] the Fracture Intervention Trial (FIT), divided into women without a history of prior vertebral fracture[2] and those with a prior vertebral fracture,[3] and the FOSamax International Trial (FOSIT).[4] The Vertebral Efficacy with Risedronate Therapy (VERT) Study[5] looked at the effect of risedronate (Actonel) on fractures.

All of these studies showed that bisphosphonates increase BMD and reduce the risk of vertebral fracture in women with osteoporosis (*t* score < –2.5). But what is the significance of a vertebral fracture? Vertebral fracture is merely defined as a reduction of the height of the vertebra by 20% on radiological tests like MRIs. To have a vertebral fracture defined this way, you don't have to have pain, a change in posture, or anything at all that would make you aware of any problem. In fact, most of the time the only person who knows you have a vertebral fracture is your radiologist. Even the term *fracture* is misleading; it's really just a loss of bone mass. For the 50% or so of women who do not have pain, there are no implications to having a vertebral fracture, other than the fact that it might make you a little shorter. In other words, these medications probably won't help you; they don't reverse the problem, if you even have one.

What about fractures that matter? Alendronate Phase III, FIT (without past fracture), and FOSIT either didn't report the results, or showed no reduction in painful vertebral fractures (i.e., the ones that matter, unless you are only worried about getting short). The Alendronate Phase III and the FIT (both with and without past fracture) showed no benefit of medication on fractures of bones, like the wrist or collarbone, that are outside the vertebra; these are collectively called nonvertebral fractures. These are more serious than vertebral fractures but don't necessarily lead to lasting disability. Alendronate Phase II, FIT (without past fracture), FOSIT, and VERT showed no benefit for the more important hip fractures, which, as I mentioned before, can lead to lasting disability. There were marginally statistically significant reductions in nonvertebral fractures in the FOSIT study (nineteen vs. thirty-seven after one year) and VERT (5% vs. 8% after three years). In the FIT study of women with past fractures treated with Fosamax, eleven had a hip fracture over four years, compared with twenty-two on placebo, a marginally statistically significant difference that represented a reduction in risk of 0.3% per year.

The Hip Intervention Program Study[6] assessed the effects of three years of risedronate or placebo in 9,331 women over age seventy with dramatic losses of bone mineral density (t score < -4, with -2.5 indicating regular osteoporosis) or t score less than -3, with a risk factor for hip fracture, like the propensity to fall. Overall, 2.8% of women on risedronate suffered hip fracture vs. 3.9% on placebo, a difference of 1.1% that was statistically significant.

In the only study of men to date,[7] 241 men with osteoporosis ages thirty-one to eighty-seven were randomly assigned to alendronate or placebo treatment for two years. There were no differences between alendronate and placebo groups in painful vertebral fractures (one vs. three) or nonvertebral fractures (six vs. five).

In summary, for postmenopausal women with osteoporosis there is no evidence that up to three years of treatment with bisphosphonates affects what we are most concerned about, hip fractures, since that is what can lead to lasting disability. The only studies that did show such protection were in women who had extreme levels of bone mineral density loss, far beyond osteoporosis, or a past history of fracture. Therefore, treating women with risk factors for hip fracture is not useful.

And what about the side effects? In the VERT study mentioned above, three patients were saved from hip fracture, but ten times as many patients had an adverse event related to the drug, most commonly stomach and esophagus complaints. This isn't a very good trade-off of risks and benefits.

One primary concern related to these medications is gastrointestinal problems related to the stomach and the esophagus. In fact, in the FIT trial of women with past fractures, twice as many patients on the medication (nineteen vs. ten on placebo) developed erosive esophagitis, an inflammation of the esophagus. That means that nine patients developed esophagitis from the drug who didn't have to, while only five patients were saved from a clinically significant hip fracture. In the FIT trial of women without past fractures, sixteen patients taking the medication developed a stomach ulcer compared to seven on placebo; that means that nine patients developed an ulcer on the medication that they would haven't had otherwise, while only eleven patients were saved from a life-threatening hip fracture. Other side effects included nausea, diarrhea, abdominal pain, and dizziness. All of these side effects can be treated with proton pump inhibitors (PPIs) (see Chapter 9); only rarely do ulcers or esophagitis progress to the point of medical emergencies (e.g., when a peptic ulcer perforates).

And what about long-term treatment? The implication of the educational campaigns for osteoporosis is that it is a disease for which you have to be treated for the rest of your life. Is there really evidence for long-term benefit? Is there any risk of harm? This issue was looked at by extending treatment for women beyond the initial five years of the original studies I described above. In the Alendronate Phase III study there was no difference in nonvertebral fractures in the first two years of the extension period,[8] and from years three to five of the extension period (i.e., after up to ten years of treatment) the medication no longer prevented any type of fracture, including vertebral fracture.[9] In the FIT study, an extra five years of treatment showed no differences in total vertebral, nonvertebral, and hip fractures.[10]

In response to these studies Susan Ott, M.D., associate professor in the department of medicine at the University of Washington and a specialist in the area of bone physiology and osteoporosis, wrote a letter to the *Journal of Clinical Endocrinology & Metabolism* in which she said, "There is no doubt that alendronate increases bone strength and decreases fracture rate during the first four years of use, but after that the profound suppression of the bone formation rate may begin to have a negative effect." In other words, after five years they seem to stop working. How could this be?

Again, bisphosphonates act by inhibiting osteoclasts, the cells that break down bone. So although they increase BMD for a few years, in the long run they decrease bone turnover. Animals treated with bisphosphonates show a decrease in bone turnover. Women on alendronate were found to take up to two years to heal after a fracture and had markedly suppressed bone formation on biopsy. It looks like bisphosphonates have a modest effect in reducing fractures during the first five years of treatment. However, after five years the inhibition of bone turnover tilts from net protective to neutral or maybe even net negative. In the long run, bisphosphonates may decrease the ability of bones to resist fracture, making bones *more brittle*. They also are not metabolized, meaning that the bisphosphonates you take now will remain in your bones for life, resulting in a long-term reduction in bone turnover.

This decrease in bone turnover is the underlying cause of the scariest potential side effect of bisphosphonates: osteonecrosis. Osteonecrosis is a degeneration of the bone in the jaw that may require surgery. Examples of osteonecrosis include "fossy jaw" or "phossy jaw," which developed in nineteenth-century workers who were exposed to phosphorus in factories where matches were made. The phosphorus would get into the bone of the jaw, much like the bisphosphonates do, and stop bone turnover, eventually killing the bone tissue. The outcome was so painful and disfiguring that it sometimes led people to kill themselves. Most of the recent cases of osteonecrosis have occurred in patients with myeloma and breast cancer who were treated with intravenous bisphosphonates zoledronic acid and pamidronate.

Dr. Cesar Migliatori[11] of NOVA Southeastern University in Ft. Lauderdale, Florida, has reported five cases of cancer patients who were treated with intravenous zoledronic acid or pamidronate and developed osteone-crosis of the jaw after a tooth extraction (related to the impaired bone heal-ing caused by the decreased bone turnover with bisphosphonate treatment). All patients developed infections of the bone that would not respond to antibiotics or surgery. They had chronic pain and problems with eating, speaking, and dental hygiene. In another review 10% of patients treated for cancer with zoledronic acid and 4% treated with pamidronate devel-oped osteonecrosis of the jaw after three years of treatment. Most of the patients had dental problems, with dental surgeries that resulted in non-healing bone.

Although most of the cases of osteonecrosis of the jaw have been re-ported in patients with bone metastases or myelomas treated with intrave-nous bisphosphonates, there are now cases of patients who have taken the medication only for the "prevention of osteoporosis." This shows that there are those out there for whom there is little potential benefit and unfortu-nately much to lose in taking bisphosphonates.

A total of fifteen cases of osteonecrosis have been reported with oral alendronate, one with oral risedronate, and one with ibandronate, which is taken for the treatment of osteoporosis or Paget's disease (a disease that makes bones weak and fragile). It is recommended that any dental work be done before going on these medications.

Nonbisphosphonates

Nonbisphosphonate medications for the treatment of osteoporosis mimic various hormonal systems involved in the regulation of bone formation, including estrogen, calcitonin, and parathyroid hormones. As I will show you, they don't work any better than bisphosphonates in preventing the fractures that matter, and they have their own problems in terms of side effects.

RALOXIFENE

Raloxifene (Evista), a drug that acts at the estrogen receptor, has been touted as having the beneficial effects of estrogen for osteoporosis without the increased risk of uterine and ovarian cancer. However, Evista has other side effects that are similar to those of estrogen, including increased blood clotting. Like the bisphosphonates, Evista does increase bone mineral density and reduce risk of vertebral fracture in postmenopausal women. However, each year it saves only about one or two women out of a hundred from a vertebral fracture. It has not been shown to prevent nonvertebral fractures.

In the Multiple Outcomes of Raloxifene Evaluation (MORE) study, 7,705 postmenopausal women with osteoporosis received raloxifene or placebo in a randomized placebo-controlled trial.[12] Although raloxifene decreased vertebral fractures and increased bone mineral density, it did not decrease nonvertebral fractures. Also, only twenty-two women out of 7,705 were saved from a hip fracture, which translates into one out of a thousand each year, a difference that isn't statistically significant. And raloxifene has other side effects, like hot flashes, that result in a significant number of women stopping its use. As many as two out of a hundred women stopped their medication because of hot flashes and other side effects like depression, insomnia, rash, leg cramps, upset stomach, cough, and headaches.

Of more concern is the finding that one out of a hundred women on Evista developed deep-vein thrombosis, a condition that can lead to pulmonary embolism, an event that kills one out of four people affected. Risk of deep-vein thrombosis was increased threefold. In other words, for every woman saved from a hip fracture, there are ten who have a life-threatening blood clot in their leg.

In the Raloxifene Use for the Heart (RUTH) study, which was designed to assess the drug's ability to prevent heart disease, 10,101 postmenopausal women with risk factors for heart disease were randomized to raloxifene or placebo for five years of treatment. There was no reduction in heart-disease events (533 vs. 553). There was a reduction in breast cancer (40 vs. 70) and vertebral fractures (64 vs. 97), but an increase in stroke (59 vs. 39) and blood clots in the leg (103 vs. 71).[13] In other words, overall this drug causes as many diseases as it prevents. Given this finding, I don't recommend using this medication.

CALCITONIN

Calcitonin (Miacalcin, Calcimar), medication that mimics a hormone secreted by the parafollicular cells of the thyroid, is derived from salmon. In the body it inhibits osteoclasts, promotes osteoblasts, and increases bone mineral density, which is why it was developed for the treatment of osteoporosis. Miacalcin was approved by the FDA only on the basis of its ability to increase bone mineral density, which went against its rules of approving only those drugs for osteoporosis that reduce fractures. It promised to do more studies, but the studies showed no benefit. The only dose that affected bone density was the high dose, and that had no effect on vertebral fracture, let alone hip fracture. I do not recommend use of this medication.

TERIPARATIDE

Teriparatide (Forteo) is a form of parathyroid hormone, the hormone that regulates calcium and phosphate metabolism in the bone and kidneys. It is given by daily injection and has been approved for women with new vertebral fractures, albeit with restrictions, because it causes bone cancer in laboratory animals. At best it can reduce the risk from 0.7% to 0.2%. These differences are not statistically significant. By my calculations, it would cost $2.5 million to prevent a single hip fracture with this drug.

Alternative Medicines and Vitamins

Given the modest outcomes and risks of the bisphosphonate drugs it is natural that women would look to alternative approaches to prevent the loss of bone density. For a long time estrogen replacement therapy was hailed as a natural way to prevent bone loss associated with the loss of estrogen after menopause. The Women's Health Initiative (WHI) indeed showed that hormone replacement therapy (HRT) prevented bone loss and reduced the risk of osteoporotic fracture.[14] In this controlled trial, however, HRT was found to have unacceptable risks, including increasing the risk of breast, ovarian, and uterine cancer as well as stroke, heart attack, and gallbladder disease. Overall the risks were greater than the benefits.[15] (See Chapter 12 for more information on HRT.)

Studies have shown modest increases in bone mineral density with soy but as yet have not evaluated its effects on fractures. Observational studies have found a relationship between BMD and magnesium, which may be low in the diet of some elderly people, but as yet no randomized controlled studies of the effects of magnesium on bone density and fracture have been reported.

CALCIUM AND VITAMIN D

Doctors routinely recommend supplementation with calcium and vitamin D to prevent osteoporosis and bone fractures in postmenopausal women. Taking calcium increases calcium in the blood, making more available for uptake into the bone. With normal aging, there is a decrease in calcium absorption by the stomach. Vitamin D (cholecalciferol) is known to increase calcium absorption in the gut as well as to act synergistically with calcium to promote bone density. This has led to the common practice of prescribing calcium and vitamin D supplementation for the prevention of hip fractures. It sounds so good and logical, and it can't hurt, so why not go ahead and do it?

Just because you become deficient in something with aging, however, doesn't mean that supplementation will correct the problem. Studies have shown that calcium and vitamin D supplementation in people over age sixty-five increased total bone density but not necessarily in areas that matter, like the femoral neck, where low bone density can cause hip fracture.[16] Moreover, the changes in bone mineral density in areas like the femoral neck were present only for men and not women. This is important since osteoporotic fractures primarily affect women. The only studies that showed that calcium and vitamin D prevented hip fractures involved French women who had osteoporosis and were living in nursing homes.[17] However, these women may have had a calcium and/or vitamin D deficiency due to diet or lack of sunlight as a result of their environment.

Other studies of individuals outside nursing homes found that vitamin D and calcium supplementation had no beneficial effects in terms of hip-fracture prevention.[18] One study of patients who had had a fracture and became immobile did not find any benefit from vitamin D and calcium in the prevention of secondary fractures.[19] The Women's Health Initiative (WHI) followed 36,282 premenopausal women ages fifty to seventy-nine who were randomly assigned to receive 1,000 mg of calcium with 400 IU of vitamin D_3 or placebo daily for seven years to assess bone fracture. Supplementation did not reduce the risk of hip fracture. Although there was an increase in hip-bone density, there was also an increase in kidney stones.[20] Since increasing hip-bone density has no practical benefit and is not related to reducing the risk of hip fracture, whereas increasing kidney stones is definitely negative, I do not recommend these supplements.

Diet and Exercise

Eat a well-rounded, balanced diet with fruits, vegetables, and a moderate amount of cheese, yogurt, and other dairy products, and you should get enough calcium in your diet to minimize bone loss with aging. In the wintertime take long walks in the sun to stimulate vitamin D production. (Most vitamin D is generated internally after exposure to the sun.) If someone in your family is elderly and doesn't get out much or is confined, wheel him or her outdoors for some sun exposure.

Physical activity and exercise play a dramatic role in the prevention of fractures. Studies have shown that the process of aging itself is ten times more important in terms of fracture risk than bone mineral density. The most critical thing to do to prevent fractures is to keep active. Loss of muscle strength is part of aging, but we can profoundly delay this effect through active exercise. It is clear from the studies that the people who get hip fractures are those who become frail and inactive and thus more likely to fall. In fact, osteoporotic fractures of the hip are inversely related to exercise. Furthermore, although bone thinning contributes to the risk of fracture, the risk is primarily related to a loss of balance, which often results in falls. Exercise helps elders maintain their balance. In fact, there is no difference in bone density between those with and without fractures.

The best exercise for increasing bone mass is strength training. Numerous studies demonstrate that engaging regularly in resistance exercises increases bone mass, especially spinal bone mass. A research study by Ontario's McMaster University found that a yearlong strength-training program increased the spinal bone mass of postmenopausal women by 9%. And it found that women who do not participate in strength training *lose* bone density.

The good news is that you do not have to become an Iron Man to derive benefit from resistance and weight training. A whole variety of exercises yield bone-building benefits, although working with weights at a gym with a trained professional is one safe way to engage in this form of activity, especially if you have never done it before. Weight lifting, even with as little as two-, five-, or ten-pound weights to start, dancing, stair climbing, walking on an incline (uphill), and brisk walking are all weight-bearing exercises that promote mechanical stress in the skeletal system and thereby contribute to the placement of calcium in bones.

How does this work? When you are engaged in weight-bearing exercise, you are exerting force on parts of your bones. The body reacts to this by stimulating osteoblasts, those cells that are responsible for laying down calcium in the bone and building up the bones. The body is in effect responding to the message that more bone strength is needed, much as it does when it increases muscle mass and tone with exercise. And the good news is that it builds up bone strength more effectively than bisphospho-nates. Rather than randomly laying down calcium in parts of the bone that may not greatly enhance the strength of the bone, as bisphosphonates do, this type of exercise results in a laying down of calcium in the parts of the bone that matter. And what's more, the effects don't wear off after five years.

While good for your cardiovascular system and overall health, aerobic exercises such as biking and swimming do not strengthen the bones. If you can incorporate both forms of exercise into your routine, good for you! If not, and you are heading toward menopause or are menopausal, focus on strength training; it does give you some aerobic benefits. A moderate in-vestment of time is all that's needed: fifteen to thirty minutes of weight training two to three times per week provides the bone density you need to prevent osteoporosis if you work all your different muscle groups and let your muscles rest for a day between workouts. Of course, it's great if you can start resistance training before you enter menopause, but even if you start later you will avoid the usual bone loss and even increase bone density slightly.

The Bottom Line

First and foremost, I cannot emphasize enough the importance of a healthy diet and exercise for maintaining strong bones and thus good mobility and a better quality of life.

Based on the available evidence I do not recommend getting bone-mineral density (BMD) or screening X-rays for vertebral "fractures" you don't know about, since I don't think these represent fractures in the way you and I think of them. Rather, they are simply a settling of the vertebrae, which is part of normal aging. If you don't have a history of fracture, you shouldn't get your bone-mineral density checked and you shouldn't consider treatment for osteoporosis. (Men should not be treated for osteoporosis.) Instead of getting screenings, I recommend that you follow my advice for prevention.

Don't ever use raloxifene, teriparatide, or calcitonin for osteoporosis treatment; the risks outweigh the benefits.

Women who have had a painful fracture can consider getting their bone-mineral density checked. Women who have been diagnosed with osteoporosis can talk to their doctors and consider taking bisphosphonates.

Use the information I have presented to assess your own situation and then make your own decision. Don't feel as though you have to take drugs. If you do take them, don't do so for more than five years.

Drug	Use	Common, Benign Side Effects	Serious Side Effects	Life-threatening Side Effects	Reasons Not to Take
Bisphosphonates					
High Risk					
Alendronate Sodium (Fosamax)	Osteo-porosis	Nausea, diarrhea, dizziness	Stomach pain, esophagus complaints	Blood clots, erosive esophagitis, stomach ulcer, osteonecrosis	Low calcium, renal disease, hyper-sensitivity, pregnancy, breast-feeding, *no* history of fracture
Risedronate (Actonel)	Osteo-porosis	Nausea, diarrhea, dizziness	Stomach pain, esophagus complaints	Blood clots, erosive esophagitis, stomach ulcer, osteonecrosis	Low calcium, renal disease, hyper-sensitivity, pregnancy, breast-feeding, *no* history of fracture

Drug	Use	Common, Benign Side Effects	Serious Side Effects	Life-threatening Side Effects	Reasons Not to Take
Etidronate (Didronel)	Osteoporosis	Nausea, diarrhea, dizziness	Stomach pain, esophagus complaints	Blood clots, erosive esophagitis, stomach ulcer, osteonecrosis	Low calcium, renal disease, hyper-sensitivity, pregnancy, breast-feeding, *no* history of fracture
Tiludronate (Skelid)	Osteoporosis	Nausea, diarrhea, dizziness	Stomach pain, esophagus complaints	Blood clots, erosive esophagitis, stomach ulcer, osteonecrosis	Low calcium, renal disease, hyper-sensitivity, pregnancy, breast-feeding, *no* history of fracture
Pamidronate (Aredia)	Osteoporosis	Nausea, diarrhea, dizziness	Stomach pain, esophagus complaints	Blood clots, erosive esophagitis, stomach ulcer, osteonecrosis	Low calcium, renal disease, hyper-sensitivity, pregnancy, breast-feeding, *no* history of fracture

Drug	Use	Common, Benign Side Effects	Serious Side Effects	Life-threatening Side Effects	Reasons Not to Take
Zoledronate (Zomeda)	Osteoporosis	Nausea, diarrhea, dizziness	Stomach pain, esophagus complaints	Blood clots, erosive esophagitis, stomach ulcer, osteonecrosis	Low calcium, renal disease, hypersensitivity, pregnancy, breast-feeding, *no* history of fracture
Estrogen-Receptor Modulators					
High Risk					
Raloxifene (Evista)		Rash, insomnia, leg cramps, headaches	Hot flashes, depression, cough, stomach pain	Increased blood clotting, deep-vein thrombosis	Thrombophlebitis, pregnancy, breast-feeding, *no* history of fracture
Calcitonin Hormone					
High Risk					
Salmon calcitonin (Miacalcin, Calcimar)	Osteoporosis	Irritation at site of application			No history of fracture
Parathyroid Hormones					
High Risk					
Teriparatide (Forteo)				Bone cancer (possible)	Cost-prohibitive

12.

Oral Contraceptive Pills and Hormone Replacement Therapy

The history of hormone therapy for both birth control and treatment of the symptoms of menopause is so rich with drama and includes such a wide assortment of eccentric characters that several Hollywood screenplays could be written about it. Since this chapter starts with oral contraceptives, it's worth taking a very brief look at the history of what is popularly known as "the pill," because it provides a framework for my discussion about its uses, side effects, and risks.

The condensed version of the pill's development starts with Gregory Pincus, an early-twentieth-century American physician, biologist, and researcher who studied hormonal biology and steroidal hormones. At a meeting in 1953, feminist and birth-control activists Margaret Sanger and Katherine McCormick encouraged the scientist to create an oral contraceptive that would give women more freedom over their reproductive and sexual choices. The idea struck him as a good one, so Pincus sought out the pharmaceutical company Searle, thinking they would share his enthusiasm and fund his research. Unfortunately, the firm turned him down because at that time laws against birth control were strict.

Through a series of experiments on another drug, a Searle chemist named Frank Colton inadvertently developed an early version of the pill that Pincus was permitted to use for his work. The resulting drug, made primarily from synthetic estrogen and progesterone, known as progestin, was made available in 1957 as a treatment for gynecological disorders. Then, in 1960, the FDA approved it as a birth control pill, and just three years later more than 1 million women were using it.

Today about 35 million women use some type of contraception, about 17 million of whom take one of the several kinds of oral contraceptive pills (OCPs) currently available, and new types are regularly introduced. For example, in May 2007 the FDA approved the first pill, called Lybrel, that if taken daily halts women's menstrual periods indefinitely and prevents pregnancies. Because so many women use oral contraceptives, it is especially important to consider the side effects and consequences. What on the surface looks like an easy choice (to take "the pill") may not be for all women.

How They Work

The female reproductive cycle is a complex monthly choreography of hormonal and physical changes whose purpose is to maximize a woman's capacity to conceive a child during the years when she is most likely to successfully bear that child and raise it to adulthood. If no conception takes place, the cycle repeats itself about every twenty-eight days.

The goal of nature and the body, conception, is not the goal of many young women in college or out there starting their careers. That is where the pill comes in.

Oral contraceptives, including the early version refined by Pincus, provide a steady supply of the female hormones estrogen and progesterone for twenty-one days, followed by seven days of nothing (usually an inert pill) during which a woman usually has her period. (An exception is the mini pill, which provides a continuous dose of progesterone only.) This steady supply of hormones shuts down the reproductive system and by so doing prevents the normal concert of events that lead to ovulation. The theoretical failure rate of OCPs is 0.1%, and the true failure rate, which is usually the result of incorrect use, is 3%.

First Generation

The earliest version of the pill contained a whopping 10 mg of progestin and 100 mcg of estrogen. First-generation oral contraceptive pills were high in estrogen and had a high risk of heart attack and stroke. This high dosage also caused several other unpleasant side effects, such as nausea, blurred vision, bloating, weight gain, depression, and blood clots. Doctors heard about and saw these reactions but generally dismissed them as female hysteria until the 1980s. Eventually researchers and drug companies took these concerns more seriously, and in the 1980s lower-dosage versions of the pill were created, many with 1 mg of synthetic progestin (lynestrenol or norethindrone), along with 100 mcg of estradiol, the synthetic estrogen, which is still considered high by many scientists. (The most recent forms of the pill contain 20 mcg of estradiol.)

Second Generation

As researchers learned more about the pill they realized that such high doses of estrogen and progesterone were not necessary. The earlier versions of the pill, called monophasic pills, also kept the dose of estrogen and progesterone fixed during the first twenty-one days, followed by seven days off. Second-generation OCPs involved lowering the dosage of these hormones, and varying the dose at different phases of the cycle: for instance seven days of 0.5-mg progesterone, seven days of 0.75-mg, and seven days of 1-mg. Pills with two doses of progesterone during the cycle are called biphasic; those with three different doses are triphasic.

Second-generation OCPs include norgestrel/ethinyl estradiol (Low Ogestrel), norethindrone/estradiol/mestranol (Ortho Novum), and levo-norgestrel/estradiol (Alesse, Triphasil, Trivora). Later-generation OCPs typically have lower concentrations of hormones, which result in fewer side effects like hypercholesterolemia, blood clotting, and mood changes. First-generation OCPs and second-generation OCPs with levonorgestrel have double the risk of heart attacks as third-generation OCPs, which I discuss next.

Third Generation

Third-generation OCPs like norgestimate/ethinyl estradiol (Ortho Tri-cyclen), and desogestrel/ethinyl estradiol (Apri, Ortho-cept) were developed to contain progesterone with less androgenic (i.e., stimulating hormones like testosterone) activity, thereby reducing problems like weight gain, acne, and increased lipids. Third-generation OCPs with the progesterones gestodene and desogestrel, however, increase the risk of blood clots twofold compared to the second-generation OCPs. Drospirenone and estradiol (Yasmin) carry a greater risk of dangerous increases in potassium in the blood, which can lead to symptoms of malaise, palpitations, and muscle weakness and, if severe, to cardiac arrhythmia or sudden death.

The FDA is set to approve Lybrel, the first OCP that eliminates periods altogether. Lybrel contains 90 mcg levonorgestrel and 10 mcg ethinyl estradiol. Lybrel is taken every day and there is no seven-day window to allow menses to occur. Breakthrough bleeding can occur during the first few months. The risks and benefits are similar to those of other OCPs. The long-term effects of eliminating the menses, of course, are not known.

Mini Pills

Mini pills, which contain progesterone only, are given as a continuous dose of hormone throughout the cycle [e.g., 350 mcg norethindrone (Nor-QD, Micronor) or 75 mcg norgestrel (Ovrette)]. They have a theoretical 99% efficacy in preventing pregnancy, which, although not as good as that of regular OCPs, is still pretty good. Unlike regular OCPs, which block all ovulations, mini pills block only 60% to 80% of ovulations, and there is more breakthrough bleeding with mini pills than with regular pills. Women who are heavy smokers, have uncontrolled high blood pressure, or have a history of breast cancer, or those who shouldn't be exposed to estrogen for some other reason, can take the mini pill.

Long-Acting Contraceptives

The injectable long-acting contraceptive medroxyprogesterone (Depo-Provera), which is administered by intramuscular injection by a physician or nurse, provides three months of contraceptive protection. Depo-Provera eliminates menstrual bleeding and is advantageous for woman who experience painful periods or want to stop the menses for other reasons. It is also more convenient and can be beneficial for women who can't remember to take a pill every day. This compound, however, has been associated with an increase in bone-mineral loss when given to teenagers. The best predictor of bone strength in later life is bone buildup in childhood; therefore, these depot forms of contraceptive are not recommended for adolescents. Other serious but uncommon side effects are liver damage and allergic reactions.

Progestasert is a long-acting intrauterine device that releases progesterone that is inserted in the uterus and provides one year of contraceptive protection. Mirena is another intrauterine device that releases levonorgestrel for up to five years. These devices are 97% to 98% effective in preventing pregnancy.

The Patch

The Ortho-Evra patch has been marketed as a convenient form of birth control that doesn't require women to remember to take a pill every day. However, the FDA has issued a warning about an increased risk of blood clots that can lead to potentially fatal clots in the lungs. The risk of blood clot is double that of OCPs. The FDA has registered twelve deaths to date in young women on Ortho-Evra. Given these facts, I do not recommend the Ortho-Evra patch for birth control.

The Morning-After Pill

Mifepristone (Mifeprex, RU-486), one of the newest and most revolutionary contraceptives, is used to terminate early pregnancies, which are defined as 49 days or less since the start of the last menstrual period. Mifepristone inhibits the activity of progesterone, which results in termination of the pregnancy. It can, however, result in an incomplete abortion or increased vaginal bleeding, both of which may require surgical intervention. So far, 1% to 5% of women have required some surgical intervention. For this reason it is only available through a physician. Two days after the drug is administered, the woman returns to the doctor's office for treatment with another medication, called misoprostol, which is a synthetic prostaglandin.

Prostaglandins are hormones that have a wide range of functions, including causing the contraction of blood vessels in the endometrium at the end of the menstrual cycle, which causes the endometrium to sluff off from the uterus as menses. In this case misoprostol facilitates passage of material from the uterus. Because of the risk of bleeding, infection, or incomplete abortion, all of which are potentially fatal, this drug should not be used unless there are follow-up appointments with a physician. After several recent deaths of several women who used the drug unsupervised, Planned

Parenthood has reversed its policy of allowing women to administer miso-prostol at home; they now must return to the physician.

Are OCPs Safe?

After the introduction of OCPs in the '60s, doctors noticed that women taking them were developing blood clots in their legs and having heart attacks and strokes at higher rates. As I mentioned above, the newer generations of OCPs, with reduced doses of hormones, have lessened these risks.

So at this point in OCP history, how safe and effective are these pills? For nonsmoking women ages fifteen to thirty, who use a comparable form of contraception, the IUD, there is no increase in death rate. Because of the health risks of pregnancy, the death rate among women ages fifteen to thirty-four who are on the pill is actually lower than that for women who do not use any form of birth control.

OCPs can be unsafe for older women who smoke. The risk of heart attack more than doubles for women over forty or women who smoke or have diabetes or high cholesterol. They also should not be used by women with a history of blood clots, untreated high blood pressure, breast or uterine cancer, migraine headaches with focal neurological symptoms, known pregnancy, or liver or cardiac disease. Some of the women taking the newer pills experience the same side effects—headaches, nausea, bloating, breast tenderness, and weight gain—as those who took the early pills. Your OCP should have low estradiol (less than 50 mcg) to decrease the risk of blood clots.

For young, nonsmoking women without hypertension or diabetes the health benefits of OCPs balance the health risks. For these women there is no increased risk of heart attack or stroke. There is a 28% increased risk of blood clot in the leg, but since this is rare, the risk that any one particular woman will get one from an OCP is still very low. For smokers there is a greater risk with OCPs that increases with age. For instance, the risk of death is one in two hundred thousand per year in nonsmoking women under the age of thirty-five. However, risk increases with age and smoking to one in seven hundred per year for smokers over age thirty-five.

The risk of cervical cancer doubles after ten years of oral-contraceptive therapy in women with a history of human papillomavirus infection (HPV). It is not clear if the risk is from the OCP or the increased risk of being infected with HPV for women on OCPs who may not use barrier protection. However, since the risk of getting cervical cancer is 0.008%, in any given year a doubling of risk means increasing your risk by another 0.008% per year. OCPs increase the risk of liver cancer, but this risk is rare. OCPs increase the risk of breast cancer by 10% to 20%.

In women of childbearing age, breast cancer is rare, and any increased risk is eliminated after OCPs are stopped. In addition, the types of breast cancers that develop in women on OCPs respond better to treatment; therefore the overall risk from breast cancer is not increased. OCPs reduce the risks of ovarian and uterine (endometrial) cancers. They also reduce the risk of anemia by reducing the loss of iron in menses, pelvic inflammatory disease, and osteoporosis (since estrogen promotes the laying down of calcium in the bones). The pill has no long-term effect on fertility.

OCPs are safe for teenage girls to use, with the exception of Depo-Provera, which I mentioned on page 238.

The Bottom Line on Contraceptives

Use an OCP with low doses of estradiol (< 50 mcg). Taking an OCP is safe for women who don't smoke. Women over age thirty-five who smoke or who should not take the regular pill for other reasons (e.g., history of blood clots) should consider the mini pill, another all-progesterone pill, or one of the alternatives to the pill I describe below.

Alternatives to the Pill

For an alternative form of birth control, consider the use of intrauterine devices (IUDs), which are 99% effective and safe. There is a rare risk of pelvic inflammatory disease in the first twenty-six days. One objection to these devices is that an embryo might be fertilized and implant itself for a day in the uterine wall before the IUD rejects it. However, the overwhelming majority of fertilized eggs do not implant themselves in the uterine wall of women with an IUD. We don't know if any fertilized embryos *can* implant themselves in women with IUDs. In my opinion this is nothing more than hand-wringing. Let's worry about things for which there is evidence to warrant concern.

Diaphragms are not as effective as OCPs (about 90%) and come with the disadvantage of having to be inserted within two hours of intercourse and left in for six hours afterward. On the other hand, they do not disrupt a woman's natural hormonal cycle to prevent fertilization. Cervical caps can be left in for several days. Both diaphragms and cervical caps are fitted by a doctor.

Hormone Replacement Therapy

At about the age of fifty, women go through menopause, which is associated with the cessation of ovulation and menstrual cycling, and a decline in estrogen and progesterone levels. The conclusion that women need to "replace" their female hormones after menopause has a long history driven by the idea that a decline in hormones leads to unnatural and unwanted effects on libido, memory, and cardiovascular health, none of which has any basis in fact.

It all started forty years ago with a book called *Feminine Forever,* by Dr. Robert A. Wilson. It was a national best seller when it was published. Wilson, a British-born gynecologist who practiced in Brooklyn, New York, and later, on Park Avenue in Manhattan, persuaded the public that "Many physicians simply refuse to recognize menopause for what it is—a serious, painful and often crippling disease."

His solution was to give women over the age of forty hormone replacement therapy (HRT). The FDA had actually approved HRT back in 1942 to treat the hot flashes, difficulty sleeping, mood swings, and other symptoms that can accompany menopause. Wilson argued that HRT was a near-miracle remedy that could stem a woman's aging process and improve her sex life. By defining a natural process as a disease he helped the pharmaceutical industry convince healthy women that they needed to take a drug every day for the rest of their lives. For the pharmaceutical industry this notion created a dream situation of finding a huge segment of the normal population to whom it could sell its pills. No matter that there were no controlled trials to support industry claims. This idea was very popular for many years, before real controlled trials showed that HRT was very bad and had caused the deaths of tens of thousands of women as well as other problems.

Hormone replacement therapy involves replacing the body's natural hormones after normal or surgically induced menopause. Common brand-name examples of HRT include Premarin (estrogen from a horse), Provera (progesterone), and Prempro (combination). About 20% of women will develop uncomfortable, and sometimes unbearable, hot flashes during the perimenopausal period. Some women develop other or additional symptoms, such as problems with rational thinking or depression, all of which can be treated successfully with HRT. Other hormones, like testosterone, can be used for purposes such as treating low libido in women.

Although HRT has a role in treating hot flashes for a limited time, or occasionally depression or insomnia, it has been marketed to a much larger number of women. For much of the history of HRT, it was believed that HRT prevented heart disease, stroke, and osteoporosis and that it improved well-being, sexuality, memory, and mood. However, there were some early indications from the Nurses' Health Study, published in 1995, that there was a 32% increase in breast cancer with HRT. Nevertheless, a great deal of marketing was done on behalf of HRT, and pharmaceutical companies made billions of dollars by arguing that all postmenopausal women needed to take it to maintain their good health. HRT was also purported to improve a woman's looks as well as her sex life.

None of this, however, held up to the test of time. The original evidence that HRT prevented heart attacks was based on what are called observational studies. Women who chose to take HRT were compared to those who didn't and were found to have fewer heart attacks. It turned out that the women who took HRT also were more proactive in matters concerning their health. They did other things, like exercise and diet, that helped to prevent heart attacks; the HRT was superfluous. Yet from 1995 to 2003 eight years went by with major marketing to women and billions of dollars in sales. The pharmaceutical companies had hit on the mother lode of all markets: not just patients with a disease but all women over age fifty.

The observational study design, however, is inherently flawed; it's easy for a systematic factor to creep in and skew the results. The only way to answer the question of whether HRT does indeed prevent heart attacks is to set up a controlled study in which women get either HRT or a sugar pill, they don't get to choose which one, and they (and their doctors) don't know what they are on. At the end of five years, you compare outcomes (i.e., heart attacks) between the two groups. It took so long to do such studies because it was argued that it would be unethical to give a sugar pill to women when HRT had such obvious benefits.

Controlled trials have since been performed. The Women's Health Initiative (WHI) involved the random assignment of 16,608 postmenopausal women to estrogen and progestin (equine estrogen and medroxyprogesterone, or Prempro) vs. a placebo from 1993 to 1998. Women on Prempro had a statistically significant 24% increase in their risk of heart attack or cardiac death. HRT also increased the risk of breast cancer by 24%,[1] and doubled the risk of pulmonary embolus (blood clot in the lung). There was about a 50% increase in ovarian cancer that was not statistically significant, mainly because ovarian cancer is much less common than breast cancer, and no increase in uterine cancer. HRT had no effect on cancer when all cancers were combined, and it reduced the risk of osteoporotic fracture.[2] It did, however, increase the risk of stroke by 31%.[3]

The Heart and Estrogen/Progestin Replacement Study (HERS) involved randomized blinded treatment of 2,768 postmenopausal women with a history of heart disease for four years with estrogen plus progestin (conjugated estrogens and medroxy-progesterone, or Prempro) or placebo and two years of follow-up. HRT had no protective effect against recurrence of heart disease.[4] There was a 10% increase in mortality with HRT, which was related in part to a doubling of the risk of blood clots that can lead to deadly pulmonary emboli (blood clots that travel to the lungs and have up to a 50% mortality rate)[5] and a 48% increased risk of gallbladder disease requiring surgery.[6] HERS also showed a pattern of increased cancer risk that was not statistically significant.

Other studies of estrogen replacement have shown increased rates of uterine and ovarian cancer. For every hundred women treated with HRT in the WHI, one woman developed a serious adverse event directly related to HRT.

Other studies showed that HRT actually accelerated the progression of thickening of the coronary arteries and doubled the risk of dying of heart disease.[7, 8] A recent meta-analysis showed a 29% increase in the risk of stroke. Based on these findings, there is no role for HRT in disease prevention.

Estrogen alone (Premarin), given to women with a hysterectomy, was shown, like estrogen and progesterone, to increase the risk of stroke, decrease the risk of bone fracture, and have no effect on cardiovascular disease. A recommendation from this research (NIH Advisory for Physicians, March 1, 2004) was that estrogen alone should not be used for the prevention of heart disease.

HRT had no effect on sexual function when analyzed on the basis of controlled trials. When I say no effect, I don't mean some effect that was not statistically significant; I mean zero effect. There was also no effect on mood. After one year women on HRT reported minuscule improvements in sleep and pain, but those were back to zero after three years.

So what could explain all the fuss about how HRT helped women's sex lives? It was all a placebo effect. You could give a woman HRT, and she would have a 25% improvement in her sex life. But you could give a woman a sugar pill, and it would have the same effect—plus it wouldn't give her a heart attack.

There has been a lot of interest in whether memory and cognition are affected by HRT. Both men and women experience the decline in memory that normally occurs with aging. Estrogen affects brain areas involved in memory like the hippocampus, which has led to the idea that the decline in estrogen after menopause is associated with a decline in memory function. Based on observational studies, it was originally believed that HRT prevented the development of Alzheimer's disease and other dementias and improved memory function or delayed the normal decline of memory with aging in women without dementia. However, at that time "smart" women were doing things that they thought were good for their health, like taking HRT, which could have led to obvious biases in these types of studies.

In fact, although HRT was originally hypothesized to prevent dementia, when carefully assessed it was found to actually double the risk of dementia.[9] HRT also resulted in a small, but not clinically significant, reduction in cognition in one study.[10]

The largest study, the Women's Health Initiative, which did not find an effect on cognition,[11] used a measure called the Mini Mental Status Exam, which asks questions like "What year is it?" or "What is this object?" You can see that this is a fairly gross measure of memory and cognition that might not pick up subtle changes. However, combining results from women treated with estrogen alone and estrogen plus progesterone showed that hormones caused a decline in cognition.[12]

A number of studies have looked at more subtle and specific memory functions. Studies of women without depression or dementia found no change in a variety of specific memory tests, including the ability to learn word pairs, find words, remember a paragraph, or connect numbered dots. Most important, the studies that used random assignment of postmenopausal women to HRT or placebo and also eliminated the kind of self-selection of educated women to take HRT that can influence the results of these studies showed no effect of HRT on memory.

Many women justifiably concerned about the risks of HRT or other things such as side effects stop taking them after they have received a prescription. Dierdre Hill, Ph.D., and colleagues at the University of Washington in Seattle conducted a phone interview study of 204 women one year after they had received a prescription for HRT. They found that 40% of these women were no longer taking HRT as originally prescribed. Reasons commonly given by the women included vaginal bleeding, anxiety, and nervousness. And this was before the large studies of the past few years showed the major health risks and lack of health benefits of HRT.

What about women with surgically induced menopause? Studies of women with hysterectomy and bilateral oopherectomy (removal of uterus and ovaries) initially showed an improvement in memory function with HRT, although these studies were uncontrolled. However, the Women's Health Initiative (WHI) study showed that estrogen alone in women with hysterectomy was associated with a decline in cognition as measured with the Mini Mental Status Exam.

In terms of benefits, HRT does reduce the loss of bone-mineral density that occurs with normal aging and reduces the risk of osteoporotic fracture. There is also minimal evidence that it improves sleep. However, these benefits are far outweighed by the risks of HRT. Women who have discomfort from hot flashes benefit from HRT. HRT leads to an 80% reduction in symptoms with an associated improvement in quality of life. HRT also improves memory and cognition in women with highly symptomatic hot flashes. If used for a short time, there is a good chance that the hot flashes will come back when HRT is stopped.

The major studies comparing HRT to placebo did not include women with mental disorders. HRT has been shown to be better than placebo in the treatment of depression in women who develop depression around the time of menopause.[13] Stressed postmenopausal women who were caring for a spouse with depression reported less hostility when compared to those on placebo.[14] Replacement of estrogen and testosterone in women who had their uterus and ovaries removed also resulted in an improvement in mood.

Non–HRT Drug Treatments for Hot Flashes

There are a number of alternatives to HRT that are safer and that have been shown to be effective for hot flashes. Selective serotonin reuptake inhibitors (SSRIs) like Paxil and Prozac block reuptake of serotonin in neurons in the brain. Clonidine stimulates the norepinephrine alpha-2 receptor, which has the effect of decreasing norepinephrine ("adrenaline") function in the brain. Gabapentin, which is used for the treatment of epilepsy, acts on the GABA neurotransmitter system in the brain. All three of these types of medications have been shown to reduce hot flashes. SSRIs and gabapentin are discussed in Chapter 15, the chapter on antidepressants. Clonidine was discussed in Chapter 5, the chapter on antihypertensives.

Alternative Medicines

NATURAL PREPARATIONS

HRT uses synthetic hormones or hormones from animals that are similar but not chemically identical to human estrogen, 17-beta-estradiol. Recently, "natural" preparations of estrogen, progesterone, and testosterone have been developed. They are usually prepared from plants, and are also known as phytoestrogens. Since they are natural, pharmaceutical companies cannot patent them. For this reason the natural hormones have not been studied, although they are available for use. They are probably preferable to the synthetic and animal preparations and might have fewer negative health consequences; however, we can't say that they don't cause the cancers and other negative health consequences that have been shown with HRT. Since they are the same thing, I suspect they do.

HERBS AND SUPPLEMENTS

Studies of herbs and supplements for the treatment of hot flashes have not shown consistent results. Soy, black cohosh, dong quai root, and evening primrose oil have all been promoted for hot flashes. In an initial study of 104 postmenopausal women randomized to 40g daily of soy or a placebo the number taking soy showed a statistically significant reduction in the number of hot flashes compared to the women taking placebo. In another study 351 women ages forty-five to fifty-five who had two or more hot-flash symptoms per day were randomly assigned to black cohosh, multibotanicals, multibotanicals plus dietary soy counseling, placebo, or hormone therapy for one year. Only hormone therapy was associated with significant reductions in hot flashes. Taking dietary soy actually turned out to be less effective at stopping hot flashes than taking a placebo for one year.

Other placebo-controlled trials did not find any efficacy of soy extract for hot flashes. Therefore I do not recommend use of soy extract for hot flashes. However, there are no major safety issues with soy, so if you want to try it, that's fine. Placebo-controlled trials have not shown dong quai or evening primrose oil to be effective in the treatment of hot flashes.

Alternative medicines that are commonly promoted for symptoms related to menopause include St.-John's-wort, flaxseed oil, fish oil, omega-3 fatty acids, red clover, ginseng, rice bran oil, wild yam, calcium, gotu kola, licorice root, sage, sarsaparilla, passionflower, chaste berry, ginkgo, and valerian root. None of these have been subjected to controlled trials. However, since they are not associated with major health risks, it is okay to try them.

Heidi Nelson, M.D., a professor of medicine at Oregon Health Sciences University in Portland, Oregon, and colleagues recently reviewed the literature for nonhormonal therapies for hot flashes, looking at the reduction in the number of hot flashes per day with different treatments. They found that hot flashes were reduced with SSRIs by 1.3 per day, with clonidine by 0.95 per day, and with gabapentine by 2.5 per day (all statistically significant). By comparison, HRT reduced hot flashes by 2.5 to 3 per day. Red clover extract had no effect, and results were mixed for soy. Other natural remedies for hot flashes were found to lack sufficient controlled trials to make a determination.

Diet and Behavior

Studies have shown that women who exercise during menopause develop hot flashes one third as often as women who do not. These findings are not based on controlled trials, however, and other factors could explain the difference. However, exercise, especially weight and strength training, have other beneficial effects, like preventing osteoporosis-related fractures, helping to make up some of the benefit lost from not taking HRT.

High-fat, low-fiber diets are associated with higher estrogen activity. Since Asian women tend to have lower levels of estrogen before (and after) menopause, the drop in estrogen levels they experience in menopause may be less dramatic, resulting in milder symptoms at menopause or none at all. Fiber increases fecal excretion of excess estrogen, which may account for the protective effect of a high-fiber diet against a variety of hormone-sensitive conditions, including breast cancer. Other foods that are recommended specifically for hot flashes include flaxseed, high-lignan flaxseed oil, fennel, celery, and parsley. Both flaxseed and high-lignan flaxseed oil are rich in lignans, which can help normalize estrogen levels. Fennel, celery, parsley, and all legumes are excellent sources of phytoestrogens (natural estrogens found in plants).

Hot flashes can be treated with several commonsense noninvasive approaches. Keep cool. Drink ice water throughout the day. Even a slight increase in your body's core temperature can trigger a hot flash. If you dress in layers you can remove and add clothing as your feelings of warmth rise and fall. Simple as it sounds, opening windows and using fans or air conditioners, even in the winter and especially at night when you are sleeping, helps keep you cool. Hot, spicy foods, caffeinated beverages, and alcohol can trigger hot flashes in some women. Avoid these or any other foods or drinks that raise body temperature.

Relaxation techniques help some women fight off hot flashes. Meditation, deep-breathing exercises, and yoga are all worth trying. Even if they don't end up preventing hot flashes, you will get other benefits from these activities, such as improved sleep and general calmness. Slow, controlled, deep rhythmic breathing or "paced respiration" practiced twice a day has been shown to decrease hot flashes. Take a slow, deep breath, hold it for a few seconds, and exhale just as slowly. They say that the paced-respiration technique can help relieve a hot flash if begun at the onset.

Finally, if you smoke, entering menopause is a good time to quit. There is never a bad time to quit smoking, of course, but smoking is linked to increased hot flashes. Quitting also improves your health in other ways, such as lowering your risk of heart disease, stroke, and cancer.

RELATIONSHIPS

Another issue related to menopause, one that makes many women reach for pharmaceutical help, is that they and the significant others in their lives worry that they will lose their libido (the premise of *Feminine Forever*, and the cause of the entire mess), but in my family that didn't seem to happen at all. I think that hormone "replacement" is really a bad idea.

Finally, many women say that once the hot flashes are over and done with and they enter their "second stage," they feel liberated, free, and happy. No more periods and no more worrying about whether sex with a hunky stranger will lead to an unwanted pregnancy (practice safe sex, ladies!). In fact, my women friends tell me that there are many advantages to being a healthy, happy, fabulous postmenopausal woman—more independence for one.

The Bottom Line on HRT

In summary, HRT should not be used for disease prevention. It increases the risk of blood-clot formation, heart attack, stroke, and breast cancer. Although it slows bone loss and osteoporosis, this does not offset the risks. In fact, HRT users experience five times as many adverse health effects as nonusers. HRT does not prevent memory loss or loss of libido in postmenopausal women. In women with depression and/or significant hot flashes with menopause, HRT improves mood, memory, libido, and quality of life. HRT should therefore not be used by postmenopausal women without depression or disabling vasomotor (hot-flash) symptoms. If you do develop depression or disabling hot-flash symptoms, you can talk to your doctor and go over the risks and benefits of your particular situation.

Furthermore, on the basis of herb and supplement studies I do not recommend the use of soy, black cohosh, dong quai, evening primrose oil, or any other supplement for hot flashes. So called "natural" female hormones, like estrogenlike compounds derived from plants, if they have any active properties, will also have the negative properties of HRT and therefore should not be used. I *do* recommend use of SSRIs, clonidine, or gabapentin for hot flashes if needed, since these drugs are safe and nonaddictive and have been shown in clinical trials to reduce hot flashes.

Drug	Use	Common, Benign Side Effects	Serious Side Effects	Life-threatening Side Effects	Reasons Not to Take
Hormone Replacement Therapy (HRT): Estrogens					
Moderate Risk					
Conjugated estrogen (Premarin)	Hormone replacement therapy	Breakthrough bleeding, dysmenorrhea, headache, nausea, vomiting, cramps, breast tenderness	Jaundice, colitis, pancreatitis, depression, change in libido	Breast cancer, endometrial cancer, heart attacks, dementia, gallbladder disease	Breast cancer, heart disease, history of blood clotting, pregnancy
Transdermal estradiol (Vivelle, Estraderm, Climara)	Hormone replacement therapy	Breakthrough bleeding, dysmenorrhea, headache, nausea, vomiting, cramps, breast tenderness	Jaundice, colitis, pancreatitis, depression, change in libido	Breast cancer, endometrial cancer, heart attacks, dementia, gallbladder disease	Breast cancer, heart disease, history of blood clotting, pregnancy
Oral estradiol (Estrace)	Hormone replacement therapy	Breakthrough bleeding, dysmenorrhea, headache, nausea, vomiting, cramps, breast tenderness	Jaundice, colitis, pancreatitis, depression, change in libido	Breast cancer, endometrial cancer, heart attacks, dementia, gallbladder disease	Breast cancer, heart disease, history of blood clotting, pregnancy
Estradiol valerate in oil (Gynogen, Delestrogen, Estra-L, Valergen, Dioval)	Hormone replacement therapy	Breakthrough bleeding, dysmenorrhea, headache, nausea, vomiting, cramps, breast tenderness	Jaundice, colitis, pancreatitis, depression, change in libido	Breast cancer, endometrial cancer, heart attacks, dementia, gallbladder disease	Breast cancer, heart disease, history of blood clotting, pregnancy

Drug	Use	Common, Benign Side Effects	Serious Side Effects	Life-threatening Side Effects	Reasons Not to Take
Diethylstilbestrol (DES)	Hormone replacement therapy	Breakthrough bleeding, dysmenorrhea, headache, nausea, vomiting, cramps, breast tenderness	Jaundice, colitis, pancreatitis, depression, change in libido	Breast cancer, endometrial cancer, heart attacks, dementia, gallbladder disease	Breast cancer, heart disease, history of blood clotting, pregnancy

Hormone Replacement Therapy (HRT): Progestins

Moderate Risk

Drug	Use	Common, Benign Side Effects	Serious Side Effects	Life-threatening Side Effects	Reasons Not to Take
Progesterone (Gesterol)	Hormone replacement therapy	Breakthrough bleeding, amenorrhea, weight gain, nausea, breast tenderness	Photosensitivity, depression, jaundice, loss of eyesight (rare)	Thrombophlebitis	Thrombophlebitis, hypersensitivity, hemorrhage, liver disease, breast cancer, pregnancy, breastfeeding
Medroxyprogesterone Acetate (Provera)	Hormone replacement therapy	Breakthrough bleeding, amenorrhea, weight gain, nausea, breast tenderness	Photosensitivity, depression, jaundice, loss of eyesight (rare)	Thrombophlebitis	Thrombophlebitis, hypersensitivity, hemorrhage, liver disease, breast cancer, pregnancy, breastfeeding

Drug	Use	Common, Benign Side Effects	Serious Side Effects	Life-threatening Side Effects	Reasons Not to Take
Megestrol (Megace)	Hormone replace-ment therapy	Breakthrough bleeding, amenorrhea, weight gain, nausea, breast tenderness	Photosensitivity, depression, jaundice, loss of eyesight (rare)	Thrombo-phlebitis	Thrombo-phlebitis, hyper-sensitivity, hemorrhage, liver disease, breast cancer, pregnancy, breast-feeding

Implantable Contraceptives

Moderate Risk

Drug	Use	Common, Benign Side Effects	Serious Side Effects	Life-threatening Side Effects	Reasons Not to Take
Levonorgestrel implants (Norplant)	Pregnancy prevention	Breakthrough bleeding, amenorrhea, weight gain, nausea, breast tenderness	Photosensitivity, depression, jaundice, loss of eyesight (rare)	Thrombo-phlebitis, infection, uterine perforation	Thrombo-phlebitis, hyper-sensitivity, hemorrhage, liver disease, breast cancer, pregnancy, breast-feeding
Intrauterine progesterone (Progestasert)	Pregnancy prevention	Breakthrough bleeding, amenorrhea, weight gain, nausea, breast tenderness	Photosensitivity, depression, jaundice, loss of eyesight (rare)	Thrombo-phlebitis, uterine perforation	Thrombo-phlebitis, hyper-sensitivity, hemorrhage, liver disease, breast cancer, pregnancy, breast-feeding

Drug	Use	Common, Benign Side Effects	Serious Side Effects	Life-threatening Side Effects	Reasons Not to Take
Abortion Pills					
Moderate Risk					
Mifepristone (Mifeprex, RU-486)	Early pregnancy termination	Bleeding, cramps, abdominal pain, nausea, vomiting, diarrhea	Heavy vaginal bleeding	Incomplete abortion, continued bleeding, infection	Ectopic pregnancy, term more than 49 days, IUD in place, adrenal failure, steroid therapy, bleeding disorders, allergy
Second-Generation Oral Contraceptive Pills (OCPs)					
Moderate Risk					
Norgestimate/ ethinyl estradiol (Ortho Tri-cyclen)	Pregnancy prevention	Headaches, nausea, bloating, breast tenderness, weight gain	Gallbladder disease, increased lipids, increased glucose	Heart attack (rare), stroke (rare), cervical cancer	Increased risk in smokers, HPV+, hyper-tensives, cancer, liver disease, cardiac disease
Norgestrel/ ethinyl estradiol (Low Ogestrel)	Pregnancy prevention	Headaches, nausea, bloating, breast tenderness, weight gain	Gallbladder disease, increased lipids, increased glucose	Heart attack (rare), stroke (rare), cervical cancer	Increased risk in smokers, HPV+, hyper-tensives, cancer, liver disease, cardiac disease

Drug	Use	Common, Benign Side Effects	Serious Side Effects	Life-threatening Side Effects	Reasons Not to Take
Norethindrone/ Mestranol (Ortho Novum)	Pregnancy prevention	Headaches, nausea, bloating, breast tenderness, weight gain	Gallbladder disease, increased lipids, increased glucose	Heart attack (rare), stroke (rare), cervical cancer	Increased risk in smokers, HPV+, hyper-tensives, cancer, liver disease, cardiac disease
Levonorgestrel/ estradiol (Alesse, Triphasil, Trivora)	Pregnancy prevention	Headaches, nausea, bloating, breast tenderness, weight gain	Gallbladder disease, increased lipids, increased glucose	Heart attack (rare), stroke (rare), cervical cancer	Increased risk in smokers, HPV+, hyper-tensives, cancer, liver disease, cardiac disease

Third-Generation OCPs

Moderate Risk

Drug	Use	Common, Benign Side Effects	Serious Side Effects	Life-threatening Side Effects	Reasons Not to Take
Desogestrel/ ethinyl estradiol (Apri, Ortho-cept)	Pregnancy prevention	Headaches, nausea, bloating, breast tenderness, weight gain	Gallbladder disease, increased lipids, increased glucose	Blood clotting (worse than second genera-tion), stroke, heart attack	Increased risk in smokers, HPV+, hyper-tensives, cancer, liver disease, cardiac disease

13.

Diabetes Drugs

Diabetes is one of those conditions that must be treated for life and requires changes in lifestyle and constant monitoring. Diabetics are in for the long haul, no matter which of the two major types of diabetes they are living with. Both type 1 and type 2 diabetes are associated with elevated glucose levels in the blood and an inability of the cells to take up the sugars that have the energy they need to perform the tasks they have to perform every day. A third type of diabetes, gestational diabetes, develops only during pregnancy and occurs more often among African Americans, American Indians, Hispanic Americans, and women with a family history of diabetes. Women who have had gestational diabetes also have a 20% to 50% chance of developing type 2 diabetes within five to ten years.

All forms of diabetes increase the risk of heart attack, stroke, eye disease, and kidney failure. Symptoms of elevated blood sugar include light-headedness, confusion, weakness, and, if untreated, seizures, coma, and death. Insulin is a hormone produced by the pancreas that stimulates uptake of glucose or sugar, the body's food, into cells. Unregulated glucose in the blood can lead to a hospital-room emergency.

Type 1 (juvenile) diabetes is a genetic disease that usually occurs in childhood but can also occur in adults, normally those under age forty. It is an immune-system disorder that is related to an insulin deficiency caused by an autoimmune attack on pancreatic β-cell islets; treatment with daily insulin shots is required. Type 1 diabetes is a condition that needs to be treated for life, and at this time it is not preventable. However, it is actually fairly uncommon: Only 10% of people who have diabetes have type 1. Those dealing with type 1 diabetes treat it with insulin therapy, meal planning (carbohydrates need to be carefully balanced), regular exercise (because activity lowers the amount of sugar in the blood), and careful monitoring of overall health. This last because diabetes alters the body's immune system and decreases the body's ability to fight infection. Foot injuries in particular have to be watched, since diabetes causes damage to the blood vessels and nerves that can decrease a person's ability to sense trauma to or pressure on the foot. An unnoticed foot injury can lead to severe infection and, if untreated, amputation.

For those who have type 2 diabetes, or "adult-onset diabetes" (about 90% of those with diabetes; 10% have type 1 or gestational), insulin shots are not necessarily required for treatment. Ten million Americans have impaired glucose tolerance, putting them at risk for the development of type 2 diabetes. From 2000 to 2010 the prevalence of type 2 diabetes is projected to increase by 46%, from 151 million to 221 million worldwide. And calling the disease "adult-onset" is fast becoming a misnomer, since more and more children and young adults are being diagnosed with type 2 diabetes each year. According to The Children's Hospital of Philadelphia, type 2 diabetes in children has risen dramatically since 1994, when less than 5% of new childhood diabetes cases were type 2. By 1999, type 2 diabetes was accounting for 8% to 45% of new childhood diabetes cases, depending on geographic location. That's because type 2 is closely linked to lifestyle, most especially obesity and lack of physical exercise, and is associated with resistance to insulin at the cell level and/or impaired insulin secretion.

The growing prevalence of type 2 diabetes over the last twenty years has led to terms such as *diabesity* (obesity plus diabetes) and *metabolic syndrome* (abdominal fat, insulin resistance, increased lipids, and hypertension). Once again, we see a modern disease caused by modern living, in this case, a bad diet and lack of exercise. Massive doses of fats and sugars that are part of our everyday food lead to diabetes because large doses of sugar in the blood lead to a spike in insulin release. High-fat diets add to the problem, as fat-filled cells release fats into the bloodstream, triggering insulin release that can lead to insulin resistance and eventual diabetes.

The U.S. is not alone in this unabated increase in type 2 diabetes; dramatic increases have also occurred in developing nations. For instance, on the Pacific island of Nauru, where diabetes was virtually unknown forty years ago, 40% of the adult population is now afflicted with the disease. The prevalence of diabetes among Chinese ranges from 2% among those who live in China to 15% among the ethnic Chinese in Mauritius, which illustrates how an increase in the rate of diabetes among ethnic Chinese may correspond to a move to another country. These changes in rates of diabetes in countries where little or no diabetes previously existed have been directly correlated with the introduction of Western diets, specifically with the arrival of American fast-food restaurants like McDonald's and Wendy's.

In fact, in 2006 A. Hauber, an economist from Bear Stearns International, and E. Gale, a doctor at the University of Bristol in England (an unusual collaboration between the world of finance and that of medicine and science), wrote:

There are two dimensions to each new treatment for diabetes. The first is the impact it will have upon glucose control, measured in terms such as clinical trial outcomes, risk vs benefit, patient satisfaction and cost. The other dimension, rarely considered in clinical journals, is that of the market place. Diabetes has been a major driver of the worldwide pharmaceutical market over the past ten years, and this sector has grown at an annual rate of just below 20%, from U.S. $3.8 billion in 1995 to U.S. $17.8 billion in 2005. Growth in the diabetes market remained at a solid double-digit level even when growth of the world pharma market slowed from 11% in 2002 to 5% in 2005. Diabetes is common—and rapidly becoming more so—and current therapies are only partially effective in controlling glucose levels and preventing late complications. It is therefore expected to remain one of the most attractive growth areas in the global pharmaceutical market. This was not always the case, for ten years ago the market in diabetes was limited to insulin, sulfonylureas and metformin, medications that were well established, largely generic and relatively inexpensive. In contrast, the past decade has seen the introduction of a wide range of new therapies that have varied in their clinical and commercial success but have invariably been more expensive than the previously available options."[1]

Treatments for Type 1 Diabetes

Type 1 diabetes is treated with injectable insulin. If you have type 1 diabetes you have no choice but to take this medication for a lifetime. This may also be true for some cases of type 2 diabetes, but this is a decision that must be made with your doctor. Taking insulin is inconvenient because it requires daily injections and checking of blood-sugar levels.

One of the major issues surrounding insulin today is its cost. Regulation of insulin production is different from that of normal drugs because it involves the production of something that the body itself makes, and it is for this reason that it is subject to a different set of FDA rules. Because of this, manufacturers of insulin have been able to keep the makers of generic insulin at bay with the argument that their methods of manufacture cannot be replicated, effectively making it very difficult for cheaper generic versions to reach the market and keeping the cost of available insulin high. I believe that regulations permitting more production of insulin by generic manufacturers will greatly benefit patients with diabetes. This issue continues to be debated in Congress.

Treatments for Type 2 Diabetes

The majority of doctors, scientists, and other health-care professionals agree that the first line of treatment for adult-onset, or type 2 diabetes, is weight loss. Even a 10% weight loss can be associated with an improvement in diabetes in a significant number of people. So, for example, if you have type 2 diabetes, weigh two hundred pounds, and are overweight by fifty pounds but manage to lose twenty, you have made dramatic gains in health, including a potential reversal of your diabetes. The second line of treatment is oral medication. If there is no response to this you may need injected insulin in addition to oral medications.

FIRST-GENERATION DIABETES MEDICATIONS

The first generation of medications for type 2 diabetes were the sulfonylureas, including glyburide (Micronase, Diabeta), tolbutamine (Orinase), glipizide (Glucotrol), and glimepiride (Amaryl). These medications, which are still on the market, are as effective as the newer medications, cost a lot less, and have a better safety profile. These first-generation diabetes medications act by promoting release of insulin from the pancreas. Side effects include dangerously low blood sugars, which can cause anxiety, nervousness, and slurred and/or staggered speech, all of which can lead to a visit to the emergency room. Other side effects include loss of appetite, nausea, and vomiting. These medications very rarely cause liver problems. Studies in the 1970s showed that patients treated with sulfonylurea drugs had higher rates of death from heart disease than did patients treated with insulin or a placebo. No studies have been performed since that time to refute or support that finding.

Another older diabetes drug still on the market is metformin (Glucophage), whose mechanism of action is different from that of the sulfonylureas. Metformin decreases the amount of glucose produced by the liver, reduces glucose absorption, and promotes glucose uptake by cells. Metformin rarely causes lactic acidosis, a buildup of lactic acid in the blood, which makes the blood more acidic and which can be fatal. The signs of lactic acidosis include deep and rapid breathing, vomiting, and abdominal pain. Side effects of metformin include diarrhea, vomiting, nausea, bloating, and loss of appetite. Rare side effects include a metallic taste in the mouth and reductions in vitamin B_{12}. Glucovance is a combination of glyburide and metformin.

The known side effects and limited efficacy of these drugs led to a search for more-effective drugs with fewer side effects. Although the new-generation diabetes drugs were introduced with great fanfare, in some cases their side-effect profile turned out to be troubling and in some cases even more deadly than the older drugs.

SECOND-GENERATION TREATMENTS

When sulfonylureas went off patent, the next generation of diabetes drugs, the thiazolidinediones, entered the scene. Thiazolidinediones, also called glitazones, act on peroxisome proliferator-activated receptors (PPARs) sitting on the DNA of cells. These drugs have a number of effects, including regulation of metabolism. Glitazones reduce sugar production by the liver and increase the sensitivity of cells to insulin. Side effects include infections, headaches, anemia, fluid retention, weight gain, and, more rarely, liver failure or cardiac events.

The first of these medications was troglitazone (Rezulin). Troglitazone was found to be effective in the prevention of type 2 diabetes in at-risk patients but was associated with high rates of liver toxicity. In one trial, 7 out of 585 treated patients had liver elevations ten times that of normal levels, high enough to be potentially associated with fatal liver damage.[2] Based on these results, the study was concluded in 1998 and the drug was taken off the market in 2000.

After the withdrawal of troglitazone because of its liver toxicity, pioglitazone (Actos) and rosiglitazone (Avandia) were the only glitazones used for treating patients with type 2 diabetes, either alone or in combination with metformin or with sulfonylureas. Avandamet is a combination of rosi-glitazone and metformin. Many doctors use glitazones in combination with insulin, which improves glucose control while decreasing the amount of insulin required.

Although the glitazones were never shown to be superior to the sulfo-nylureas and cost ten times as much, successful marketing led to their domination of the playing field for type 2 diabetes. And some of the side effects of these medications can be outright harmful. Important side effects of glitazones are weight gain and fluid retention. Fluid retention can be particularly harmful to patients with heart failure and seems to be worse when glitazones are used in combination with insulin. Metformin can also cause fluid retention and heart failure.

For these reasons the FDA recommends that patients who have diabetes and heart failure should not take glitazones or metformin. In spite of this, these medications are prescribed for 24% of patients with diabetes and heart failure. This was described by Dr. Hannele Yki-Javrinen in an edito-rial in *The Lancet* in 2005 as being due to "the power of marketing over evidence-based medicine in guiding treatment practices." The number of prescriptions for these drugs for heart-failure patients has doubled over the past five years.

A new glitazone, called Muraglitazar, which has been shown to increase the risk of death, heart attack, and stroke by more than twofold,[3] has not been approved by the FDA. Another glitazone, called Rezulin, has been taken off the market because of lethal side effects related to liver damage. There is always concern that whenever there is a major side effect with one drug in a class, other drugs of the same type will have the same side effect. Therefore there is concern that other glitazone drugs have the potential to cause fatal liver damage, although so far the glitazone drugs still on the market have not been associated with an increased risk.

Concerns about the glitazones include the possibility of an increased risk of heart disease and increased weight gain. For instance, in the A Dia-betes Outcome Progression Trial (ADOPT)[4] 4,360 patients with poorly controlled type 2 diabetes were randomly assigned to four years of treatment with rosiglitazone, metformin, or glyburide. Compared to metformin, rosiglitazone had only a minimal increase in the number of patients who maintained glucose control at four years (40% vs. 36%), results that, although statistically significant, were described as "not clinically significant" in a commentary on the article. Rosiglitazone, however, caused more heart failure than glyburide and was associated with more weight gain (+10.6 lb vs. –6.4 lb for metformin) and fluid buildup, or edema (the probable cause of the heart failure). Twenty-two rosiglitazone patients developed heart failure, compared to nineteen with metformin and nine with glyburide.

In the PROspective pioglitAzone Clinical Trial In macroVascular Events (PROactive) Study,[5] 5,238 patients with type 2 diabetes and evidence of vascular disease were randomly assigned to treatment with pioglitazone or placebo as part of their typical treatment regimen. Compared to 572 on placebo, 514 of the pioglitazone patients had a vascular event, including heart attack, stroke, or surgical intervention for vascular disease, which was not a statistically significant difference. Of those who took pioglitazone, 281 developed heart failure, compared to 198 on placebo, a highly statistically significant 42% increase possibly related to the fact that glitazones are known to cause fluid retention. In other words, the drug saved fifty-eight patients from a heart attack or stroke but caused heart failure in 117 (overall not a good trade-off).

Steven Nissen, M.D., and Kathy Wolski, MPH, reported in 2007 in the *New England Journal of Medicine* a 43% increase in heart attacks with Avandia compared to other treatments for diabetes. In other words, a drug given to prevent the consequences of diabetes (including cardiovascular events) actually increases them.

GLITAZONES AND WEIGHT GAIN

Weight gain is one of the most troubling side effects of medications for the treatment of type 2 diabetes. Studies have consistently shown that glitazones cause weight gain. Pioglitazone has been associated with a nine-pound increase in weight as well as an increase in bladder cancer, which was marginally statistically significant. The glitazones inhibit the release of free fatty acids from cells, which can make you, well, more *fatty*. In some cases, these drugs can cause a weight gain of up to a hundred pounds. Since type 2 diabetes is *worsened* by weight gain, this means that the medications that are supposed to treat the condition may be doing just the opposite. Overall there is an eight-pound weight gain with glitazones.

Glitazones actually create fat cells, which may be part of the way they increase weight. Glitazones also cause fluid buildup, a side effect that is at least twice as common when given with insulin, which probably explains why the insulin-glitazone combination has been banned in Europe. For instance, in the Rosiglitazone Clinical Trial, 319 patients with type 2 diabetes were treated with insulin and placebo or with insulin plus rosiglitazone for twenty-six weeks. Of those patients on high-dose rosiglitazone 16% had edema (fluid buildup) vs. 13% on low-dose rosiglitazone and 5% of placebo-treated patients.[6]

STATINS

Diabetics are most definitely at an increased risk for heart disease. This increased risk has led the American Heart Association and the National Cholesterol Education Panel of the National Institutes of Health to call them "heart-disease equivalents," a label that has been used to justify a push for more treatment of diabetics with statins for the prevention of heart attacks as well as their recurrence in diabetics with a history of heart disease. But just because they have a greater risk of heart attacks doesn't mean they will get extra benefit from taking cholesterol-lowering drugs.

Much has been made of a few studies that have shown a reduction of heart attacks in diabetics without heart disease who have been treated with statins.[7, 8] However, more studies have shown no benefit for diabetics without heart disease,[9–11] and some studies in heart-disease patients show that diabetics get *less* benefit from statins than do nondiabetics.[12, 13] Other studies show that patients with heart disease and diabetes derived no more benefit than did patients without diabetes; in fact, when considered alone, the diabetic group did not have a reduction in major cardiovascular outcomes (heart attack, cardiac death, strokes).[14]

Diabetes is one of several risk factors for heart disease, including smoking, diet, high cholesterol, high blood pressure, family history, depression, and stress. I recommend first addressing the risk factors by changing your lifestyle, and by looking at diabetes as one piece of the puzzle in terms of your risk of heart disease. If you have diabetes and heart disease you may benefit from a statin; however, I do not recommend taking statins to treat diabetes if you do not have heart disease. For more on statins, see Chapter 4.

Alternative Medicines

A handful of supplements have been promoted as treatments for diabetes. Study results on these products are inconclusive at best.

CHROMIUM

Chromium, a trace mineral, is an essential nutrient that has been promoted for the prevention and treatment of diabetes based on the fact that chromium deficiency is associated with glucose intolerance. Ten million Americans spend $150 million a year on chromium supplements, making it the best-selling mineral supplement after calcium. However, the mechanism by which chromium relates to glucose is unknown. Chromium concentrations in the body cannot be measured with accuracy, and the amount of normal dietary intake of chromium is uncertain, since such a small amount of chromium is absorbed from food that the actual uptake from food is very difficult to measure.

One uncontrolled study showed improvement on a test that is a marker of the stages leading up to diabetes (called the glucose tolerance test) in three out of six diabetics given 1,000 mcg of chromium and no effect on nondiabetics. Another study compared placebo to trivalent chromium at 200 mcg/day for six weeks, followed by a crossover (placebo patients then took chromium). There was no effect on results of the glucose tolerance test. Another study randomized seventy-six patients with atherosclerotic disease to 250 mcg of chromium chloride or placebo for seven to sixteen months. In the patients with diabetes, there were no differences between the chromium-treated patients and the placebo group.

One study randomly assigned 180 Chinese subjects with type 2 diabetes to two doses of chromium picolinate or placebo for four months. Glucose control was improved with the higher dose of 1,000 mcg/day of chromium, as were measures of blood glucose and insulin levels. This is the only controlled study of chromium, however, that showed any benefit; more controlled studies need to be done to confirm these early results. Also, the fact that this was a Chinese sample means that the results aren't necessarily valid for Americans or Europeans, since there may be differences in nutritional status (i.e., chromium supplementation may be replacing a chromium deficiency in the Chinese). For instance, prior studies showing beneficial effects of selenium, another trace metal, in Chinese could not be replicated in the U.S.

GARLIC

Garlic has been shown to improve glucose control in rat models of diabetes; studies in humans, however, have not shown that garlic improves glucose control. Although garlic was initially promoted for its cholesterol-reducing effect, subsequent research has not confirmed it.

ALA

Alpha lipoic acid (ALA), which is found in liver, potatoes, and broccoli, has no effect on glucose levels. It is, however, prescribed in Germany for diabetic neuropathy. In a three-week German study, 328 patients with type 2 diabetes and diabetic neuropathy received either intravenous ALA or a placebo. The study found a statistically significant improvement in the pain, tingling, and disability related to neuropathy in those who got the ALA. This study also looked at seventy-three of the participants who had type 2 diabetes and cardiac neuropathy and who had taken either oral ALA or placebo. Those who had taken ALA showed an improvement in measures of cardiac heart-rate conductance.

In an attempt to replicate these promising results, a multicenter study was conducted in which 509 patients with diabetic neuropathy received three weeks of intravenous ALA followed by six months of oral ALA or placebo. This time there were no statistically significant differences in ALA vs. placebo in changes in overall symptoms. After three weeks of intravenous ALA or placebo use, however, 120 patients showed a statistically significant change in symptoms. So although there appears to be some benefit from ALA, study results vary, and it is not clear that it has lasting benefit in the case of diabetic neuropathy.

Diet and Behavior

Type 2 diabetes, yet another disease caused by modern living, can be treated by changing the way we live. It might seem like everyone knows that lifestyle changes are important, but many of us just find it too difficult to implement them. In in the course of researching this chapter, I came across a "case study" in a professional medical book that made me think that even professionals can't see the forest for the trees when it comes to treating diabetics. The book, *Psychology and Sociology Applied to Medicine*, 2nd ed. (Churchill Livingstone, 2004, p. 123), which was edited by a group of doctors and health-care workers, tells the story of type 2 diabetic "Stacey," a sixteen-year-old living in the U.K. who loves clubbing with her friends. When she goes dancing (at least she's getting a bit of exercise) and drinks too much, her blood-glucose levels drop, and sometimes the next morning, she has to be rushed, unconscious, to the hospital. If she hasn't passed out, she's described as bad-tempered and uncooperative.

Instead of suggesting that Stacey get some help for her drinking problem (by the way, the legal drinking age in the U.K. is twenty-one; so I am not sure what clubs Stacey frequents), the authors recommend encouraging the young woman "to attend sessions specifically for groups of teenagers with diabetes where they can discuss how to overcome the lifestyle challenges posed by their self-management." As for Stacey's doctor, the writers say that he or she "may be able to suggest an adjustment to her insulin injections on evenings when she is going out." On the other hand, Stacey's dietician "may be able to recommend certain foods Stacey should eat before going out, and snack foods or soft drinks that she could have while clubbing." Finally, "Stacey or her mother could leave a favorite snack conveniently by her bed for when she returns home late." And these words of wisdom end the section: "Parents should not relinquish responsibility for their teenage children's diabetes too soon." Indeed. Stacey should probably stay home instead of engaging in underage, illegal drinking and would be better served by doctors and dieticians (and book authors) who cared more about her future as an alcoholic diabetic. As far as I can tell the authors are serious.

At any rate, teenager or not, it doesn't make sense to up your insulin dosage so you can binge drink or, for that matter, take a pill or inject insulin to treat or prevent a disease that is caused by eating too much. The most important factor in the development of type 2 (adult-onset) diabetes is diet and weight. One important study looked at patients who had what is called impaired glucose tolerance, a condition that often progresses to full-blown type 2 diabetes. At-risk individuals who met with a nutritionist who helped them change their diet and lifestyle (more exercise, less fat and saturated fat, more fiber) *cut their risk of developing diabetes by 58%,* even though they only lost eight pounds on average. Prevention of diabetes with lifestyle intervention was more effective than medication (metformin), with a 58% reduction in new-onset diabetes in at-risk patients, compared to 31% for those taking metformin. Eleven percent of patients on placebo developed diabetes in one year, compared to 8% of those on metformin and 5% of those with the lifestyle intervention.[15] Patients on metformin had more gastrointestinal side effects than those in the other groups.

Diet and exercise are *critical* to the prevention and treatment of type 2 diabetes. If you are overweight, have your doctor give you a glucose tolerance test, which involves measuring the glucose level in your blood before and after you have drunk a glucose (sugar) drink. If your level is too high, that means your body is not processing glucose efficiently and is putting you at risk for diabetes. If the test is positive, you should take it as a serious wake-up call to change your diet and exercise. Remember, even a 10% decrease in weight can have dramatic positive effects.

Finally, if you are at risk for developing type 2 diabetes or have already been diagnosed as having this disease, you should lose weight by replacing simple carbs (like white bread and pasta) with those that take longer to digest, such as whole-wheat noodles and whole-grain bread, legumes, and whole grains. Cut out sugary sodas, candy, and processed and fast foods. Eat lots of leafy greens, colorful vegetables, and fresh fruit. Limit your intake of red meat to once per week and choose only lean cuts. Eat fish or chicken twice a week. Exercise for thirty minutes at least three times a week. First-generation diabetes medications are the least expensive, work just as well as the newer medications, have a better safety profile, and are preferrable to the glitazone medications.

The Bottom Line

The first-line treatment for type 2 diabetes is diet and exercise. If that doesn't work, you should start with the first generation of diabetes medications. They work just as well as the glitazone drugs, are less expensive, and appear to have fewer cardiovascular side effects. If you have a history of heart failure you should not take glitazones or metformin, as they are associated with excessive retention of fluids, which can exacerbate heart failure. I don't see much value in alternative medicine for diabetes treatment, so there are none that I recommend.

Drug	Use	Common, Benign Side Effects	Serious Side Effects	Life-threatening Side Effects	Reasons Not to Take
Sulfonylureas					
Medium Risk					
Glyburide (Micronase, Diabeta)	Diabetes	Nausea, vomiting, metallic taste	Headache, weakness, blurred vision, muscle weakness, weight gain, confusion	Low blood sugar (slurred speech, coma), liver damage, increased death from heart attack	Liver disease, hyper-sensitivity
Chlorpropamide (Diabenese)	Diabetes	Nausea, vomiting, metallic taste	Headache, weakness, blurred vision, muscle weakness, weight gain, confusion	Low blood sugar (slurred speech, coma), liver damage, increased death from heart attack	Liver disease, hyper-sensitivity
Tolbutamine (Orinase)	Diabetes	Nausea, vomiting, metallic taste	Headache, weakness, blurred vision, muscle weakness, weight gain, confusion	Low blood sugar (slurred speech, coma), liver damage, increased death from heart attack	Liver disease, hyper-sensitivity
Glipizide (Glucotrol)	Diabetes	Nausea, vomiting, metallic taste	Headache, weakness, blurred vision, muscle weakness, weight gain, confusion	Low blood sugar (slurred speech, coma), liver damage, increased death from heart attack	Liver disease, hyper-sensitivity
Glimepiride (Amaryl)	Diabetes	Nausea, vomiting, metallic taste	Headache, weakness, blurred vision, muscle weakness, weight gain, confusion	Low blood sugar (slurred speech, coma), liver damage, increased death from heart attack	Liver disease, hyper-sensitivity

Drug	Use	Common, Benign Side Effects	Serious Side Effects	Life-threatening Side Effects	Reasons Not to Take
Biguanides					
Medium Risk					
Metformin (Glucophage)	Diabetes	Bloating, metallic taste	Diarrhea, vomiting, nausea, loss of appetite	Lactic acidosis (may be fatal), vitamin B_{12} deficiency	Liver disease, renal impairment, alcoholism
Glyburide and Metformin (Glucovance)	Diabetes	Bloating, metallic taste	Diarrhea, vomiting, nausea, loss of appetite	Lactic acidosis, vitamin B_{12} deficiency	Liver disease, renal impairment, alcoholism
Thiazolidinediones (glitazones)					
High Risk					
Pioglitazone (Actos)	Diabetes	Headache	Fluid retention, weight gain	Liver failure, anemia, heart failure	Liver disease, heart failure
Rosiglitazone (Avandia)	Diabetes	Headache	Fluid retention, weight gain	Liver failure, anemia, heart failure	Liver disease, heart failure
Rosiglitazone & metformin (Avandamet)	Diabetes	Headache	Fluid retention, weight gain	Liver failure, anemia, heart failure	Liver disease, heart failure

14.

Drugs for Dementia

Alzheimer's disease (AD), a condition associated with memory loss, confusion, spatial orientation problems, mood swings, delusions, and language difficulties, among other symptoms, affects 4 million people in this country alone. Most common in older patients, Alzheimer's lasts on average ten years (largely related to the effect Alzheimer's has on limiting survival). Before the age of sixty-five one in a thousand people will develop Alzheimer's. After sixty-five, it affects one in fifty, and after age eighty the risk is one in five. Nursing-home care is necessary at some point, often at the six-year mark. Risk factors for AD are family history, age, and Down's syndrome.

The condition is caused by the development of plaques in the brain that are filled with something called amyloid. These plaques are concentrated in the parts of the brain that are involved in learning and memory, including the hippocampus, frontal lobe, cingulum, temporal lobe, and parietal cortex. On a chemical level, there is damage to the acetylcholine system, which plays a role in memory vis-à-vis a loss of receptors for this chemical in the hippocampus and other areas.

While AD is present in 60% of patients with dementia, it must be differentiated from mild cognitive impairment (MCI), which may or may not progress to Alzheimer's. Alzheimer's must also be differentiated from frontotemporal dementia, vascular dementia (from small strokes, seen in 15% of patients), and depression, which are not necessarily associated long term with the development of Alzheimer's. Unlike Alzheimer's, dementia is often caused by deficiencies of vitamins B_{12} and folate, which can be treated with vitamin supplementation. However, diagnosing Alzheimer's in its early stages is often difficult.

One of the factors weighing most heavily on families dealing with a loved one who suffers from Alzheimer's is its cost: $16,000 per year for the care of affected patients, including the costs of nursing homes, doctors, and medications. Once a patient with Alzheimer's loses the ability to care for him- or herself, the disorder quickly progresses to a total loss of function and eventual death. Alzheimer's takes a particularly heavy toll on the families of affected patients: Studies show that 80% of caregivers are under heavy stress, and 50% suffer from depression. Given these grim statistics, it is no wonder that families, patients, and their doctors are desperate for treatments for this disorder.

In spite of the fact that there is no cure for Alzheimer's and that there is no hope for a reversal of symptoms if the diagnosis is accurate, patients and their families spend billions of dollars on medications each year in an attempt to do what they can to combat the inevitable onslaught of the decline. At best, the available meds can push memory up a few points on the scale and perhaps buy a year of time, but they can't change the rate of decline or its inevitable conclusion. For some, however, one more year with a loved one can be worth it. I can understand that completely. One year might make all the difference when it comes to a relationship with a parent or spouse. However, I also want you to understand what study results really show for Alzheimer's drugs, so that you understand the limits of what these drugs can really accomplish and for how long.

All of the studies, as discussed here, consistently show about a five-point change on the Alzheimer's Disease Assessment Scale–Cognitive Subsection (ADAS-Cog, a 70-point measure of memory and cognition), a measure of

Alzheimer's-related cognitive impairment, which translates into about a 7% increase in cognition. Let's take a look at what this really means. Here's an example: If I asked you to buy ten items at the grocery store, you would remember seven with the drug and six without it. The increase is just a tweak of the chemical system and doesn't do anything to stop the underlying disease. To paraphrase a colleague's observation, "I don't think it's worth two hundred and fifty dollars per month to name eleven animals in a minute vs. ten animals."

The Medications

Memory loss is one of the most, if not *the* most, devastating results of Alzheimer's. Scientists have been able to pinpoint one of the causes, a loss of acetylcholine function, that is, function of the neurotransmitter involved in learning and memory, and this has led to a rush to develop drugs to counter its decline.

TACRINE

Tacrine (Cognex), the first result of these efforts, inhibits the enzyme (acetylcholine esterase) that breaks down acetylcholine in the brain. In a thirty-week trial of tacrine vs. placebo, 653 patients with AD started treatment, but only 263 finished the study. ADAS-Cog scores started at 29 in both groups, improved two points with tacrine, and lost 2 points with placebo, a statistically significant difference.[1] Another study randomized 663 Alzheimer's patients to thirty weeks of treatment with tacrine or placebo, after which patients were treated with tacrine and were so informed (placebo comparisons were stopped), then followed up for two years or more. At two years there was a threefold increase in the risk of nursing-home placement for those in the placebo group vs. the patients treated with tacrine.[2]

The widespread use of tacrine has been hindered by its liver toxicity, which requires patients to undergo repeated blood tests to measure liver function. Elevations in liver enzymes usually occur in the first few weeks after starting the medication. Half of patients will have elevations of liver function, with a third of those having elevations that are three times normal. This is usually the point where doctors stop the drug and allow enzyme levels to return to normal. Tacrine-induced liver elevations do not appear to lead to chronic liver problems if the medication is stopped.[3] When most patients resume taking the medication, they don't experience a repeat elevation of liver enzymes. Other common side effects of the drug are nausea, which occurs in a third of patients, and stomach upset. In the first study mentioned above, nausea, liver-enzyme elevations, and stomach upset caused about 70% of patients to stop using tacrine within the first few months of treatment.

DONEPEZIL

Tacrine's impact on the liver and the accompanying inconvenience of repeated blood testing led researchers to create a drug that eliminated both problems. The result, donepezil (Aricept), is now the best-selling Alzheimer's drug, with close to $1 billion per year in annual sales. Donepezil inhibits acetylcholinesterase without causing liver toxicity.

In one study, 431 patients with AD were randomized to one year of donepezil or placebo. Compared to placebo, donepezil was shown to delay symptoms of cognitive-function decline in Alzheimer's patients by five months. After one year, Mini Mental Status Exam (MMSE), a thirty-point scale that measures memory and cognitive function scores went from 17 to 18 with donepezil and remained at seventeen with placebo, a difference that was not statistically significant.[4] Most common side effects were diarrhea (17%), nausea (9%), headache (9%), and runny nose (12%). There were no patients with liver abnormalities. About a quarter of the study group dropped out from both the placebo and donepezil groups because there was no improvement in their memory. MMSE scores went from 18 to 20 with donepezil and 18 to 17 with placebo, a statistically significant difference.

In another study 286 patients who possibly or probably had Alzheimer's were randomized to take either donepezil or placebo for one year. Patients were assessed with the Gottfries-Brane-Steen Scale, a measure of dementia severity with scores ranging from 0 to 162. Their GBS score went from 30 to 17 with placebo and 30 to 22 with donepezil, a difference that wasn't statistically significant. Also, their MMSE (a thirty-point scale) went from 19 to 17 with placebo and remained at 19 with donepezil, which is also not statistically significant.[5] In another study, 290 patients with Alzheimer's were randomized to take either donepezil or placebo for twenty-four weeks. The donepezil-treated patients went from 12 to 13, while the placebo-treated patients remained at 12 on the thirty-point MMSE.[6] Alzheimer's patients did not show a decline in mental function for the first thirty-eight weeks of treatment.[7] Other studies, however, have not shown a delay in the onset of nursing-home care or disability. One recent study showed a delay in cognitive decline from mild cognitive decline to Alzheimer's in the first year but no effect after three years.[8]

Based on the evidence, in 2006 the British National Institute of Clinical Excellence (NICE) recommended that donepezil not be used for the treatment of severe or mild Alzheimer's because its modest efficacy did not justify its side effects and expense. This naturally stirred up a firestorm of controversy, with the pharmaceutical industry arguing that NICE was advocating withholding medication from patients with severe Alzheimer's to save money for the British health-care system.

In response to the controversy about whether patients with severe Alzheimer's should get medications, a study of 248 patients with severe Alzheimer's disease living in nursing homes was performed. Patients were randomized to take donepezil or placebo for six months. On the Severe Impairment Battery, which is a one-hundred-point measurement of cognitive impairment, donepezil-treated patients went from 54 to 57, while placebo patients went from 57 to 55, a statistically significant difference. On the Alzheimer's Disease Cooperative Study–Activities of Daily Living (ADCS-ADL) scale, a fifty-four-point measure of complex abilities, donepezil-treated patients went from 14 to 13 and those on placebo from 14 to 11, also statistically significant.[9] Although these results are statistically significant, they are along the lines of being able to name eleven animals instead of ten; in other words, not that meaningful in light of the severe side effects that have to be endured and the fact that these drugs have no effect on the trajectory of the disease.

RIVASTIGMINE

Another drug in this class is rivastigmine (Exelon), which inhibits both acetylcholinesterase and butyrylcholinesterase enzymes. In one study, 345 patients were randomized to take either rivastigmine or placebo for twenty-six weeks, followed by twenty-six weeks of open-label treatment, meaning the patients knew they were getting the medication. Rivastigmine delayed the cognitive decline of AD and led to a five-point difference from placebo on the seventy-item ADAS-Cog.[10] These results are no better than those of donepezil or any of the other Alzheimer's drugs. Side effects are headache, nausea, diarrhea, insomnia, and dizziness.

GALANTAMINE

Galantamine (Reminyl) is an acetylcholinesterase inhibitor that modulates the nicotinic acetylcholine receptor. This receptor binds the neurotransmitter acetylcholine, which plays a critical role in learning and memory. In one study, 978 patients with Alzheimer's were randomized to take either placebo or galantamine at different doses for five months. The ADAS-Cog (with a range of 0 to 70), which measures memory and cognition, showed a two-point improvement with galantamine and a two-point decline with placebo. There were also improvements (or lack of deterioration) in the study doctors' judgment of overall function and behavior.[11]

Another study randomized 636 Alzheimer's patients to galantamine or placebo for six months, followed by six months of open treatment. ADAS-Cog scores, which were 26 at baseline in both groups, improved two points with galantamine and declined two points with placebo, a four-point difference on the seventy-point scale that measures memory and cognition.

Galantamine basically pushed patients up a notch in terms of function, but then they continued to deteriorate over a year at the same rate as patients on placebo. At the end of the year, they were back to where they started, while the placebo group was worse, but both were continuing to get worse at the same rate.[12] Galantamine did not have a better effect on cognition than that of other previously studied Alzheimer's drugs. As with Cognex, a third of patients developed nausea or vomiting, and about a third of patients dropped out because of side effects. Galantamine was not associated with liver abnormalities, unlike Cognex.

WEIGHING THE RISKS

Study results that are just now emerging are cause for more concern regarding Alzheimer's-specific drugs. The *New York Times* reported on March 17, 2006, on a study which at that time had not yet been published (Gardner Harris, "Study for Alzheimer's Drug Revives Questions on Risk"), which showed that of 974 patients with Alzheimer's who were treated with donepezil (Aricept) or placebo, eleven in the Aricept group died, but there were no deaths in the placebo group. This difference was statistically significant. A similar significant increase in deaths was previously reported for Reminyl.

Overall the efficacy of acetylcholinesterase inhibitors, a two- to four-point change on a seventy-point scale, is questionable for these drugs, which also have potential side effects. They also do not prevent the progression of the disease. Based on these findings, Hanna Kaduszkiewicz, M.D., and colleagues at the University of Hamburg Medical Center, have written in *BMJ* that "because of flawed methods and small clinical benefits, the scientific basis for recommendations of cholinesterase inhibitors for the treatment of Alzheimer's disease is questionable."[13]

HORMONE TREATMENT

For many years people believed that estrogen and progesterone prevented the development of Alzheimer's disease, benefited the cognitive dysfunction of AD patients, and improved memory function in normal people or delayed the normal decline of memory with aging. However, when carefully assessed in the Women's Health Initiative (WHI) study, a placebo-controlled randomized trial (the best way to resolve this in my opinion), estrogen and progesterone were found to actually double the risk of dementia.[14] In other studies, estrogen and progesterone resulted in no changes,[15] a small but not clinically significant reduction in cognition,[16] or a worsening of cognition.[17, 18] At this time estrogen is not recommended for the treatment or prevention of AD.

PSYCHOTROPIC MEDS

Recently there has been a disturbing trend of prescribing antipsychotics for the elderly. In fact, statistics show that antipsychotic medications are being prescribed for one quarter of the Medicare beneficiaries in nursing homes. In spite of the fact that these drugs should not be used to treat dementia in the absence of a psychotic disorder, only one quarter of elderly patients on antipsychotics actually have a psychotic disorder. In other words, the majority of those antipsychotic prescriptions currently being written are inappropriate for elderly patients without an indication for treatment with an antipsychotic, namely hallucinations or delusion. In addition, the risk of side effects like diabetes and lipid elevations is greater for older patients using these powerful drugs. The FDA recently warned that the use of atypical antipsychotic medication doubles the risk of death in the elderly.

In some cases Alzheimer's patients can experience symptoms of aggression, hallucinations, delusions, disorganized thoughts, and bizarre behavior, all of which may be treatable with antipsychotic medications. However, antipsychotic medications should only be used for Alzheimer's patients who are psychotic. Despite this caveat, they are still being used to calm or in other ways control Alzheimer's patients or other elderly people with a dementia condition.

The typical antipsychotic medications block the dopamine-2 receptor in the brain, which is believed to be one of the factors involved in the symptoms of psychosis. Probably more important is the sedating effect of anti-psychotics (previously known as "major tranquilizers"), which makes their use for Alzheimer's patients with agitated behavior very seductive.

The antipsychotic drugs developed for schizophrenia are actually used just as much or more in elderly patients with dementia. One study of all the studies of antipsychotics for the treatment of behavioral problems in demented patients found data on 3,353 patients randomized to an antipsychotic and 1,757 randomized to placebo that revealed a 1.2% absolute increase in the death of those patients on antipsychotics. The authors concluded that treatment of demented patients with antipsychotics may be associated with an increased risk of death.

The first generation of antipsychotic medications, which includes thorazine, haloperidol, mellaril, and trilafon, is associated with troubling extrapyramidal side effects, including twitching, jerking movements, and lip smacking. They also have anticholinergic side effects and may interfere with memory in the elderly.

The second generation of atypical antipsychotic meds—newer, more expensive antipsychotics—blocks a range of different dopamine receptors in addition to others like the serotonin receptors. It is thought that this mechanism of action is the reason they are not associated with extrapyramidal side effects. The first atypical, clozaril, has been associated in rare cases with agranulocytosis, a fatal condition in which the body stops making blood cells and immune cells. For this reason, patients on clozaril have to have their blood checked frequently. Other atypicals, including olanzepine, risperidal, and quetiapine, have fewer neurological side effects. These medications have not, however, been without their own problems: They can interfere with glucose metabolism, increasing the tendency to develop adult-onset (type 2) diabetes and in rare cases ketoacidosis;[19] they also increase lipids and cause weight gain, all of which can increase the risk of heart disease. Use of olanzepine, clozaril, risperidal, and the atypical antipsychotics has been associated with an increase in diabetes but less so with risperidal. There are conflicting results for quetiapine.[20]

The risk of death when using typical antipsychotics was even higher than that with atypical antipsychotics. Risperidal and quetiapine were associated with a twofold increase in stroke in patients with dementia. Moreover, neither quetiapine nor risperidal were effective for the treatment of agitation in elderly demented patients, and quetiapine was associated with a more rapid cognitive decline over time than was placebo. As I mentioned above, antipsychotic drugs should not be used to control the behavior of elderly people unless they are really suffering from psychosis (e.g., seeing or hearing things that aren't there); they have not been shown to be helpful, and they increase the risk of death.

The increased risk of stroke in elderly patients with dementia who take olanzepine prompted the Canadian Drug Regulatory authorities to send a letter to doctors in Canada warning them of this potential danger. The FDA, however, has sent no such letter to American doctors, many of whom are unaware of the risks and the recommendation to cease using atypical antipsychotics for behavioral symptoms in demented elderly patients. I recommend that patients with Alzheimer's or other forms of dementia should not be given antipsychotic drugs unless they have clear forms of psychosis (e.g., seeing or hearing things that are not there or having frank delusions or incorrect beliefs) as outlined in the *Diagnostic and Statistical Manual of Mental Disorders.*

NONSTEROIDAL ANTI-INFLAMMATORY DRUGS

There is some question about whether nonsteroidal anti-inflammatory drugs (NSAIDs) prevent the development of Alzheimer's. With risks of their own, these medications should not be used for Alzheimer's prevention or treatment.

ANTIDEPRESSANTS

Patients with Alzheimer's often have symptoms of depression that can be treated with antidepressant medications. An antidepressant drug in the monoamine oxidase inhibitor (MAOI) class that is often used is selegiline

(Eldepryl). Overall, studies have not shown this medication to be effective for treating mood or cognitive problems in AD. Side effects include hypertensive crisis (the blood pressure suddenly becomes very high, to the point at which it can become a medical emergency) when patients eat high-tyramine foods like cheese, wine, or beer. Pretty much all classes of psychotropic medications, including all antidepressants, antipsychotics, and mood-stabilizing drugs, have been used for Alzheimer's, although none have been shown to have specific efficacy.

The anticholinergic side effects of the tricyclic antidepressants are especially bad for patients with dementia and the elderly, since they are more susceptible to the memory-impairing effects of these medications. For this reason the tricyclics amitriptyline and doxepin should not be prescribed for the elderly. In spite of this, these two medications make up the most common inappropriately prescribed medications for the elderly, making up 23% of all such medications (21% of the medications prescribed for the elderly are considered to be inappropriate based on criteria outlined by Paton and Ferrier in the *British Medical Journal* in 2005).

Alternative Medicines

A variety of herbs and supplements, including an assortment of vitamins and gingko biloba, have been touted as improving memory and cognition or the ability to concentrate.

VITAMINS

Early on, vitamin E and its antioxidant properties were thought to lessen the inflammatory effects of plaque formation in the brains of Alzheimer's patients. However, studies have not found vitamin E to be beneficial for arresting the progression of cognitive impairment due to Alzheimer's.

The use of B vitamins has also been advocated as a way to improve cognition because high levels of the amino acid homocysteine have been seen in patients with Alzheimer's disease. Since homocysteine is involved in vitamin B pathways, it was felt that lowering homocysteine with vitamin B therapy would lead to an improvement in cognition. In one study, 276 healthy people over age sixty-five with elevated homocysteine concentrations were given folate and vitamins B_{12} and B_6 or a placebo. Neither folate nor vitamin B supplementation resulted in an improvement in scores of cognition after two years.[21]

GINKGO BILOBA

Ginkgo biloba, a supplement derived from the ancient ginkgo tree of China, has long been believed to increase memory, energy, and concentration. It is also used to treat tinnitus and vascular disease. Many consider ginkgo a neuroprotective agent as well as an antioxidant. In Germany, more than 5 million prescriptions for ginkgo are written every year, and sales in the U.S. are $240 million per year. Studies have shown some benefit in patients with dementia, although the effects on cognitive test scores were no greater than the modest effects of anticholinesterase inhibitors and were not associated with a subjective impression of improvement by families and doctors.[22] The manufacturers, however, promote ginkgo for the enhancement of memory in normal individuals or for prevention of the normal decline of memory with aging. A recent large controlled trial using a large battery of tests found no effect of ginkgo on memory function in normal individuals.[23] Ginkgo can have serious side effects, including coma, bleeding, and seizures. It should not be used with medications that are used to decrease blood clotting, like warfarin. Minor but more common side effects include nausea, vomiting, diarrhea, headaches, and dizziness.

THE BOTTOM LINE

I don't think any of the medications currently available, including vitamins and supplements, are worth giving to anyone affected by Alzheimer's or other types of dementia. It's just not going to make a substantial difference in their condition, and will not stop its progression. Only in severe cases of actual psychosis (which is very rare) would there be a need for antipsychotic treatment. If your family member is uncontrollable at home, you may need to consider a nursing home. If the nursing home staff feels your loved one is uncontrollable, they will most likely want to give him or her antipsychotics; you may need to put your foot down and insist that they not do so. I also urge you to join one of the many groups and organizations for families dealing with Alzheimer's; sharing frustrations and experiences with those who can relate and sympathize can provide some comfort and support.

Drug	Use	Common, Benign Side Effects	Serious Side Effects	Life-threatening Side Effects	Reasons Not to Take
Acetylcholinesterase Inhibitors					
Moderate Risk					
Tacrine (Cognex)	Dementia	Nausea, vomiting	Stomach upset, diarrhea, rash	Liver damage, seizures, irregular heart rate	Liver dysfunction
Donepezil (Aricept)	Dementia	Nausea, vomiting, headache, runny nose, muscle cramps, drowsiness	Diarrhea	Irregular heart rate, fainting	Allergy to drug

Drug	Use	Common, Benign Side Effects	Serious Side Effects	Life-threatening Side Effects	Reasons Not to Take
Acetylcholinesterase and Butyrylcholinesterase Inhibitors					
Moderate Risk					
Rivastigmine (Exelon)	Dementia	Headache, nausea, diarrhea, insomnia, dizziness	Vertigo, agitation, rash, confusion	Arrhythmias, stomach bleeding, depression, hallucinations	Hyper-sensitivity, pregnancy, breast-feeding, ulcer
Acetylcholinesterase Inhibitors and Nicotinic Modulators					
Moderate Risk					
Galantamine (Reminyl)	Dementia	Nausea, vomiting, loss of appetite	Diarrhea, dizziness	Fainting, irregular heart rate, stomach bleeding	Allergy to drug
Antidepressants					
Low Risk					
Selegiline (Eldepryl)	Depression in dementia	Nausea, vomiting, sore throat	Headache, blurred vision, dizziness, hallucinations, agitation	Wine and cheese hypertensive crisis, allergic reaction	Allergy to drug

15.

Antidepressants

The urban psychiatrist's office is quiet and comfortable: a brightly colored Turkish kilim on the whitewashed wide plank floors and creamy yellow walls soften the clean lines of the modern leather sofa-and-chair set. The patient is soothed by the surroundings, and chats calmly with the doctor. In the corner of this iconic, upscale shrink's office sits a woman, listening intently, observing, and taking notes. Is she a graduate student learning from a mentor? A newly minted doctor absorbing therapeutic technique from an experienced pro? None of the above. In fact, this scenario is one example of the drug-company practice of paying doctors to allow their salespeople to sit in on doctor-patient sessions in what they call "shadowing." Although ostensibly the purpose of this practice is to "train" the product representatives, the real reason is to find out why patients are not being prescribed their medicines and to influence prescribing behavior.

Shadowing is a required part of the job of drug sales representatives, and while it involves being intimately involved in the therapy of a patient, former salespeople confirmed that there was no oath or directive protecting any patient confidences. Dr. David Fassler, who testified about the practice in front of a governing committee of the American Medical Association, said, "As child and adolescent psychiatrists, we were also particularly concerned when we learned that this kind of shadowing was occurring in situations involving young children, since issues of informed consent are even more complex with younger patients."

Fassler introduced Barbara Felt-Miller, a former drug company sales rep who had been required to engage in shadowing. As quoted in the *Psychiatric Times* on July 18, 2003, she said, "I was never trained to view a human body like a physician does. I personally found sitting in on an exam embarrassing."

The pharmaceutical industry has wiggled its way into psychiatrists' offices in more ways than one. Steve Sharfstein, M.D. (*Psychiatric Times*, August 19, 2005), the president of the American Psychiatric Association, now bemoans the fact that the "bio-psycho-social" model has given way to the "bio-bio-bio" model, where there is a total focus on medication to the exclusion of other treatments, such as various forms of talking therapy; exercise, which works for depression, as I describe later; or working with families.

Consequently, it's not surprising that the market for antidepressants is fast growing and currently brings in $14 billion a year to the pharmaceutical industry. With managed care limiting the time and visits available for people with depression, it has become increasingly easier to whip out a prescription pad than to take the time required for psychotherapy. Other pressures are also behind the increase in antidepressant prescriptions. Direct-to-consumer advertising in the U.S. is also driving up antidepressant usage. Interestingly, by making consumers more likely to talk to their doctors about going on a medication, when patients ask for an antidepressant, they get it 76% of the time compared to patients with the same symptoms who don't ask to go on antidepressants, who are given antidepressant prescriptions only 31% of the time.

Antidepressants are approved by the FDA for the treatment of several disorders in addition to depression. These include posttraumatic stress disorder (PTSD), obsessive-compulsive disorder (OCD), panic disorder, and social phobia as well as the depressed stage of bipolar disorder. Some anti-depressants are also approved for smoking cessation and premenstrual syndrome. Symptoms of depression that are responsive to medication include decreased interest in things, persistent sadness or feelings of depression that occur most of the day over weeks at a time, thoughts of suicide, hopelessness, feelings of worthlessness, decreased energy, loss of appetite, agitation, sleep disturbance, problems concentrating, and low self-esteem.

Antidepressants and How They Work

Theories of how the brain mediates depression involve alterations of the serotonin and norepinephrine systems. Drugs that increase brain levels of the neurotransmitters serotonin and norepinephrine have both been shown to work for depression. Antidepressants typically bind to proteins, called transporters, that are responsible for taking the neurotransmitters back up into the neurons after they have been released into the spaces between the neurons, called the synapses. Drugs that block uptake of the neurotransmitters by the transporter result in an increase in the neurotransmitters in the synapses, which is believed to account for at least part of the reason these drugs work. Many of the antidepressant drugs block the serotonin transporter, the norepinephrine transporter, or a combination of the two. The original drugs, the tricyclics, had a more general effect on blockage of neurotransmitter uptake.

EARLY TREATMENT

The first medication found to work for the treatment of depression was discovered by accident. A drug called imipramine (Tofranil), developed in the 1940s for the treatment of tuberculosis, helped a number of the depressed patients on the tuberculosis wards in terms of their depression (if not their tuberculosis). This led psychiatrists in France, and later the U.S., to try this drug on patients hospitalized for depression. This was the birth of the tricyclic medications.

Tricyclics, which include doxepin (Sinequan), amoxapine (Asendin), and amitriptyline (Elavil), increase norepinephrine and serotonin levels in the synapses (the spaces between the nerve cells in the brain). The main problem with the tricyclics is their anticholinergic side effects: dry mouth, constipation, memory problems, confusion, blurred vision, sexual dysfunction, and decreased urination. Other problems include heart arrhythmias and blood pressure drops. Elavil is associated with the worst of these problems and probably shouldn't be used.

The anticholinergic side effects of the tricyclics are especially bad for the elderly, who are more susceptible to the memory-impairing effects of these medications. Anticholinergic side effects include dry mouth, trouble urinating, cognitive problems, vision problems, and decreased perspiration. Despite these serious side effects, doctors commonly prescribe the tricyclics amitriptyline and doxepin for the elderly. Twenty-one percent of the medications given to the elderly are believed to be inappropriate, and one out of every four of these inappropriate medications is amitriptyline or doxepin.

NOREPINEPHRINE REUPTAKE INHIBITORS

Other drugs that have been developed specifically to block reuptake of norepinephrine into the synapses include desipramine (Norpramin) and nortriptyline (Aventyl, Pamelor). They have less-severe anticholinergic side effects and effects on the heart and blood pressure than newer medications like the SSRIs.

MAOIs

Drugs that block the monoamine oxidase inhibitor enzyme (MAOI drugs) and therefore boost the monoamines (serotonin, norepinephrine) include phenelzine (Nardil) and tranylcypromine (Parnate). Because they can cause a "wine-and-cheese reaction" of potentially life-threatening elevations of blood pressure if taken with foods that are high in tyramine content, which include wine, cheese, chocolate, and beer, they are not used much anymore.

ANTIDEPRESSANTS WITH NOVEL MECHANISMS OF ACTION

Some drugs act on various neurotransmitter systems or in general are poorly understood in terms of mechanism of action. These include bupro-prion (Wellbutrin), which acts primarily on dopamine systems and is used for both depression and smoking cessation (under the brand name Zyban, which is identical to buproprion, which can be bought in generic form for a lower price). Side effects include weight loss and restlessness. There are rare cases of seizures with high doses of Wellbutrin.

Drugs with mixed actions are trazodone (Desyrel) and maprotiline (Ludiomil), which have less-severe anticholinergic side effects and effects on the heart and blood pressure than Desyrel. In rare cases Desyrel can cause priapism (extended painful erection that requires emergency treatment).

Nefazodone (Serzone) has both serotonin reuptake inhibition and post-synaptic serotonin receptor blockade properties. It blocks the reuptake of serotonin into the neuron, and it also blocks a receptor for serotonin on the neuron on the receiving end. It therefore has a chemically unique mode of action. Nefazodone has been associated with several cases of liver failure, which can be fatal. It also affects the fetus in animal studies; humans should not take it during pregnancy. Other side effects include dry mouth, nausea, headache, and upset stomach. Given the alternatives of antidepressants that do not cause liver failure and are just as effective, Serzone should not be used except as a last resort.

Mirtazapine (Remeron) is a quatrocyclic antidepressant that acts on a number of different receptor systems and increases release of norepineph-rine and serotonin. Side effects include sweating and shivering, tiredness, strange dreams, elevation of lipids, weight gain, upset stomach, anxiety, and agitation. Mirtazapine works well for depression and is safe.

Selective Serotonin Reuptake Inhibitors (SSRIs)

As the tricyclics went off patent, a new generation of drugs called selective serotonin reuptake inhibitors (SSRIs) was pushed as being better, since they acted specifically on the serotonin transporter and therefore didn't have many of the side effects that were said to result from the effects of nonspecifics on many neurochemical systems.

These medications, which include fluoxetine (Prozac, Sarafem), paroxetine (Paxil), fluvoxamine (Luvox), citalopram (Celexa), and sertraline (Zoloft), act by blocking the transporter that brings the serotonin back from the spaces between the neurons (synapses) into the neurons, effectively increasing the levels of serotonin in the synapses. Fluoxetine, paroxetine, sertraline, and other SSRIs are free of anticholinergic side effects as well as effects on blood pressure and the heart. Contrary to popular belief, however, the newer generation of antidepressants doesn't work any better than the old ones, with the possible exception of the dual reuptake inhibitors, which may work better but have their own problems, which I discuss later.

The primary advantages of SSRIs are a questionable decrease in the number and severity of side effects and the fact that you can't take a fatal overdose. However, dropout rates are no greater than with the old drugs, which suggests that the new side effects can be just as bad as the old ones. In general the sexual dysfunction and jitteriness that come with the SSRIs can be just as bad as the sedation and dry mouth that come with the old drugs. The success of the SSRIs has been mainly a triumph of marketing.

All SSRIs work in the same way and differ only in properties such as how strongly they bind to the serotonin transporter, how long they remain in the bloodstream, and how they are metabolized. Escitalopram (Lexapro), which is essentially the same as citalopram (Celexa), was brought on the market in 2002 because Celexa was going off patent. It costs much more than generic citalopram, and there is no reason why it should be used instead of the less-expensive and equally effective citalopram.

EFFICACY

The SSRI medications have not been shown to work better than the older tricyclics. In fact, they are actually less effective than is commonly believed.[1] The Danish Study Group found that the older tricyclic medication clomipramine worked better for severe depression than paroxetine, although it had more side effects. A review from fifteen years ago showed that fluoxetine was only modestly more effective than placebo, with more than 80% of the improvement accounted for by a placebo effect.[2] A more recent meta-analysis from data submitted to the FDA showed that 80% of the improvement with antidepressants comes from the placebo response. When the data from all of the studies performed on venlafaxine (Effexor), fluoxetine (Prozac), and nefazodone (Serzone) were lumped together, there was only about a two-point improvement on a fifty-six-point scale (the twenty-one-question Hamilton Depression Scale) above and beyond the placebo response. The conclusion was that the effects of antidepressants are modest, if even real, but that it is not ethical to give a placebo.

It was also pointed out that the efficacy of SSRIs is greater than that of medications used for other purposes, like statins. Others have argued that SSRIs may not be much better than placebo but that the relapse rate is much higher on placebo. However, studies following patients who were treated with antidepressants did not show that they did better over the long haul. In fact, they may have done worse, even accounting for baseline differences in symptom severity.[3] There are no studies showing that in the long run people treated with antidepressants are better off. It might be questioned whether a two-point increase on a fifty-six-point scale that may not be sustainable is a clinically meaningful improvement.

Worry over the efficacy of SSRIs prompted a reexamination of the efficacy of antidepressants in general as well as a reconsideration of the theory that placebos may work just as well. A meta-analysis showed that there was a highly variable response to placebos, up to 50%, and that the placebo-response rate in studies of depression seemed to be growing over the years. In addition, studies by private research firms seemed to be showing higher placebo-response rates than those in studies by universities, suggesting that there were differences in populations, assessments, or inducements for participation.

SIDE EFFECTS

Side effects of SSRIs include nausea, diarrhea, headache, insomnia, and agitation. One of the most troubling side effects of the SSRIs is sexual dysfunction, which affects about a third of patients. This includes loss of libido, delayed ejaculation, and erectile dysfunction. The antidepressants that don't have this side effect, like Wellbutrin, can be given in addition to an SSRI or substituted for it. Other antidepressants without sexual side effects include Remeron and Desyrel, drugs not in the SSRI class.

SSRI treatment is also associated with about a threefold increase in the risk of gastrointestinal bleeding. Although for the average patient there typically is not an increased risk of bleeding, if you are taking aspirin or another NSAID you should be on another medication like Prilosec to protect your stomach.

In my clinical experience as a psychiatrist, I have found there to be a real but small risk of a condition called akathisia, a feeling of internal restlessness and agitation, associated with changes in doses of SSRIs, which can lead to suicidal thoughts and behavior. No one has yet shown that SSRIs increase the rates of *completed* or "successful" suicides in either adults or children. But one reason for the increased agitation is that the recommended starting dose is often too high. I recommend starting at half the recommended dose and moving patients up very gradually.

Akathisia is also treatable with Valium and other benzodiazepine drugs (sedatives), and I don't think that doctors should be afraid to use them for a limited time. In addition, the risk of suicidal thinking and suicide appears to be much higher for those with conditions other than isolated major depression, so it is important to not use SSRIs too freely. Unfortunately we live in an era in which SSRIs are handed out like candy at the general practitioner's office, and we need to change that. If SSRIs are prescribed, I think it should be done under the careful monitoring of a psychiatrist and in conjunction with regular talking sessions.

A more troubling problem is the potential for suicide that is associated with SSRIs. The FDA has recently warned that SSRI antidepressants may increase the risk of suicidal thoughts or suicide. A recent meta-analysis of studies of adults taking SSRIs showed no increase in suicidal thoughts or attempts, while there was a 57% increase in nonfatal self-harm with SSRIs that was of borderline statistical significance. However, another meta-analysis showed a greater than twofold increase in fatal and nonfatal suicide attempts in patients on SSRI vs. placebo, and in those on SSRIs compared to other nonmedication treatments. The risk was 5.6 per 1,000 patient years (the number of years people take the drug times the number of patients). In other words, if one hundred people each took an SSRI for ten years, about five of them would make a suicide attempt that they wouldn't have if they hadn't been on an SSRI.

There was no difference, however, between SSRIs and the older tricyclic antidepressants, suggesting that *all* antidepressant medications may carry an increased risk of suicide. Questions about suicidal thinking with antidepressants have been around for years, and occurred with the tricyclics. Some doctors, including my father (who is a retired psychiatrist), offer the explanation that the increase in energy that antidepressants experience often gives the suicidal patient enough stamina to go through with the act.

Another disturbing trend that came from this analysis was the change in suicidal thoughts over time. In the U.S. there are 24.5 million doctor visits for depression per year, a 70% increase from fifteen years ago. Sixty-nine percent of these visits result in a prescription for an antidepressant. The analysis showed that the risk of suicidal thinking and suicide itself has been gradually increasing over the years. It is unclear whether this is the result of an increase in the number of antidepressant prescriptions by primary-care physicians or other causes.

Antidepressants and Pregnancy

The use of antidepressants during pregnancy is controversial, to say the least. In one study of 228 pregnant women who had been exposed to fluoxetine and compared to matched controls, there was no difference in pregnancy loss or major birth anomalies. There was an increase in minor birth anomalies in the women who were treated with fluoxetine (16% vs. 7%). However, exposure to fluoxetine in the third trimester was associated with a ninefold increase in jitteriness (tremors, irritability, agitation, and respiratory distress) as well as an increase in premature delivery.

Another study of 377 women compared those who each had a baby with primary pulmonary hypertension (PPH) to those women with non-PPH babies. Compared to the controls, the women with babies with PPH had a sixfold increase in the use of SSRI antidepressants after the twentieth week of pregnancy. The SSRIs (which included paroxetine, fluoxetine, sertraline, and citalopram) most often associated with the PPH were paroxetine and sertraline (fluoxetine did not show an effect). Women who stop their medication, however, have a greater than threefold increased risk of suffering a relapse of depression.

Dual Reuptake Inhibitors (SNRIs)

The latest group of antidepressants, the serotonin and norepinephrine, or dual, reuptake inhibitors (SNRIs), includes venlafaxine (Effexor) and duloxetine (Cymbalta), which generally have shown a better treatment response for depression than have the SSRIs and tricyclics. In one study, investigators looked at data from a number of randomized, placebo-controlled trials of Effexor, tricyclic antidepressants, and SSRIs for the treatment of depression. Treatment response was defined as a 50% reduction in symptoms of depression. Forty-four studies with 4,033 patients were included. Overall, venlafaxine had a success rate of 74%, which was statistically significantly better than that of the SSRIs, which had only a 61% success rate, and the tricyclics, which had only a 58% success rate. The difference in the efficacy of tricyclics and that of SSRIs was not statistically significant. However, it is worth noting that a larger number of patients dropped out of treatment while on tricyclics because of side effects. Other studies have shown better responses for venlafaxine and duloxetine than for tricyclics and SSRIs.

Both venlafaxine and duloxetine can cause dizziness, constipation, dry mouth, headache, changes in sleep, and, more rarely, a serotonin syndrome with restlessness, shivering, and sweating. A decrease in saliva can cause cavities. Venlafaxine has also been associated with a dose-dependent increase in blood pressure. And venlafaxine seems to carry the greatest risk of suicide of all the antidepressants, with a threefold increased risk of attempted or completed suicides.

Mood-Stabilizing Agents

Mood-stabilizing agents are used conventionally in the treatment of epilepsy, but they may also be effective in the stabilization of mood in patients with psychiatric disorders, especially patients with bipolar disorder.

Bipolar disorder (formerly known as manic-depressive disorder) is a condition that affects more than 2 million Americans. People who have this illness tend to experience extreme mood swings, along with other specific symptoms and behaviors. These mood swings, or "episodes," can take three forms: manic episodes, depressive episodes, or "mixed" episodes. The symptoms of a manic episode often include elevated mood (feeling extremely happy), extreme irritability and anxiety, talking too fast and too much, an unusual increase in energy, and a reduced need for sleep. It's also very common for someone to act impulsively during a manic episode and to engage in behaviors that are risky or that they later regret, like spending sprees. And in more than half of all manic episodes, people are troubled by delusions or hallucinations. For example, they may think they have a relationship with someone famous, claim to be an expert in an area they really know nothing about, feel paranoid (unusually fearful), or hear voices that are not there. The symptoms of a depressive episode often include an overwhelming feeling of emptiness or sadness, a lack of energy, a loss of interest in things, trouble concentrating, changes in normal sleep or appetite, and/or thoughts of dying or suicide.

It is not known exactly how mood-stabilizing drugs work for bipolar disorder, but many of them modulate the function of the excitatory amino acid glutamate, a brain neurotransmitter that plays a critical role in memory and has been implicated in both epilepsy and mood and anxiety disorders. Mood-stabilizing agents, which include valproic acid (Valproate), carbamazepine (Tegretol), topiramate (Topomax), lamotrigine (Lamictal), phenytoin (Dilantin), and neurontin (Gabapentin), are commonly used in clinical practice, often in combination with SSRI medications, since psychiatrists commonly add psychotropic medications from different classes of drugs if patients don't respond to treatment. Valproate can cause potentially fatal liver failure, although it very rarely does so.

Lamictal, which has been shown to be helpful in cases of bipolar disorder, can cause Stevens-Johnson's syndrome, a potentially lethal disease that involves a rash that spreads over the body and causes the skin to shed. (It clears up when the medicine is stopped.) This side effect is *very* rare. Lithium (Eskalith, Lithobid, Lithonate), an important treatment of bipolar disorder, is a primary mineral that has been shown to stabilize the mood of patients with bipolar disorder. Within the right levels, this drug is safe but blood levels need to be checked. Signs that the dosage is too high include diarrhea, increased thirst, nausea, trembling, rash, and fatigue. Adjustments of the dosage can eliminate these symptoms.

The Talking Cure

With all the talk of neurotransmitters and chemical changes we have lost sight of the true nature of affective disorders. The serotonin hypothesis of depression has been overplayed in the direct-to-consumer advertising as a way to link the "one pill to one chemical imbalance" idea. There never was much evidence that a deficiency of serotonin underlay depression, or that this deficiency could be fixed with a medication that boosts serotonin. If that were the case, then why don't you get better right away with an antidepressant, since it boosts serotonin right away? The academic psychiatry community never believed this hypothesis, although it never said much about it. Now it has moved on to other theories of how antidepressants work, one of which is that it is through the promotion of nerve growth, although the marketing teams of the pharmaceutical companies still use diagrams of brains and serotonin imbalances, since it's a theme that consumers seem to relate to.

The fact is that for many (if not most) people the symptoms of depression they experience are related to things that happen in their lives and how they deal with them emotionally. Early-life stress plays an important role in the development of depression for many people. Relationships and stress in the workplace are also important contributors, and often these factors combine. These are things that need to be dealt with through psychotherapy, exercise, diet, journaling, spiritual growth, and/or a change of circumstances if necessary, which includes getting out of dysfunctional relationships or jobs. If you have severe major depression, medication alone may not suffice; psychotherapy plus medication is better than taking medication alone.

During psychotherapy you meet regularly with a trained professional who will help you identify and work through the factors that may be causing your depression. Psychotherapy helps people with depression understand the behaviors, emotions, and ideas that contribute to depression; regain a sense of control and pleasure in life; and learn coping skills. Psychodynamic therapy is based on the assumption that a person is depressed because of unresolved, generally unconscious conflicts, often stemming from childhood. Interpersonal therapy focuses on the behaviors and interactions a depressed patient has with family and friends, the primary goal of which is to improve communication skills and increase self-esteem in a short period of time. Cognitive behavioral therapy involves examining thought patterns that can be negative and self-defeating, and going over the basis of such thoughts and how they contribute to emotions. Psychotherapy has been shown to be as effective in the treatment of depression as medication, and some people, especially those with early-life-stress issues, may not respond to medication without it.

Electroconvulsive Therapy (ECT)

My grandfather (who is now deceased) had several episodes of depression during which he was completely unable to function and had ideas that people were trying to steal his money as well as other delusions. Every time he was treated unsuccessfully with several different antidepressants before receiving ECT, which shocked him right out of his depression, as he described it. It worked like a charm every time.

I think ECT has gotten a bad rap. With new procedures for inducing anesthesia (they don't strap you down and shock you like they do in the movies), it is a much simpler and better-tolerated procedure than it used to be. And up to 80% of people experience improvement, which is a better response rate than that for medication. Many of those who respond to ECT, like my grandfather, don't respond to medications, and the long-term effects on memory are slight at worst. The fact is, ECT is the most effective treatment for depression available. So if you or someone you know has been on several medications and has not responded, you might want to consider it.

Vagal Nerve Stimulation

Vagal nerve stimulation (VNS), a new technique that involves the surgical placement of a stimulating device on the vagal nerve in the neck, sends rhythmic pulses of electricity that stimulate the vagal nerve, by which means it is thought to influence brain function and treat depression. VNS is a new treatment, although there is some evidence that it can help people who don't respond to medication. Like ECT it is a treatment of last resort.

Alternative Medicines

There are some natural remedies that have been recommended for depression.

ST.-JOHN'S-WORT

St.-John's-wort (*Hypericum perforatum*) is a popular medication for the over-the-counter treatment of mild depression; 12% of Americans report using it at least once a year. The mechanism of action of St.-John's-wort, which is similar to that of antidepressants, includes monoamine oxidase inhibition, serotonin reuptake inhibition, and actions on sigma receptors. In some earlier controlled studies St.-John's-wort was shown to be better than placebo and just as effective as tricyclic antidepressants in the treatment of depression. However, most of the early studies were poorly controlled and did not use standard definitions of depression, making it difficult to draw conclusions about the efficacy of St.-John's-wort.[4]

More recently there have been several large controlled trials as well as meta-analyses that have provided information on the efficacy of St.-John's-wort. A large placebo-controlled randomized trial using appropriate methodology in patients with severe cases of major depression showed no difference between St.-John's-wort and placebo.[5] However, a direct head-to-head comparison of St.-John's-wort to the SSRI paroxetine showed it was better in reducing symptoms of depression in patients with severe major depression; 71% of patients treated with St.-John's-wort had a 50% reduction in symptoms compared to 60% of those on paroxetine.[6] In this study, headache was the only side effect with St.-John's-wort that was more common than with placebo.

A second study funded by the NIH and performed by the Hypericum Depression Trial Study Group (HDTSG) showed that St.-John's-wort was no more effective than placebo but no worse than an antidepressant. In fact, the placebo did best: It was effective in 32% of patients, compared to 25% for sertraline and 24% for St.-John's-wort. However, patients taking St.-John's-wort experienced fewer side effects than those who took the antidepressant. St.-John's-wort caused an increase in swelling, frequent urination, and sexual dysfunction, while sertraline caused diarrhea, nausea, sexual dysfunction, forgetfulness, frequent urination, and sweating.

Critics of these studies said that selecting only patients with severe depression obscured the potential benefits for patients with mild depression. One recent meta-analysis of patients with severe depression did not show consistent effects for St.-John's-wort: There was only about a 15% increase in efficacy over placebo for severe depression. Another meta-analysis of St.-John's-wort for both major and minor depression was consistent with greater efficacy: about a 60% increase over placebo.

Overall, St.-John's-wort probably is effective for the treatment of minor depression, and, based on its biological activity, there is a plausible mechanism that explains why. The surprising thing is that the limited research evidence suggests that it is just as effective as the SSRIs for mild depression. St.-John's-wort can also interact with a number of medications, including digoxin (heart medication), theophylline (asthma medication), protease inhibitors (IHV medications), and cyclosporine (used for organ transplant patients), and for that reason should not be used or should only be used with caution and under a doctor's supervision by patients taking these meds.

SAMe

S-Adenosylmethionine (SAMe), a molecule that is found in all human cells, is promoted as a supplement for the treatment of depression. It plays a role in methylation reactions, including gene expression, maintenance of cell membranes, and neurotransmitter synthesis. Administration of SAMe has been shown to increase levels of serotonin in the brain. A meta-analysis from Italy that pooled data from several small studies concluded that SAMe was better than placebo and equal to tricyclic antidepressants in efficacy with fewer side effects. However, there was considerable variability in the studies conducted. Studies have also not had adequate long-term follow-up to determine the long-term benefits of SAMe for depression, although it does not appear that SAMe has potential long-term toxicity.

KAVA

Kava (or Kava-kava) is an extract of the roots of the Polynesian plant *Piper methysticum*, which is used in the South Pacific as a sedative, aphrodisiac, and stimulant. Active compounds include the kava pyrones, which may have effects on the brain. Several controlled trials have shown that kava reduces anxiety in patients with anxiety disorders. In one study twenty-four subjects with stress-induced insomnia were treated for six weeks with 120 mg of kava daily followed by two weeks with no treatment and then valerian for another six weeks. Both kava and valerian improved sleep (decreased onset, lengthened sleep time) and reduced stress severity. Side effects of kava include dizziness, dry mouth, gastric disturbance, diarrhea, drowsiness, depression, and more rarely, liver failure, which has caused it to be banned in some countries. (although not, unfortunately, in the U.S., thanks in part to the Dietary Supplement Health and Education Act (DSHEA) of 1994, which I describe in more detail in Chapter 18 (Vitamins and Supplements). Because of the very real risk of liver failure and possible death I do not recommend kava for the treatment of mood disorders. Kava is potentially lethal and should not be used.

OMEGA-3 FATTY ACIDS

There is one study I know of that has examined the effects of omega-3 fatty acids on symptoms of bipolar disorder.[7] Thirty patients with bipolar disorder were randomized to receive four months of omega-3 fatty acids in the form of fish-oil capsules or placebo. There was a significantly longer period before remission of bipolar symptoms in the omega-3 patients than in the patients on placebo. It is possible, however, that because patients on omega-3 treatment could detect the "fishy" smell of their supplements while those on placebo would not get the fish smell (a problem that cuts across many studies of herbs and supplements), there was a placebo effect. Although interesting, this study is an isolated one, and little else has been done to look at the relationship between omega-3 fatty acids and mood.

Diet and Exercise

A number of studies dating from the mid-1990s to more recently show that cardiovascular and resistance or weight training combat mild to severe depression. It turns out that exercise results in a surge of serotonin, the neurotransmitter that makes us feel good right after working out, as well as in a long-term mood shift once we've started exercising regularly, effects that may be related in part to an increased growth in brain cells. Regular exercise also has favorable effects on the immune system, which may promote health, especially in stressed and/or depressed individuals.

A study of 12,028 randomly selected individuals ages twenty to seventy-nine showed that increasing physical activity was associated with a 70% reduction in self-reported stress as well as a decrease in life dissatisfaction. Even two to four hours of walking per week was associated with significant improvements. Another study of a group of employees showed reductions in stress levels and depression, and improvements in feelings of health and vitality after a twenty-four-week program of aerobic exercise when compared to a control group. In a 1985 study, forty-three patients with depression, about half of whom were being treated for the condition with antidepressants, were randomized to receive nine weeks of exercise training (aerobic for one hour, three times a week at 50% to 70% maximum aerobic capacity) or occupational therapy. Exercise was associated with statistically significantly greater decreases in depression as measured by the Beck Depression Inventory (a measure of symptoms of depression). In another study, eighty-six patients with depression who were treated with antidepressants but did not have a therapeutic response were randomized to exercise or health-education classes. Exercise involved weight-bearing exercise for forty-five minutes twice a week for ten weeks. More patients treated with exercise experienced improvement as measured by a 30% improvement on a scale for the measurement of depression called the Hamilton Depression Scale (55% got better with exercise vs. 33% without, a difference that was statistically significant). In another study, eighty-three patients with major depression underwent aerobic exercise training vs. not changing what they were doing before. Exercise training was associated with better symptom improvement in terms of anxiety and general symptoms but not in depression.

Other studies have shown the impressive results of exercise in fighting or reducing symptoms of depression. For example, researchers at Freie University in Berlin also found that thirty minutes of exercise a day significantly improved the moods of patients who had been suffering from depression for nine months. In a report published in the *British Journal of Sports Medicine,* twelve patients with depression underwent ten weeks of training on a treadmill for thirty minutes a day. There was a statistically significant six-point drop in depressive symptoms as measured on the Hamilton Depression Scale. The authors concluded, and I agree, that exercise could be at least as effective as drugs in treating mild to moderate depression.

In one study, 156 patients over age fifty with major depression were randomly assigned to aerobic exercise, antidepressants (sertraline), or a combination of the two for sixteen weeks. All patients showed an improvement in symptoms of depression, with an essentially identical response among the groups.[8]

A 2005 report explained the results of a three-year-long study of eighty patients that was designed to test whether exercise is an efficacious treatment for mild to moderate major depressive disorder and what amount would be needed to see a positive difference in depressed people. The report, published in *The Journal of Preventive Medicine* (January 2005), found that a half hour a day of exercise six days a week is the ideal "dosage" to improve the mood of people who have mild to severe depression. Researchers compared two groups of depressed patients and found that while the group that performed eighty minutes of exercise a week received little to no mental-health benefit (a 30% reduction vs. 29% in a "placebo exercise" group), the three-hour-a-week group had a substantial (47%) reduction in symptoms.

Exercise may also complement the effects of antidepressant medication in depressed patients. One study added exercise to antidepressant treatment for seventeen patients who did not have a complete response to antidepressant medication. Exercise was prescribed according to currently recommended public-health guidelines—at least thirty minutes of aerobic activity a day—with both supervised and home-based sessions. There was a ten-point decrease in the Hamilton Depression Scale (a clinically significant change) in the eight patients who completed the study.

Exercise is far less expensive and more accessible than medication and psychotherapy. Plus it has none of the side effects, such as the sexual dysfunction seen with some antidepressants. Indeed, the "side effects" of using exercise as an antidepressant are beneficial to general well-being: improved cardiovascular health, increased strength, and weight loss.

Proper diet is also critical for preventing depression. Studies have shown that high-fat foods lead to changes in mood. You may have seen Morgan Spurlock wolf down multiple cheeseburgers in supersized portions at McDonald's in the *Supersize Me* documentary film and then complain about a feeling of depression that could be relieved only by going back to McDonald's. Experimental studies have shown that a large intake of fats leads to feelings of sleepiness that are not related to the food alone. Diets deficient in folate and vitamins B_6 and B_{12} are also associated with depression.

Part of living a happy, healthy life is eating the right food. If you get your meals from fast-food restaurants, you are going to be getting high-fat, high-sodium, and high-sugar meals. What you eat influences how you feel.

Cook your own meals and eat a lot of fresh fruits and vegetables, fresh fish, and not too much other meat or fatty foods. When you do eat out, go to a high-quality (which does not mean expensive) place that cares about the food it serves and cooks it to order. Eating well will help your physical as well as your mental and emotional health; a good meal is a pleasure, especially when enjoyed with family and friends.

The Bottom Line

If you suffer from depression you should adopt a regular exercise and nutrition regimen, since these have been shown to help relieve depression, and are free of side effects. Give psychotherapy a try. If this doesn't work and you are suffering from mild depression, it is reasonable to try St.-John's-wort. Results of studies done on St.-John's-wort suggest that it may not be that good for severe major depression, but SSRIs might not be that great either.

Beyond that, antidepressant medications *are* useful in the treatment of depression. In general the SSRIs have fewer of the side effects that are typical of the older-generation tricyclics, like dry mouth. However, they can also be associated with a significant inhibition of libido, which can be a real problem if you are in a relationship. If you do take SSRIs, start out at half the dose that the manufacturer recommends, and increase and decrease the dose in very small increments to avoid the mood swings and suicidal thoughts that seem to be associated with overly rapid changes in medication. Atypical antidepressants like Wellbutrin can overcome those sexual side effects.

The MAOIs work well, especially for atypical depression (increased sleep and appetite), but most people don't like the fact that while taking them it is necessary to avoid wine and cheese. In general all antidepressants are equally effective, so the choice of antidepressants is based on side effects and costs. The dual reuptake inhibitors venlafaxine and duloxetine do seem to have a slight advantage in terms of efficacy over SSRIs and the other antidepressants like the tricyclics, but at least in the case of venlafaxine the suicide risk may negate the added efficacy.

For severe depression, especially for those who have no response to an SSRI, some of the tricyclics, like imipramine or clomipramine, may work better and are worth a try. For bipolar (manic-depressive) disorder, lithium is useful for preventing a return of manic episodes. Other medications, like lamotrigine, are also effective, although not necessarily better. For changes in mood that are related to depression or bipolar disorder, medications like tegretol or valproic acid can be added on.

If you have tried several medications and have severe depression, you might consider ECT or VNS as a last resort.

Drug	Use	Common, Benign Side Effects	Serious Side Effects	Life-threatening Side Effects	Reasons Not to Take
Tricyclics					
Moderate Risk					
Imipramine (Tofranil)	Major depression	Dry mouth, constipation, memory problems, blurred vision, urination problems, sexual dysfunction	Blood pressure changes	Heart arrhythmias, overdose	Heart condition
Doxepin (Sinequan)	Major depression	Dry mouth, constipation, memory problems, blurred vision, urination problems, sexual dysfunction	Blood pressure changes	Heart arrhythmias, overdose	Heart condition

Drug	Use	Common, Benign Side Effects	Serious Side Effects	Life-threatening Side Effects	Reasons Not to Take
Amoxapine (Asendin)	Major depression	Dry mouth, constipation, memory problems, blurred vision, urination problems sexual dysfunction	Blood pressure changes	Heart arrhythmias, overdose urination,	Heart condition seizures, glaucoma
Amitriptyline (Elavil)	Major depression	Dry mouth, constipation, memory problems, blurred vision, urination problems, sexual dysfunction	Blood pressure changes	Heart arrhythmias, overdose	Heart condition seizures, glaucoma

Norepinephrine Reuptake Inhibitors

Low Risk

Drug	Use	Common, Benign Side Effects	Serious Side Effects	Life-threatening Side Effects	Reasons Not to Take
Desipramine (Norpramin)	Major depression	Dry mouth, constipation, memory problems, blurred vision, urination problems, sexual dysfunction	Blood pressure changes	Heart arrhythmias, seizures	Heart condition seizures, glaucoma
Nortriptyline (Aventyl, Pamelor)	Major depression	Dry mouth, constipation, memory problems, blurred vision, urination problems, sexual dysfunction	Blood pressure changes	Heart arrhythmias, seizures	Heart condition seizures, glaucoma
Amoxapine (Ascendin)	Major depression	Dry mouth, constipation, memory problems, blurred vision, urination problems, sexual dysfunction	Blood pressure changes	Heart arrhythmias, seizures	Heart condition seizures, glaucoma

Drug	Use	Common, Benign Side Effects	Serious Side Effects	Life-threatening Side Effects	Reasons Not to Take
Clomipramine (Anafranil)	OCD	Dry mouth, constipation, memory problems, blurred vision, urination problems, sexual dysfunction	Blood pressure changes	Heart arrhythmias, seizures	Heart condition seizures, glaucoma
MAO Inhibitors					
Moderate Risk					
Phenelzine (Nardil)	Major depression	Constipation, blurred vision, urination problems, sexual dysfunction	Dizziness, headache, insomnia	Wine-and-cheese hypertensive crisis, liver damage, anemia	Liver disease, heart failure, pheochromocytoma; should not be taken by children
Tranylcypromine (Parnate)	Major depression	Constipation, blurred vision, urination problems, sexual dysfunction	Dizziness, headache, insomnia	Wine-and-cheese hypertensive crisis, liver damage, anemia	Liver disease, heart failure, pheochromocytoma; should not be taken by children
Quatrocyclics					
Low Risk					
Mirtazapine (Remeron)	Major depression	Shivering, fatigue, nightmares, weight gain, anxiety, dry mouth, constipation	Lipid elevations, swelling, muscle pain	Trouble breathing, sore throat	Kidney or liver disease; if you are taking MAOIs
Maprotiline (Ludiomil)	Major depression	Dry mouth, drowsiness, nausea, vomiting	Rash, swelling	Seizures, hallucinations, irregular heart rate, jaundice	Liver disease; if you are taking MAOIs

Drug	Use	Common, Benign Side Effects	Serious Side Effects	Life-threatening Side Effects	Reasons Not to Take
Selective Serotonin Reuptake Inhibitors (SSRIs)					
Low Risk					
Paroxetine (Paxil)	Major depression, panic, OCD, PTSD, General-ized Anxi-ety Disorder (GAD)	Nausea, diarrhea, headache, insomnia	Decreased libido, akathisia	Suicidal thoughts, mood swings with dose change	Allergic reaction; if you are taking MAOIs
Sertraline (Zoloft)	Major depression, panic, OCD, PTSD, General-ized Anxi-ety Disorder (GAD)	Nausea, diarrhea, headache, insomnia	Decreased libido, akathisia	Suicidal thoughts, mood swings with dose change, bleeding	Allergic reaction; if you are taking MAOIs
Fluoxetine (Prozac)	Major depression, OCD	Nausea, diarrhea, headache, insomnia	Decreased libido, akathisia	Suicidal thoughts, mood swings with dose change	Allergic reaction; if you are taking MAOIs
Citalopram (Celexa)	Major depression	Nausea, diarrhea, headache, insomnia	Decreased libido, akathisia	Suicidal thoughts, mood swings with dose change	Allergic reaction; if you are taking MAOIs
Escitalopram (Lexapro)	Major depression	Nausea, diarrhea, headache, insomnia	Decreased libido, akathisia	Suicidal thoughts, mood swings with dose change	Allergic reaction; if you are taking MAOIs

Drug	Use	Common, Benign Side Effects	Serious Side Effects	Life-threatening Side Effects	Reasons Not to Take
Fluvoxamine (Luvox)	Major depression	Nausea, diarrhea, headache, insomnia	Decreased libido, akathisia	Suicidal thoughts, mood swings with dose change	Allergic reaction; if you are taking MAOIs
Other Antidepressants					
Bupropion (Wellbutrin, Zyban)	Depression, smoking cessation	Weight loss, restlessness, dry mouth, insomnia, constipation, nausea, vomiting		Seizures	Seizure disorder, allergy to medication
Trazodone (Desyrel)	Major depression	Dizziness, constipation, dry mouth, headache	Priapism	Allergic reaction, irregular heart rate	Allergy to medication, pregnancy, acute heart disease
Nefazodone (Serzone)	Major depression	Dry mouth, nausea, headache, stomach upset, dreams	Blurred vision	Liver failure	Liver disease, pregnancy
Dual Reuptake Inhibitors					
Venlafaxine (Effexor)	Major depression	Restlessness, shivering, constipation, nausea, headache	Sexual dysfunction, hypertension, muscle cramp	Suicidality, stomach bleeding, allergic reaction	Allergy to drug; if you are taking MAOIs
Duloxetine (Cymbalta)	Major depression	Constipation, nausea, diarrhea, vomiting, dry mouth	Sexual dysfunction, blurred vision, muscle pain, dizziness	Stomach bleeding, liver damage	Allergy to drug; if you are taking MAOIs

Drug	Use	Common, Benign Side Effects	Serious Side Effects	Life-threatening Side Effects	Reasons Not to Take
Mood stabilizers					
Lithium (Lithobid)	Bipolar disorder	Nausea, tremor, weight gain, diarrhea, thirst	Blurred vision, stomach upset	Change in renal function	Heart disease, renal disease, brain damage; if you are taking diuretics
Valproic acid (Valproate, Depakene, Depakote)	Bipolar disorder	Mood change, anorexia, nausea, trembling	Rash, dizziness	Liver failure, birth defects, bleeding, pancreatitis	Liver disease, pregnancy, breast-feeding
Carbamazepine (Tegretol)	Bipolar disorder	Dizziness, drowsiness, nausea, vomiting	Confusion, depression, hallucinations	Bone marrow suppression, heart failure, liver dysfunction	Hyper-sensitivity, pregnancy, breast-feeding, allergy to medication
Topiramate (Topomax)	Bipolar disorder	Dizziness, nervousness, headache, irritability	Confusion, aggression	Low blood sugar, blurred vision	Allergy to medication
Lamotrigine (Lamictal)	Bipolar disorder	Dizziness, headache, sleepiness, nausea, vomiting	Blurred vision	Stevens-Johnson syndrome	Allergy to medication
Neurontin (Gabapentin)	Bipolar disorder	Dizziness, headache, sleepiness, nausea, vomiting	Blurred vision	Eye movements	Allergy to medication

16.

Insomnia Treatments

Modern life means that many of us are on the go 24/7—literally. We check our cell phones and BlackBerries constantly; scour the Internet at all hours of the day and night; and bring office work home with us so that after dinner we can keep right on working in an effort to "stay on top" and "ahead of the other guy." Fitting in leisure time extends a day even further into the evening, and TiVo allows us to watch favorite TV programs anytime we want, often late at night. One result of this overcharged, overbooked lifestyle is lack of sleep; all that activity during the day and into the night is stimulating, so that when we do actually get between the sheets, we can't fall asleep. Today, about one out of four Americans reports some difficulties in falling or staying asleep.

Insomnia in its most disabling form—meaning several consecutive sleepless nights—affects 10% to 15% of Americans. This problem has been a boon for the sleep-aid industry; millions are taking medications for insomnia, and the number is increasing all the time. In the past five years there has been a 100% increase in the use of sleeping pills. Older people and women have even higher rates of insomnia. Usage of sleeping pills is more worrisome for the elderly than for young people because they are more likely to have serious side effects from these drugs, like memory impairment, falls, and car crashes. Between 5% and 33% of individuals over the age of sixty are prescribed a sleeping pill in the form of a Z drug (see page 320) or a benzodiazepine. The *New York Times* reported on February 2, 2006 (Stephanie Saul, "Record Sales of Sleeping Pills Are Causing Worries"), that drug companies were spending $298 million a year on ads for these drugs, a fourfold increase over the previous five years, and in return for that investment were taking in $2 billion a year in revenue.

Primary insomnia, the most common form of insomnia, is unrelated to any other disorder or illness. Patients with primary insomnia are anxious and restless in bed, and feel pressure to go to sleep. They develop negative attitudes and expectations about their ability to go to sleep and may sleep better away from bed (e.g., in a comfortable chair or on a sofa while they're watching TV or listening to music).

There are multiple common potential causes of insomnia, including:

- Poor sleep habits (doctors call it "sleep hygiene"), including staying up too late or getting up too early, eating and drinking late at night, illness, or overstimulating ourselves with work, worry, stress, or late-night TV watching.
- Sedentary lifestyle (people who exercise regularly, but not late at night, sleep better and more deeply than those who don't)
- Menopause
- Pain
- Medical conditions such as cancer, AIDS, lung disease, musculoskeletal disorders, and degenerative brain disease.
- Medications (including bronchodilators, caffeine, theophylline, and stimulants such as Ritalin, amphetamines, steroids, antihypertensive drugs, and antidepressants)
- Snoring or restless bed partner
- Stress and anxiety
- Excessive alcohol or other drug use

- Sleep apnea, often seen in overweight individuals, where the airways become obstructed and cause the individual to wake up frequently. Sleep apnea can be accurately diagnosed and treated by a doctor using a machine called Continuous Positive Airway Pressure (CPAP), which delivers air into the airways through a mask that is worn at night.
- Shift work

Insomnia can lead to a host of other problems. For instance, about 40% of those with insomnia also suffer from anxiety or depression. It is difficult to say whether the insomnia or the mental disorder comes first. Trouble falling and staying asleep can also affect memory and cognition as well as decrease productivity and quality of life. Recent studies have shown that insomnia has an important effect on promoting a variety of poor physical health outcomes, including a link between being overweight and lack of sleep. In addition, there are some serious side effects to consider.

Pharmaceutical Sleep Solutions

A variety of medications have been either developed specifically for the treatment of insomnia or prescribed for it because of their sedative side effects. These include barbiturates, benzodiazepines, benzodiazepine subtype-specific drugs, and over-the-counter antihistamines, sedating antidepressants, antipsychotics, melatonin, and herbal remedies.

Though many of these medications do in fact help people sleep more, people who take sleeping pills say that they feel more satisfied about the extra sleep they get but that the positive effect on their ability to think and function the next day is offset by the long-lasting side effects of the drugs, such as impairments in memory and cognition, so they end up with no lasting benefit.

LUMINAL: A TRUE HOLLYWOOD STORY

Some of the first treatments of insomnia were barbiturates. Also known colloquially in the 1950s and 1960s as "mother's little helper," barbiturates have been around since the late nineteenth century, when heavy doses were found to put users out for a day and a half.

In 1912 two independent teams of chemists synthesized what became known as Luminal, or phenobarbitol, a drug to which users can easily build up a resistance. In the middle of the last century, it became obvious that with this drug there was significant potential for dependence, abuse, and death, particularly among depressed, repressed mid-century house-wives and such famous '60s and '70s icons as party girl Edie Sedgwick, guitar legend Jimi Hendrix, sex symbol Marilyn Monroe, singer Judy Garland, photographer Diane Arbus, and the beautiful actresses Inger Stevens and Jean Seberg, among others. Celebrity usage (including deliberate suicide) is one reason why the history of Luminal is tinged with undeserved glamour.

Now a tightly controlled substance, Luminal has not completely faded from the scene. Phenobarbital is still among the top three hundred drugs prescribed in the U.S. (www.rxlist.com), although much of it is used to treat epilepsy and its related seizures. Barbiturates are also used for anesthesia before surgery and for management of swelling of the brain. Barbiturates enhance the inhibitory neurotransmitter gamma-aminobutyric acid (GABA) as well as depressing nerve and muscle tissue. Aside from dependence, side effects include drowsiness, lethargy, headache, dizziness, breathing problems, and allergic reactions.

BENZODIAZEPINE MEDICATIONS

In the 1960s benzodiazepines displaced barbiturates as the most commonly used treatments for insomnia. They were originally marketed as having less potential for dependence and abuse, although this claim was not borne out over time. Benzodiazepines act on a receptor in the brain called the GABA-benzodiazepine receptor complex, the same complex that alcohol and the inhibitory neurotransmitter GABA bind to, although benzodiazepines have their own binding site. Like alcohol, they act by increasing a general inhibition on neurons in the brain that results in a calming effect.

Benzodiazepines are not widely prescribed for insomnia today. Those that continue to be prescribed include alprazolam (Xanax), which is mainly used for anxiety attacks and panic disorder; clonazepam (Klonopin), which is used for epilepsy; and temazepam (Restoril). Triazolam (Halcion) is a benzodiazepine that was widely prescribed at one time, but it is very short-acting and can cause patients to wake up in the night. It also has been associated with a number of negative psychiatric side effects (including violence and aggression, thought to be related to disinhibition), especially in the elderly, for which it received bad publicity and due to which it fell out of favor.

Other benzodiazepine medications that are longer acting and that are still sometimes used in the treatment of insomnia include oxazepam (Serax), lorazepam (Ativan), chlordiazepoxide (Librium), clorazepate (Tranxene), halazepam (Paxipam), prazepam (Centrax), quazepam (Doral), estazolam (Prosom), diazepam (Valium), and flurazepam (Dalmane). There isn't really much difference among these benzodiazepines other than their time of onset of action and how long they or their metabolites stay in the body.

The long-acting drugs can cause significant mental impairment the next day in older patients and are associated with a 50% increase in hip fracture because older people who take them do not have full use of their motor skills the following day and often fall. Serax has the least-severe effect on memory and as a result is recommended as the best benzodiazepine to use for a sleeping pill, although it should be used for less than four weeks. (All medications for insomnia are not recommended for long-term use.)

The benzodiazepines have not been shown to be better in terms of inducing sleep than diphenhydramine or promethazine. The benzodiazepines decrease the time it takes to fall asleep by just four minutes. On average, benzodiazepines increase the user's sleep time by about one hour more per night. However, individuals taking benzodiazepines report that they *feel* like they fall asleep faster than they actually do.

Side effects during the day can cause serious problems. When compared to patients on placebo, those on benzodiazepines reported 80% more daytime drowsiness, dizziness, and light-headedness. Other side effects are problems the next day with memory as well as an increase in motor vehicle accidents. Driving accidents are a potentially serious problem in patients taking sleeping pills. Use of benzodiazepine medications is associated with a 60% increase in traffic accidents. This increased safety risk is not a factor with other psychotropics, including antidepressants. Risk was increased with concurrent alcohol usage and age. There was also an increased risk with zopiclone, one of the newer-generation insomnia medications (see below).[1] The authors of this study concluded that patients taking sleep medications shouldn't drive. These risks in addition to the more serious problems of sleepwalking and even sleepdriving (see below) raise serious concerns about these drugs.

NONBENZODIAZEPINE "Z-DRUG" MEDICATIONS

The newer generation of insomnia medications, including zaleplon (Sonata), zolpidem (Ambien), eszopiclone (Lunesta), and zopiclone (Imovane), or "Z" drugs, acts on specific subsets of the GABA receptor. They are commonly called *nonbenzodiazepine* medications, but that term is misleading, since they bind to the same GABA-benzodiazepine receptor complex in the brain that the benzodiazepines and alcohol bind to. The difference is that they bind to a different part of the same receptor complex. They have been marketed as having less potential for dependency and fewer side effects than the older generation of benzodiazepine medications, and some argue that these drugs also have less potential for abuse than the benzodiazepines.

Systematic studies, however, have not shown these drugs to be more effective or safer than the benzodiazepines, although they cost several times more. For instance, pooling of data from three trials with a total of ninety-six patients showed no difference between benzodiazepines and zopiclone in terms of how much time it took subjects to fall asleep, although patients treated with benzodiazepine slept twenty-three minutes longer. Total sleep time is increased by only about twenty minutes with Z drugs. There were no differences between benzodiazepines and zopiclone in major side effects (adverse events). And no difference among the different Z drugs in safety or efficacy has been established. General side effects for all of these meds include memory impairment, drowsiness, headache, dizziness, nausea, and nervousness. There is no evidence to date that the risk of dependency on the Z drugs is any less than that for the earlier classes of insomnia medications like the benzodiazepines.

So which of the Z drugs are the best? A 2004 review by the U.K. National Institute for Clinical Evidence (NICE) showed no difference among the different Z drugs (Sonata, Lunesta, Ambien, or Imovane) in efficacy, next-day impairment, or risk of withdrawal or dependence. In addition, there were no benefits in terms of efficacy or side effects when they were compared to benzodiazepines. Sonata has a much shorter half-life (1 hour) than Ambien (2.5 hours) and Lunesta (6 hours), and is therefore promoted as being associated with less drowsiness the next day. Lunesta is a pure "mirror version" of the same molecule as its parent, zopiclone, and appears to have been developed in a marketing effort to leave behind the negative marketing that was associated with studies of zopiclone (conducted before the latest Z drugs were released), which showed an increase in traffic accidents with its use. Until studies are performed to specifically address the issue, we have to assume that all of the Z drugs will eventually be found to be associated with an increase in driving accidents.

Another serious side effect that patients taking Ambien have experienced is sleepwalking. Ambien increases slow-wave sleep, which has been associated with sleepwalking. On March 8, 2006, the *New York Times* reported several cases of people who got up, walked around the house, cooked, and even drove. Cases of people who have gotten out of bed after taking Ambien (sometimes with a glass of wine), driven, and gotten into car accidents, with absolutely no memory of what happened, have also been reported. Some people have gotten up in the middle of the night, crashed their cars into parked cars, and then tried to drive away, with no memory of what happened (remember Patrick Kennedy?).

One man on a transatlantic flight took Ambien with two glasses of wine. In his sleep, he tore off his clothes and threatened to kill himself and others. As a result, the plane had to make an emergency landing. He had no memory of the incident.

Any amount of alcohol, even a glass, greatly increases the risk of having a dangerous sleepwalking accident. Also, sleepwalking has been reported more commonly with Ambien probably because it accounts for 85% of the insomnia medication market. It is very possible that other insomnia medications can have the same side effect.

Off-Label Solutions

There are a handful of drugs that are prescribed and used "off label" for insomnia. These include drugs from allergy meds to antidepressants. Since they have active ingredients that work on other brain and body functions, even the most benign of these drugs (such as antihistamines) should be used with care if not caution.

ANTIHISTAMINES

Drugs developed for the treatment of allergies have also been found to have sedative properties that are useful for treating insomnia, and there are versions available both by prescription and over the counter. The most commonly prescribed antihistamine for insomnia is hydroxyzine (Atarax, Vistaril). Over-the-counter diphenhydramine (Benadryl, Simply Sleep, Tylenol PM, Excedrin PM, and their "store brand" counterparts), often recommended by doctors as a sleep aid, is effective for many people. These medications are relatively free of potential for addiction or abuse. Side effects are less common than those for the benzodiazepines or Z drugs and include dry mouth, urinary retention, and, more rarely, confusion, nightmares, nervousness, and irritability. If you are having trouble falling asleep I recommend cognitive or behavioral therapy (which I discuss later and which works better than drugs) for a long-term solution. Otherwise, I recommend one of these drugs as long as you don't use them for more than a week.

SEDATIVES

Sedatives are generally used to calm someone who is having an anxiety attack or to soothe extreme nervous tension. However, they are also often used to help those with insomnia, even if the sleep disorder is unrelated to nervousness or anxiety. Meprobamate (Miltown, Equanil) is a tranquilizer that can lead to addiction and should not be used for insomnia. Doctors rarely write prescriptions for it anymore.

Ramelteon (Rozerem) is a melatonin receptor agonist that is used for insomnia. Melatonin is a hormone of the body that is involved in the wake/sleep cycle. Side effects include headache, drowsiness, fatigue, nausea, dizziness, and, more rarely, diarrhea and depression. Advantages of this medication are the absence of abuse potential (it doesn't seem to have as much of a reinforcing effect as medications like benzodiazepines) and the lack of withdrawal symptoms.

Buspirone (Buspar), originally marketed as a nonaddictive treatment for anxiety, is an agonist of the serotonin 1A receptor and is relatively free of next-day drowsiness and memory impairment as well as the potential for dependence or abuse. Although sometimes prescribed for insomnia, controlled trials to evaluate its use as a sleep aid have not been performed. Side effects, which are minimal, include nausea, headache, and light-headedness.

ANTIDEPRESSANTS

Antidepressants are sometimes prescribed for the treatment of insomnia for people whose primary problem is not insomnia. This practice seems to be particularly common in elderly patients. Trazodone (Desyrel) and amitriptyline (Elavil) are two examples that are commonly used for such patients. However, their efficacy has not yet been established, and they can have negative side effects. Elavil has the most anticholinergic side effects of any of the antidepressants (confusion, dry mouth, trouble urinating). Desyrel can cause priapism (a painful and sustained erection that may require a trip to the emergency room).

Tricyclics like amitriptyline and doxepin, which are used as sleep aids for the elderly, have been specifically identified as inappropriate for their use. Tricyclics increase cardiovascular risk, decrease mobility, and increase the risk of falls for the elderly. Tricyclics make up 23% of all prescribed medications for the elderly, and in fact amitriptyline is the most common inappropriately prescribed psychotropic medicine for seniors.

Alternative Medicines, Herbs, and Supplements

A wide variety of alternative remedies, including herbs, and supplements, many of which are derived from roots and herbs that were and in some cases still are used in traditional Chinese, Indian, or Native American medicine, have been marketed for insomnia. Some plants known to have psychoactive properties, like poppy seed and Indian hemp, include almonds, chamomile, catmint, fennel, hops, lettuce, lime, marjolaine, may blossom, mullein, oats, orange flower, passionflower, rosemary, and willow. None of these have been evaluated in double-blind placebo-controlled trials for their efficacy in treating insomnia.

VALERIAN

Valerian, an extract of the valerian root (*Valeriana officinalis*), is widely prescribed in Europe for the treatment of insomnia and is available as a supplement in the U.S. In an early study, 166 volunteers were given vale-rian, a valerian-containing commercial product, or a placebo. After three doses, valerian was associated with a significant decrease in the time it took to fall asleep and improvement in sleep quality. Sleep was better for those who took the pure Valerian extract than for those who took the proprietary product Hova®, which contains valerian extract. However, this study did not measure how well the blinding worked, which is important because valerian has a strong and distinctive smell.

An uncontrolled study of fifty-four subjects showed a reduction in heart rate, blood pressure, and subjective distress caused by a stressful task after they received valerian. This study suggests that valerian may have sedative properties. In another study, sixteen patients with sleep disorders were ran-domly assigned to two doses of valerian or a placebo nightly, and EEG measures of their sleep as well as subjective reports of sleep quality were taken while patients were sleeping in a sleep laboratory. Side effects in-cluded vivid dreams in as many as 16% of cases and, less commonly, drowsiness, depression, dizziness, headaches, or blurred vision. When the patients were given a single dose of valerian, the lower dose had no effect on subjective or EEG measures of sleep. Because of inconsistent results and no clear mechanism by which valerian could treat insomnia without sig-nificant side effects I think that large, properly controlled trials are needed to determine whether valerian is useful for insomnia. However, in the meantime, since valerian does not have major side effects, I wouldn't neces-sarily discourage anyone from using it.

KAVA

Kava (or Kava-kava) is an extract of the roots of the Polynesian plant *Piper methysticum,* used in the South Pacific as a sedative, aphrodisiac, and stim-ulant. Active compounds include the kava pyrones, which may have effects on the brain. Several controlled trials have shown that kava reduces anxiety in patients with anxiety disorders. In one study, twenty-four subjects with stress-induced insomnia were treated for six weeks with 120 mg of kava daily, followed by two weeks of no treatment and then valerian for another six weeks. Both kava and valerian improved sleep (decreased onset, lengthened sleep time) and reduced stress severity. Side effects of kava include dizziness, dry mouth, gastric disturbance, diarrhea, dizziness, drowsiness, depression, and, more rarely, liver failure, which has caused some countries to ban it. Because of the very real risk of liver failure and possible death, I would not recommend kava for the treatment of insomnia.

MELATONIN

Melatonin, a hormone that occurs naturally in the body, is involved in the regulation of the wake/sleep cycle. Melatonin can decrease the time it takes to fall asleep but overall has no effect on sleep time. It is popular with travelers. By taking melatonin, however, keep in mind that you are meddling with your own body's hormonal status, which can have risks. For instance, taking melatonin may affect growth or reproductive function. Other side effects include abdominal cramps, confusion, depression, drowsiness, nausea, and vomiting. I don't see that melatonin involves any major risks, so if you want to try it on your next flight across the Atlantic, feel free to do so.

Diet and Behavior

There are several nonmedication treatments that have been shown to improve insomnia.

COGNITIVE THERAPY

Studies have shown the most effective therapy for the treatment of insomnia is cognitive behavioral therapy (CBT). It is more effective than medication in treating sleeplessness and results in a significant improvement in sleep duration and quality without side effects.

A few sessions with a therapist trained in cognitive therapy is the best way to derive the most benefit. The first step is to replace negative thoughts ("I can't sleep without medications") with more positive ones ("If I take the time to relax, I can get to sleep without help from pills"). The theory is that you "retrain" your brain to learn to sleep peacefully and deeply again.

Changing sleep habits is the second step in cognitive therapy: for example, using the bed and bedroom only for sleep (no working or TV watching in bed), setting and maintaining a regular sleep schedule, eliminating daytime naps, and minimizing or avoiding altogether caffeine, alcohol, stimulants, and heavy or extremely spicy meals four to six hours before going to bed. Relaxation techniques such as progressive muscle relaxation often help. This technique involves alternately contracting individual muscles and relaxing with exhalation, progressing through the body one muscle group at a time.

Behavioral changes are highly effective and last longer than drug therapy. About 80% of patients will show improvement: The time it takes to fall asleep is reduced from sixty-five minutes to thirty-five minutes, sleep time is increased by thirty minutes, and subjective ratings of sleep quality are higher.

In a well-conducted study, forty-six patients with insomnia were randomized to receive CBT, zopiclone, or placebo medication each night for six weeks.[2] Sleep was assessed using sleep diaries and polysomnography. CBT included sleep hygiene, sleep restriction, stimulus control, cognitive therapy, and relaxation. CBT was better than zopiclone for sleep efficiency, with an increase from 81% to 90%, compared to zopiclone, which remained at 82% before and after treatment. CBT resulted in an increase in slow-wave sleep and a decrease in time spent awake at night. Six months after the end of treatment, CBT resulted in better sleep efficiency as measured using polysomnography than either placebo or zopiclone. Since long-term use of sleeping pills is not recommended, what this study shows is that people with chronic insomnia really need to make the effort to get behavioral therapy treatment, or at a minimum to educate themselves about the principles that are promoted in the types of CBT programs utilized in this study.

Meditation and gentle yoga can also help some people fall asleep more easily as part of a cognitive therapy program or on their own. Insomniacs often spend too much time in bed trying to sleep, and the best thing to do is to get out of bed and read for a while or listen to soft music.

The Bottom Line

When treating insomnia it is important to consider its impact in its proper context. The manufacturers of sleeping pills make much of the fact that one out of four people complains of insomnia, and of these, half have severe functional disturbances. In a review of all the data from studies of sleeping pills, Drs. Jennifer Glass, Usoa Busto, and colleagues from the University of Toronto, writing in the *British Medical Journal* in 2005, said that ". . . clinical benefits [of sleeping pills] may be modest at best. The added risk of an adverse event may not justify the benefits, particularly in a high risk elderly population."

While medications for the treatment of insomnia may increase the amount of sleep time you experience, it is only by about twenty minutes, and they do not lead to improvements in quality of life, cognition, daytime function, or feelings of sleepiness. They can also increase accidents, falls, fractures, and mortality, particularly in the elderly, and dependency. Based on this I do not recommend medication for the treatment of insomnia. If you do have to take a pill for sleep, I prefer over-the-counter medications like Benadryl to a prescription pill, and strongly advise you not to take medications for more than a few days. And remember, if you do take a prescription pill, you can drink *no* alcohol, not even a single glass of wine.

Overall, patients who take sleeping pills have a 25% increase in mortality.[3] Older patients are prescribed sleeping pills eight times more often than younger people, even though they have less of a tendency to be anxious. Fourteen percent of hip fractures can be attributed to confusion related to a sleeping pill or other psychotropic drug; in the elderly, hip fracture is associated with a high mortality rate. Another study found that out of 308 older adults with cognitive impairment, 11% of the cases of impairment were related to a drug they were on, and in 46% of those cases, the culprit was a sleeping pill. Often cognitive function had deteriorated slowly over the many years these patients had been on a sleeping pill. After stopping the pill, all patients had long-term improvement in cognitive function.

Most studies of these medications involve only six weeks. However, it is known that patients with chronic insomnia develop tolerance over time and lose the beneficial effects of medication. Guidelines from a National Institutes of Health Consensus Conference recommend that hypnotics not be used for more than six weeks because of problems with rebound insomnia, withdrawal, dependence, and other poor health consequences. In the real world, however, patients are treated for months or years with medication, and nothing is known about the long-term side effects or potential for dependency.

Based on objective monitoring in the laboratory, the average insomniac sleeps six hours a night. Increased mortality does not occur until sleep is less than six hours, in the range of four or five hours. The average person sleeps seven hours a night and has the best health outcomes. So it is not true that you need eight hours of sleep a night. In fact, when people started to sleep more than eight hours, they had *worse* health outcomes.[4] Six hours of sleep is adequate for most people.

A common myth is that it is abnormal to wake up in the middle of the night (something indicating that you may need medication). Sleep studies show that when people are removed from artificial light, they tend to fall asleep when it gets dark, sleep for three or four hours, wake up in the middle of the night at some random time, lie awake for several hours, then fall asleep again for three to four hours. Studies in primitive hunter-gatherer societies show that these people sleep in the same way. One hypothesis is that this has adaptive value, since if one of the clan is always awake at some particular time during the night, he or she is more likely to detect predators and wake up the rest of the clan. It is not natural to stay up until eleven o'clock every night with the help of artificial lights and then sleep eight straight hours through the night (secondary to the exhaustion of having stayed up for fifteen straight hours). Therefore, if you wake up in the middle of the night, you should not jump to the conclusion that you need to be medicated for it.

Pleasant dreams!

Drug	Use	Common, Benign Side Effects	Serious Side Effects	Life-threatening Side Effects	Reasons Not to Take
Barbiturates					
High Risk					
Phenobarbital (Luminal)	Insomnia	Drowsiness, lethargy, headache, dizziness	Problems breathing, delirium, depression	Allergic reaction, decreased blood counts (rare), respiratory depression, addiction	Allergy, addiction, depression
Butabarbital (Butisol)	Insomnia	Drowsiness, lethargy, headache, dizziness	Problems breathing, delirium, depression	Allergic reaction, decreased blood counts (rare), respiratory depression, addiction	Allergy, addiction, depression
Pentobarbital (Nembutal)	Insomnia	Drowsiness, lethargy, headache, dizziness	Problems breathing, delirium, depression	Allergic reaction, decreased blood counts (rare), respiratory depression, addiction	Allergy, addiction, depression

Drug	Use	Common, Benign Side Effects	Serious Side Effects	Life-threatening Side Effects	Reasons Not to Take
Antihistamines					
Low Risk					
Hydroxyzine (Atarax, Vistaril)	Insomnia	Dry mouth, urinary retention	Confusion, nightmares, irritability	None	None
Benzodiazepines					
Moderate Risk					
Alprazolam (Xanax)	Insomnia	Drowsiness	Dependency, memory loss, confusion	Hip fracture, driving accidents	History of addictions, memory impairment
Clonazepam (Klonopin)	Insomnia	Drowsiness	Dependency, memory loss, confusion	Hip fracture, driving accidents	History of addictions, memory impairment
Temazepam (Restoril)	Insomnia	Drowsiness	Dependency, memory loss, confusion	Hip fracture, driving accidents	History of addictions, memory impairment
Triazolam (Halcion)	Insomnia	Drowsiness early wake-up	Dependency, memory loss, confusion	Hip fracture, driving accidents	History of addictions, memory impairment
Oxazepam (Serax)	Insomnia	Drowsiness	Dependency, memory loss, confusion	Hip fracture, driving accidents	History of addictions, memory impairment
Lorazepam (Ativan)	Insomnia	Drowsiness	Dependency, memory loss, confusion	Hip fracture, driving accidents	History of addictions, memory impairment
Chlordiaze-poxide (Librium)	Insomnia	Drowsiness	Dependency, memory loss, confusion	Hip fracture, driving accidents	History of addictions, memory impairment

Drug	Use	Common, Benign Side Effects	Serious Side Effects	Life-threatening Side Effects	Reasons Not to Take
Clorazepate (Tranxene)	Insomnia	Drowsiness	Dependency, memory loss, confusion	Hip fracture, driving accidents	History of addictions, memory impairment
Halazepam (Paxipam)	Insomnia	Drowsiness	Dependency, memory loss, confusion	Hip fracture, driving accidents	History of addictions, memory impairment
Prazepam (Centrax)	Insomnia	Drowsiness	Dependency, memory loss, confusion	Hip fracture, driving accidents	History of addictions, memory impairment
Quazepam (Doral)	Insomnia	Drowsiness	Dependency, memory loss, confusion	Hip fracture, driving accidents	History of addictions, memory impairment
Estazolam (Prosom)	Insomnia	Drowsiness	Dependency, memory loss, confusion	Hip fracture, driving accidents	History of addictions, memory impairment
Diazepam (Valium)	Insomnia	Drowsiness	Dependency, memory loss, confusion	Hip fracture, driving accidents	History of addictions, memory impairment
Flurazepam (Dalmane)	Insomnia	Drowsiness	Dependency, memory loss, confusion	Hip fracture, driving accidents	History of addictions, memory impairment

Serotonin 1A Agonists

Low Risk

Drug	Use	Common, Benign Side Effects	Serious Side Effects	Life-threatening Side Effects	Reasons Not to Take
Buspirone (Buspar)	Insomnia	Nausea, headache, light-headedness	None	None	None

Drug	Use	Common, Benign Side Effects	Serious Side Effects	Life-threatening Side Effects	Reasons Not to Take
Z Drugs					
Moderate Risk					
Zaleplon (Sonata)	Insomnia	Drowsiness, headache, nervousness	Memory loss	Sleepwalking, driving accidents	Allergy to medication
Zolpidem (Ambien)	Insomnia	Drowsiness, headache, nervousness	Memory loss	Sleepwalking, driving accidents	Allergy to medication
Eszopiclone (Lunesta)	Insomnia	Drowsiness, headache, nervousness, bad taste	Memory loss	Sleepwalking, driving accidents	Allergy to medication
Zopiclone (Imovane)	Insomnia	Drowsiness, headache, nervousness	Memory loss	Sleepwalking, driving accidents	Allergy to medication
Melatonin Receptor Agonists					
Low Risk					
Ramelteon (Rozerem)	Insomnia	Headache, drowsiness, fatigue, dizziness, nausea	Diarrhea	Depression	Pregnancy or nursing

17.

Drugs for
Sexual Dysfunction

I n the past few years there has been a steady rise in the promotion, publicity, and advertising for disorders of sexual function, including most prominently erectile dysfunction (ED). ED is defined as an inability to achieve or maintain an erection sufficient for sexual intercourse. An estimated 10 to 20 million Americans, including 15% of men over age seventy, suffer from ED.

Older men who suffer from hypertension, vascular disease, and/or diabetes are the men who most commonly experience ED. These conditions lead to changes in blood vessels, which in turn cause ED. The second-most-common cause of ED is other medications, including antihypertensives, beta-blockers, antipsychotics, antidepressants, spironolactone (Aldactone), cimetidine (Tagamet), and finasteride (Proscar). Psychological or emotional concerns are the *least* common causes.

Needless to say, the pharmaceutical industry is exploiting a previously untapped market of millions of older adults with sexual difficulties as well as, and even more important, millions more younger men who have no or barely significant problems with sexual function but who use ED drugs recreationally in order to last longer during intercourse. Indeed, according to a 2003 report in the *New York Times,* "GlaxoSmithKline and Bayer, the comarketers of Levitra, boldly admit that they are focusing on men who may have successful sexual relationships but who simply want to improve the quality or duration of their erections."

This statement upset the makers of Viagra so much that Pfizer spokeswoman Janice Lipsky told *Times* reporter Gardiner Harris that Levitra had benefited from "false claims and public relations in which they inaccurately state that Levitra works faster and is better, neither of which is true." Such petulance on the part of drug companies is unusual, but it shows how competitive they are for consumer preference; after all, in 2003 after only one month of not-so-subtle advertising (including a guy in a commercial who throws a football through a circle perfectly after taking the drug), Levitra had captured half of Viagra's market share among new prescriptions, as reported by the *New York Times* on September 18, 2003 ("Levitra, a Rival with Ribald Ads, Gains on Viagra").

The Big Three

Viagra, Levitra, and Cialis, known as the Big Three, are the most widely available and commonly prescribed ED drugs; competition for market share among their makers is stiff. Unfortunately, none of them is perfect, and each has significant downsides to consider.

SILDENAFIL

Sildenafil (Viagra) has been available since the late 1990s for the treatment of ED, and currently about 7 million prescriptions for Viagra are written every year, representing $1 billion a year in sales. Like a lot of drugs, this one's journey to the pharmacist's shelf began in a quest to treat a different condition, in this case angina (heart disease). During trial studies researchers noticed that it had a positive effect on erection, which turned out to be stimulating news for Pfizer. The drug was patented in 1996, approved by the FDA on March 27, 1998, and became the first pill approved for the treatment of erectile dysfunction in the U.S.

Viagra works because it inhibits the cyclic guanosine monophosphate (cGMP) phosphodiesterase type-5 (PDE5) enzyme, thereby increasing blood flow in the corpus callosum of the penis and causing an erection. Viagra has its peak effect in one hour and lasts about four hours.

Viagra has been shown to be highly effective for ED. Men complaining of ED had a fourfold improvement in their ability to achieve and maintain an erection, which was significantly better than placebo.[1] There was also a doubling of satisfaction with intercourse.

Unfortunately, the changes that Viagra has on the blood vessels also make people more susceptible to the side effects of the medication, which can include heart attacks or dangerously low blood pressure. Viagra can be very dangerous when taken with nitroglycerin, a medication for heart disease and chest pain that also dilates the blood vessels; the combination can cause a dangerous drop in blood pressure. Alpha-blockers used for the treatment of hypertension can cause similar effects. Viagra and nitrates, or alpha-blockers, should not be taken within twenty-four hours of each other. About 120 men per year die after taking Viagra; in most cases the cause can be attributed to a cardiovascular event. Other side effects are headache, flushing, and dyspepsia. An infrequent side effect is an erection that doesn't go away.

Another rare complication of Viagra is blindness. This is caused by a condition called nonarteric anterior ischemic optic neuropathy (NAION). NAION is caused when a blood vessel is blocked by a blood clot or atherosclerosis. Similar problems elsewhere in the body lead to heart attacks and strokes. But when the blood vessel leads to the optic nerve, vision loss or blindness in the eye can be the result. The FDA has received fifty or so case reports of the drug having causing NAION. This condition often clears by itself with time.

Viagra can also lead to blue-colored vision, the exact mechanism of which is unknown. This condition also gradually improves with time.

You should not take Viagra more than once a day or use it with other drugs for ED.

VARDENAFIL

Vardenafil (Levitra) has a time effect and profile similar to those of Viagra—the one thing that the Pfizer spokesperson was right about. All ED drugs (Levitra, Cialis) have the same mechanism of action as Viagra; there is no evidence that one is more effective or safer than another, and all have the same potential side effects. Like Viagra, Levitra can also be used for one-time-only sexual intercourse. There have been no reported cases of NAION with Levitra.

TADALAFIL

Unlike Viagra and Levitra, Tadalafil (Cialis) acts for up to forty-eight hours. It is therefore marketed as enabling the user to engage in more spontaneous sexual activity over, say, the course of a weekend. Side effects of Cialis are similar to those of Viagra. There have been a few cases of blue-colored vision with Cialis.

Other Pharmaceutical Treatments

There are a couple of other drug therapies that are used to treat ED with some efficacy.

TESTOSTERONE

Testosterone is frequently used for decreased libido in both men and women. With normal aging there is a natural decrease in testosterone that may be associated with decreased libido. It is often prescribed for men who have a condition called hypogonadism, which is characterized by lower-than-normal testosterone levels and can be caused by conditions that affect the testes, pituitary gland, or hypothalamus gland or by a genetic disorder. Many doctors prescribe testosterone for older men with ED who have "low-normal" testosterone levels, especially males who have not responded to Viagra. It can be prescribed as a pill or as a gel that is applied locally to the penis. Studies of the long-term safety and efficacy of testosterone have not been done. Testosterone can cause gynecomastia (enlargement of breasts), a loss of sperm (with infertility), and excessive frequency and duration of erections—the side effect that prompts doctors to prescribe it for ED. In women there is a decrease in estrogen, progesterone, and androgens (including testosterone) on the order of 25% to 50% after menopause. Testosterone is the hormone that is most linked to libido in women. Because of this, women with decreased libido can be treated with testosterone. Testosterone should not be used by patients with serious cardiac, hepatic, or renal disease or by patients with carcinoma of the breast or prostate.

ALPROSTADIL

Two treatments for ED involve using a drug called alprostadil (al-PROS-tuh-dil) (Caverject). Alprostadil, a synthetic version of the hormone prostaglandin E, helps relax smooth muscle tissue in the penis, thereby enhancing the blood flow needed for an erection. There are two ways to use alprostadil:

* *Needle-injection therapy.* With this method, a fine needle is used to inject alprostadil (Caverject, Edex) into the base or side of the penis. This generally produces in five to twenty minutes an erection that lasts about an hour. Because the injection goes directly into the spongy cylinders that fill with blood, alprostadil is an effective treatment for many men. And because the needle used is so fine, pain from the injection site is usually minor. Other side effects may include bleeding from the injection, pro-

longed erection, and formation of fibrous tissue at the injection site. The cost per injection can be expensive. Injecting a mixture of alprostadil and other prescribed drugs may be a less expensive and more effective option. These other drugs may include papaverine and phentolamine (Regitine).

• *Self-administered intraurethral therapy.* This method's trade name is Medicated Urethral System for Erection (MUSE). It involves using a disposable applicator to insert a tiny suppository, about half the size of a grain of rice, into the tip of the penis. The suppository, placed about two inches into the urethra, is absorbed by erectile tissue in the penis, increasing the blood flow that causes an erection. Although needles aren't involved, this method may still be painful or uncomfortable. Side effects may include pain, minor bleeding in the urethra, dizziness, and formation of fibrous tissue.

Alternative Medicines

A number of herbs have traditionally been used for male impotence. They are marketed heavily today to compete in the "natural" market as "healthy" and easily available options for those who don't want to or can't get prescription-only ED pharmaceuticals. However, there is currently little in the way of controlled research studies in this area that tells us anything definitive about their efficacy or serious side effects.

HERBS

Asian ginseng *(Panax ginseng)* has traditionally been used for male impotence, though no current studies support this usage. Ginseng is safe, although the mechanism by which it is purported to work is not clear. Damiana *(Turnera diffusa)* is a flowering shrub that was traditionally used as an aphrodisiac and as a treatment for various sexual disorders; there are no current studies to confirm its effectiveness, although it is apparently safe. Ginkgo biloba increases arterial blood flow, which may have a positive effect on male sexual function. Muira puama *(Ptychopetalum olacoides)* is promoted for ED and lack of libido. There are no major toxicities, although there are no studies demonstrating efficacy. I would recommend saving your money instead of buying any of these remedies.

YOHIMBE

Yohimbe (also spelled Yohimbine) is a natural product derived from the bark of an African tree that is used for the treatment of impotence. Yohimbe does work for impotence, but like many plant products it has specific known pharmacological effects and has been absorbed into the world of pharmacology. Yohimbe is known to block certain receptors in the brain that results in a stimulation of the adrenergic system. Yohimbe does not work better than Viagra and friends, and has the same side effects (anxiety, restlessness, and the potential for cardiac events).

Diet and Behavior

Studies have shown that obese men with ED who underwent a diet and exercise program lost fourteen pounds and had an improvement of 14 to 19 on the International Index of Erectile Function. These gains were statistically significant, although not of the same magnitude as those of Viagra.[2] For heavy men with ED, losing weight has some advantages in terms of sexual function. However, there are many men, both overweight and not overweight, who have ED that will not respond to weight loss.

The Bottom Line

ED drugs do have a role in some men's health by helping those who suffer from true ED improve their relationships and sexual satisfaction. Patients with heart disease, however, need to proceed with caution when considering ED drugs, and review with their doctors all medications they are taking before they fill a prescription for any impotence pharmaceutical. I also do not recommend ED drugs for recreational use, because we don't know the long-term effects, and some of the short-term effects we do know, like blindness, can be devastating, to say the least.

Drug	Use	Common, Benign Side Effects	Serious Side Effects	Life-threatening Side Effects	Reasons Not to Take
Erectile Dysfunction Drugs					
Moderate Risk					
Sildenafil (Viagra)	Erectile dysfunction	Headache, flushing, dyspepsia	Persistent erection, blindness, blue-colored vision	Heart attack, stroke (rare in patients without heart disease)	Heart disease, treatment with nitro-glycerin or alpha-blockers
Vardenafil (Levitra)	Erectile dysfunction	Headache, flushing, dyspepsia	Persistent erection	Heart attack, stroke (rare in patients without heart disease)	Heart disease, treatment with nitro-glycerin or alpha-blockers
Tadalafil (Cialis)	Erectile dysfunction	Headache, flushing, dyspepsia	Persistent erection, blindness, blue-colored vision	Heart attack, stroke (rare in patients without heart disease)	Heart disease, treatment with nitro-glycerin or alpha-blockers

Drug	Use	Common, Benign Side Effects	Serious Side Effects	Life-threatening Side Effects	Reasons Not to Take
Androgens					
Moderate Risk					
Testosterone (Histerone, Tesamone, Delatest, Everone, Andronate, Depo, Duratest, Testoderm, Androderm)	Decreased libido	Dizziness, insomnia, headache, fatigue, acne	Gynecomastia, loss of sperm, excessive erections, accentuation of male features	Hypercalcemia, prostatic hypertrophy	Cancer of breast or prostate; severe kidney, liver, or cardiac disease
Methyl testosterone (Android, Orton, Tested, Vermilion, Meander)	Decreased libido	Dizziness, insomnia, headache, fatigue, acne	Gynecomastia, loss of sperm, excessive erections, accentuation of male features	Hypercalcemia, prostatic hypertrophy	Cancer of breast or prostate; severe kidney, liver, or cardiac disease
Fluoxymes-terone (Halotestin)	Decreased libido	Dizziness, insomnia, headache, fatigue, acne	Gynecomastia, loss of sperm, excessive erections, accentuation of male features	Hypercalcemia, prostatic hypertrophy	Cancer of breast or prostate; severe kidney, liver, or cardiac disease

18.

Vitamins and Supplements

Whenever I visit my hometown of Seattle I'm astonished at the number of local television and radio talk shows devoted to dispersing "information" on vitamins and dietary supplements. Cheerful hosts who are neither medical experts nor scientists gladly dispense testimonials on the power of vitamins and offer vitamin remedies for various ailments to their eager audiences. Almost nothing of what they are saying, unfortunately, is based on fact or hard science.

Perhaps the situation is the same across the country, and I notice the proliferation of these shows only when I'm visiting family and have more time to peruse the popular media. It could very well be the case that such programs are on all the time everywhere, since 40% of us use some type of alternative medicine, often in concert with conventional treatments, and most of those who use alternative medicines never tell their doctors. Today, the alternative-medicine industry, which includes vitamins, supplements, homeopathic remedies, and herbs, is a $46-billion-per-year business, large enough to compete with pharmaceutical companies. Sales of vitamins alone are $17 billion a year and growing because a lot of us buy into the argument that vitamins are worth the money. If you were to follow the

343

advice of one company (Life Extension), as many do, you would spend a minimum of $7,248 per year on vitamins.

There is something awfully seductive about the idea that some extra vitamin A every morning or a dose of ginseng tea twice a day can somehow change your life for the better, particularly for a country full of optimists. This is magical thinking at best, since there is little evidence that vitamins and supplements taken in a pill form are good for our health. In fact, scientific evidence shows that some vitamins are bad for us, increasing the risk of cancer and heart disease, hip fracture, and other ailments. Others, taken in high doses, can be toxic. These are the findings of well-designed controlled trials that involved tens of thousands of patients and that have been replicated several times over! In fact, people in the scientific community are now calling on researchers to stop spending money on vitamin-supplement trials because we know these products are either useless or harmful in terms of health.

For instance, Deepak Vivekananthan, Mark Penn, Shelly Sapp, Amy Hsu, and Eric Topol from the Cleveland Clinic wrote in 2003 that "the use of vitamin supplements containing beta-carotenes and vitamin A, beta-carotene's biologically active metabolite, should be actively discouraged because this family of agents is associated with a small but significant excess of all cause mortality and cardiovascular death [i.e. death from any cause or death from heart disease]. We recommend that clinical trials of beta-carotene should be discontinued because of its risks . . . we do not support the continued use of vitamin E treatment and discourage the inclusion of vitamin E in future primary and secondary prevention trials . . ."[1]

The most important fact to remember about the beneficial effects of vitamins is that they are related to the nutritional content of the foods they are found in. The nutritional value and benefits of vitamins in foods are not transferred when vitamins are put into pill form. For example, there are multiple forms of vitamin C in an orange, but vitamin tablets have only one form of vitamin C. We have no guarantee that the form of vitamin C in the pill is the helpful form we find in an orange. I understand that for those of you who may be avid vitamin takers, this information is a very hard pill to swallow. But you can get every vitamin you need by eating a variety of fresh vegetables, fruits, whole grains, legumes, and lean protein.

If you take more than you need in pill form, you may be causing yourself harm. The Danes were puzzled by the fact that there was an increase in osteoporosis among Danish women. They analyzed a number of factors and found that excessive intake of vitamins, whether through fortified foods or other sources, was associated with an increased risk of osteoporosis in their county. They found a link to the excessive intake of vitamins through American fortified foods, such as breakfast cereals. It seems the American predilection for fortifying everything with vitamins has gone haywire. As a result, the Danes banned Kellogg's vitamin-fortified cereal. On December 8, 2004, a spokesperson for that country was quoted by *nutraingredients.com* as saying that "the Danish population already has a high intake of calcium, iron, B_6 and folic acid . . . the knowledge on toxicity of vitamins and minerals is very limited and practically nonexistent for children . . . [vitamin deficiencies exist] only in small groups like immigrants who aren't getting enough vitamin D or pregnant women who need folic acid. We need to take care of all of the groups in our population." Since that time the European Union has placed a limit on the amount of vitamins and minerals that can be added to food.

And it isn't only in Europe. Feskanitch and colleagues followed 72,337 nurses from 1980 to 1998 and showed that women in the top 20% of vitamin A intake (through diet and vitamin supplements such as multivitamins) had a 48% increase in hip fracture compared with women in the bottom 20% of vitamin A intake.[2]

I don't want to leave you with the impression that vitamins and supplements are always dangerous, because they are not. Nor do I want to leave you with the impression that vitamin and nutrient supplementation of the food supply is always a bad thing. However, if you are a resident of the U.S. or Europe and have access to a variety of foods, you don't need added vitamins, minerals, or supplements, for they are more likely to cause harm than good. There are residents of Third World countries, however, who may benefit from the addition of vitamins and supplements to their foods.

We are continuously discovering more beneficial effects of the nutrients found in fruits and vegetables, so it is always better to eat these primary sources of vitamins rather than to take them in pill form.

Vitamins and Nutrition

Vitamins got their name because they are "vital to life," meaning that if you are completely deprived of them for a long enough period of time, you become sick. One hundred years ago many of our forefathers did suffer from malnutrition. That was an age of *undernutrition*. Americans are now living in an age of *overnutrition* or overeating, depending on how you look at it. Today's modern food-distribution system and the availability of a wide range of fresh foods throughout the year mean dietary deprivation is no longer an issue in this country. Except for a few isolated cases of people who can't absorb their food, we haven't seen mass cases of vitamin deficiency in this country since the pilgrims washed ashore. We've just been frightened or overly excited by vitamin manufacturers, the processed-food industry, and their supporters in the government into thinking we can benefit from supplements. We don't.

The link between health and vitamins may have gained momentum in 1962, when Linus Pauling won the Nobel Prize. He was convinced that megadoses of vitamins were good for your health. But these claims were based solely on his personal experience with vitamins; his own research had nothing to do with vitamin C. Just because one person takes a pill and feels better (even if the person is a Nobel Prize–winning scientist), that doesn't mean the pill was responsible for the effect. That is why we have placebo-controlled trials. In fact, there is no evidence to support the claim that vitamin C in pills or in fresh foods prevents colds. The best that can be said is that vitamin C reduces symptoms by 23% and may decrease the length of time you suffer from cold symptoms by about a day. The fact that vitamin C continues to be touted for the prevention of colds can only be attributed to the incredible marketing ability of the vitamin and supplement industry and the ability of the American public to suspend disbelief.

The modern-day obsession with vitamins, supplements, and nutrition can be traced back to a book from the 1960s called *Let's Get Well* by Adelle Davis, who advocated high doses of vitamins for the promotion of health and the prevention of heart disease and cancer. Davis claimed to have spent many hours in the library reading the scientific literature to find support for the statements she made in her books. Later it was found that many of the citations were grossly inaccurate or had no basis in reality. Davis died of cancer at the age of seventy. J. I. Rodale, founder of Rodale Press and the magazine *Prevention,* was another advocate of high-dose vitamins for disease prevention. He died of a heart attack at the age of seventy-two.

The USDA hedged its bets regarding vitamins when in 1941 it first came up with the Recommended Daily Allowance (RDA). The RDA determined how many vitamins and minerals we need to take in daily in our diets. (This is not to be confused with the food pyramid, developed by the USDA in the 1950s, which tells us how much of the different food groups, like fruits, vegetables, cereals, meat, and dairy products, we need.) Most of us are familiar with the RDA from our childhood days of reading the back of our cereal boxes during breakfast time. What most people don't understand is that the authors of the RDA only knew what degree of deprivation caused illness.

The USDA didn't really know the minimum of what you could take and still be healthy. For instance, pellagra, a condition caused by a deficiency of niacin (vitamin B_3) that plagued the American South in the first part of the twentieth century, was associated with mental dullness, lethargy, and other symptoms. It was related to the southern diet of fatback, corn bread and molasses. When foods with niacin and its precursor, tryptophan, such as meats and dairy products, became more available as the standard of living rose, the deficiency was eliminated along with the disease.

However, since the southern diet was previously devoid of these foods and since no clinical trials were ever conducted to determine the minimum amount of niacin required, government officials essentially hedged their bets and doubled what you probably need. Better safe than sorry. They also based the recommendation on a tall, young, healthy male who exercises on a regular basis. That means the RDA recommendations don't apply to women, children, the elderly, small people, or sedentary folks. The USDA doesn't have a clue how much those people need. In fact, if those people followed the USDA recommendations, it wouldn't be possible to eat enough food to get all the vitamins it says are needed without getting fat, unless they exercised quite a bit. Based on the fact that the RDA analysis of vitamin requirements is founded on a bogus standard related to a young, healthy male and an estimate that started out at least double the necessary requirement, the RDA nutritional requirements are at least four times the actual minimum amount of vitamins and minerals needed and probably much, much more.

A, B_{12} AND CS OF THE INDUSTRY

Largely due to the legislative efforts of Senator Orrin Hatch (R-Utah), who has been part owner of a vitamin company and an important advocate for the vitamin and supplement industry, one fifth of which is located in his home state of Utah, the vitamin and supplement industry is not regulated. Congressional passage of the Dietary Supplement Health and Education Act (DSHEA), which was sponsored by Senator Hatch in 1994, removed regulatory authority that the FDA previously had over vitamins and supplements by providing manufacturers with a very large loophole. As long as they don't claim that their products cure a *specific disease* without showing evidence, they can make general health claims without providing backup. For instance, a manufacturer can say its product "promotes liver health" and advise someone with a liver problem to take it. The fact that there is no evidence for this claim doesn't matter under the law. No wonder we get taken in by vitamin salespeople. They can and do make their products sound so good.

The FDA does not regulate quality control of vitamins and supplements in the same way that it regulates drug safety and manufacture, and as a result product quality is not particularly reliable. One quarter of vitamins and supplements have no measurable amount of the substance they purport to contain, while another quarter has less than half of the amount of the item listed on the label. Many products are manufactured in Asia, and are adulterated with chemicals, minerals, pharmaceuticals, and sometimes other harmful ingredients, such as pesticides. (Check www.consumer lab.com for details.)

The usual tactic that vitamin makers use to sell their products is to point to evidence that a vitamin has had a particular effect in laboratory studies, ignoring data related to their actual use by humans. Like the pharmaceutical companies, they have found a larger audience in healthy people by emphasizing the so-called preventative qualities of their products. Indeed, vitamin makers claim their products can prevent everything from aging to cancer.

Supplement marketers are fond of using the language of science to push products. In the case of antiaging, for example, a company typically finds a very basic scientific study about the antioxidant properties of a particular vitamin, and it will link that with research that oxidation increases with aging and contributes to age-related diseases like heart disease and cancer. However, just because something has antioxidant properties doesn't mean that taking it will prevent diseases related to oxidation. For example, vitamin E has been shown in animal studies to reduce free radicals that cause oxidative stress in animal models of atherosclerosis. Based on studies like this many scientists have had high hopes that vitamins would prevent heart disease as well as other diseases like cancer. In fact, the studies that have been done, which I discuss later in this chapter, show that, if anything, they have the opposite effect.

Most sober scientists who pay attention to the data have come to the conclusion that vitamins and supplements do not prevent heart disease and cancer. That has not, however, prevented vitamin marketers from continuing to promote the theoretical benefits of vitamins, based on animal studies that have not been extended to clinical trials in humans. As I will outline below, vitamins have no benefit and in many cases have the potential to harm. In my opinion, with vitamins and supplements we have returned to the era of the patent medicines (undocumented and potentially dangerous compounds that were promoted with outrageous health claims, which led to the passage of the Food and Drug Act in 1905).

Another aspect of vitamin marketing is the portrayal of products as wholesome and natural. They are frequently juxtaposed with conventional medications, which are portrayed as artificial, foreign, unwholesome, and potentially dangerous. And yet vitamins and minerals are no more natural than medications. They are all chemically manufactured in factories. Vitamin and supplement makers are big companies, often conglomerates, with aggressive marketing teams and big advertising budgets. They thrive on the absence of information.

Conventional doctors often look the other way, because they don't want to be accused of being out of touch with patients or too focused on technological or pharmaceutical solutions. Another factor is that patients do not typically tell their doctors what herbs, vitamins, and supplements they are taking, so doctors do not always know what they are on.

However, doctors have become increasingly concerned about the potential harm that the hawkers of vitamins can do. In the summer of 2005, the prestigious Medical Letter, a nonprofit group that studies the evidence and develops consensus statements to advise doctors about important medical issues, issued a critical report on a number of different vitamins, stressing the apparent risks that have emerged from recent studies. The Food and Nutrition Board of the National Academy of Sciences—the top U.S. authority on nutritional recommendations—has concluded that taking antioxidant supplements serves no purpose.

"People hear that if they take vitamins they'll feel better," says Edgar R. Miller, clinical investigator for the National Institute on Aging and author of an analysis that showed a higher risk of death among vitamin E users in several studies. "But when you put [vitamins] to the test in clinical trials, the results are hugely disappointing and in some cases show harm. People think they are going to live longer, but the evidence doesn't support that. Sometimes it's actually the opposite."

If the preceding argument has not convinced you to stop taking vitamins, the following look at the most commonly consumed vitamins, supplements, and herbs will show you just how potentially unsafe those benign-looking pills can be.

Multivitamins

According to the USDA's MyPyramid, we need to eat five servings of fruits and vegetables a day. Vitamin makers are quick to point out that Americans don't do that, so they need to take a multivitamin every day. For instance, the Life Extension Foundation (affiliated with the vitamin and supplement manufacturer Life Extension), reported that the number of vitamins in fruits and vegetables farmed in the U.S. has been declining over the past fifty years. In the September 2005 issue of *Life Extension* magazine, the foundation stated that "for those who find the new, unregulated world of genetically manipulated vitaminless vegetables unpalatable—or find that they don't want to eat vegetables that have absorbed . . . pesticides in the soil . . . high quality standardized supplements are one way of incorporating a standard amount of known nutrients in the diet . . ."

But do multivitamins help? Large studies have shown that a multivitamin a day or taking a suite of individual vitamins does not decrease the numbers of infections that people get. At best it may reduce the time you spend being sick by a day or so.

The multivitamin craze started with epidemiological studies showing lower rates of cancer and heart disease in people who eat lots of fruits and vegetables. It was assumed that the antioxidant properties of the vitamins in fruits and vegetables must prevent oxidative damage to LDL cholesterol and DNA. However, there never really was good evidence that vitamin pills provided helpful antioxidants in the first place. And we don't really know what it is about fruits and vegetables that is good for you, since manufactured vitamins represent only one small element of the multitude of compounds (including multiple forms of the same vitamins) present in fruits and vegetables. In addition, scientists are not sure that removal of free radicals by antioxidant agents is necessarily a good thing; one theory is that by doing so the immune system becomes less vigilant and more likely to miss cancerous cells, thereby increasing the risk of cancer.

However, once people were convinced that antioxidants could help prevent cancer and heart disease and that antioxidants could be obtained through vitamins, it became fixed in their minds. But the studies showing the link between cancer and antioxidants in produce have been out for at least ten years, so it's hard to understand why they aren't better known. Certainly vitamin manufacturers do not want the studies publicized, but public health officials should have an interest in making sure the knowledge is widely distributed to the public.

VITAMIN A

One of the most potentially toxic vitamins is vitamin A. Found naturally in the form of beta-carotenes in carrots and other bright orange, yellow, and green vegetables like sweet potato, pumpkin, asparagus, and spinach and in liver, it is vital to good vision and other physiological functions. A deficiency of this vitamin, particularly in children, causes night blindness, skin and neurological problems, and a greater risk of death from measles, diarrhea, or malaria. Almost nonexistent in the industrialized world, it is a major problem in developing countries where food is less plentiful.

When beta-carotene is broken down, it yields vitamin A. Both vitamin A and the beta-carotenes are sold as vitamins or supplements, respectively; however, they both are converted in the body to the physiologically active form of vitamin A, retinoic acid, which is the version of vitamin A that actually has an effect on the body.

Since vitamin A has antioxidant properties, it has long been assumed to have protective effects on diseases related to oxidation, like heart disease and cancer. However, years of research and large studies with tens of thousands of patients have shown that vitamins do not prevent heart disease or cancer. In fact, rather than protecting your health, unnecessary amounts of vitamin A can actually have the opposite effect. In the beta-carotene component of the Physicians' Health Study, 22,071 male physicians were randomized to either beta-carotene at doses equal to two carrots a day or to a placebo for a twelve-year period. There were no overall differences between the two groups in rates of cancer and heart disease,[3] which suggests that vitamin A and specifically its antioxidant properties did not reduce disease rates.

In the Beta-Carotene and Retinol Efficacy Trial (CARET), 18,314 smokers were randomized to either beta-carotene and vitamin A in doses equal to four carrots a day or to a placebo. There was a 28% increase in lung cancer in the supplemented group, which was statistically significant.[4] Mortality was 17% higher in the supplemented group as a result of a 28% higher rate of lung cancer and a 17% higher rate of heart disease. In other words, those who received the vitamin got *more* cancer, not less.

In the Alpha-Tocopherol, Beta-Carotene (ATBC) Cancer Prevention Study 29,133 male smokers from Finland were treated with beta-carotene, alpha-tocopherol (vitamin E), a combination of the two, or a placebo in a randomized double-blind trial. There was an 18% increase in lung cancer and an 8% increase in total mortality in the beta-carotene–supplemented group.[5] Smokers with a prior history of heart attack had a 75% increase in heart attack with beta-carotene therapy.[6] Subjects getting vitamin E had a 2% increase in mortality.

As mentioned above, Feskanitch and colleagues showed that vitamin A increased the risk of osteoporosis, or thinning of the bones, in women to the point where the risk of hip fracture was increased by 48%. These effects were seen in women *taking as little as twice the recommended daily amount of vitamin A.* For every 1 mg increase in retinol (a form of vitamin A), there was a 68% increase in the risk of hip fracture. In fact, a national epidemic of osteoporosis in Swedish women was traced to a supplementation of vitamin A in food in that country.

Megadoses of vitamin A can also cause dry skin, swelling of the brain, psychosis, depression, headache, ulceration of the colon, and a range of other toxic effects. We have known about the toxicity of vitamin A since the nineteenth century, when explorers at the North Pole became psychotic after eating polar bear liver, which has high concentrations of vitamin A.

There is also cause for concern for women who take vitamins containing vitamin A during pregnancy. Vitamin A is a retinoid, which is known to affect the development of neural tissue in utero. Rothman and colleagues reported in the *New England Journal of Medicine* in 1995 that taking high doses of vitamin A during pregnancy was associated with an increase in birth defects, primarily deformations of nervous tissue and the heart. The risk of birth defects was increased 2.6-fold in women who took supplements that when combined with food intake provided less than double the Recommended Daily Allowance (RDA). In other words, if women took *any* supplements, they increased the risk of birth defects. In fact, women who might get pregnant should not take multivitamins that have *any* vitamin A or beta-carotene in them even at lower doses, given their known association with birth defects. The average woman already gets 120% of required vitamin A from diet alone, so there is no need for supplementation. For men who eat a balanced diet that includes fruits and vegetables, there is no need for vitamin A supplementation.

Based on these studies, doctors such as Dr. Vivekananthan and his colleagues have repeatedly recommended ending the enrollment of patients in trials of vitamin A and beta-carotene and ending their use in daily practice. After looking at all the studies, it is easy to conclude that there is an increased risk of both heart disease and cancer with beta-carotene. Combining results from several studies showed that patients getting a combination of vitamin A and beta-carotene had a 29% increase in mortality.[7] These findings were very surprising to those who conducted the studies, as they were expecting the opposite.

So does that mean we should stop eating carrots? No. Don't forget that vitamin A is essential for survival. However, vitamin A is stored in the liver for long periods of time, and the amount that we get in our diet is more than adequate. As I said before, there is evidence that eating foods high in vitamin A increases the risk of osteoporosis, even in the absence of supplements. The greatest concern is in Nordic countries, where diets are high in fish oils, liver, and other foods high in vitamin A. Based on the results of the studies I've reviewed, I recommend that you not take *any* amount of vitamin A or beta-carotene in the form of *fortified* foods like breakfast cereal or vitamins and supplements.

VITAMIN C

Vitamin C is a water-soluble vitamin that is required for the growth and repair of many tissues of the body. As I discussed earlier, from the late 1960s until just before his death in 1994, Nobel Prize–winning scientist Linus Pauling was convinced that megadoses of vitamin C were not only good for you in general but specifically were able to prevent colds. But these claims were based solely on his personal experience with vitamins and not on his own research with vitamin C. There is in fact no evidence that vitamin C prevents colds. The best that can be said is that vitamin C may decrease the length of time you suffer from cold symptoms by about a day *if you take vitamin C year-round.* There is no evidence that vitamin C prevents or is beneficial for the treatment of any other diseases.

Since vitamin C is not fat soluble and therefore is excreted almost right away in the urine, there are few side effects with regular doses. Megadoses can cause diarrhea, nausea, and abdominal cramps.

VITAMIN D AND CALCIUM

As I discuss in Chapter 11, vitamin D (cholecalciferol) and calcium are frequently used for the prevention of osteoporosis and hip fracture in aging women. The manufacturers of these products have gotten women so scared that their legs will snap off that women in their twenties often take them as supplements. However, there is *no* use for these pills, even for older women.

With normal aging, there is a decrease in calcium absorption by the stomach. Calcium is the major ingredient of bones, so with the age-related decrease in calcium absorption, there is a decrease in bone density. Vitamin D (cholecalciferol) increases calcium absorption in the gut, which has led to the common practice of prescribing calcium and vitamin D supplementation together for the prevention of hip fractures.

However, just because your bones will thin when you are in your sixties doesn't mean that taking calcium in your twenties or thirties will affect that. There is no evidence that taking calcium or vitamin D when you are young will prevent bone fractures in old age. Studies have shown that calcium and vitamin D supplementation in people over age sixty-five increased total bone density but not necessarily in the areas that matter, like the femoral neck.[8] Moreover, the changes in bone-mineral density in areas like the femoral neck (which cause hip fracture) were present only for men and not women. This is important since osteoporotic fractures primarily affect women.

The only studies that showed that calcium and vitamin D prevented hip fractures involved French women who had osteoporosis and were living in nursing homes.[9] However, it is unclear whether these women had calcium and/or vitamin D deficiency due to their nursing-home diet or lack of sunlight from their environment. Other studies of individuals outside nursing homes found no beneficial effects from vitamin D and calcium supplementation in terms of hip-fracture prevention.[10, 11] In what has been the most definitive study to date, 36,282 women in the Women's Health Initiative (WHI) study were randomized to calcium and vitamin D or placebo for seven years. There were no differences between the groups in hip fracture or other types of fractures, although there was an increase in kidney stones.[12]

Based on the evidence from these studies, there is no reason to take vitamin D or calcium, ever. You can get all the vitamin D you need by taking a walk in the sunshine, especially in winter, since sunlight stimulates natural formation of vitamin D. However, if you want to take vitamin D there is no risk.

VITAMIN E

Vitamin E was shown in the laboratory to have "antioxidant" effects that should be good for a number of things from heart disease to dementia. But trials for vitamin E have not shown that it prevents heart disease or cancer. For instance, in the Heart Protection Study, 20,536 patients with heart disease or diabetes were randomized to receive vitamins (a combination of vitamin E, beta-carotene, and vitamin C) or a matched placebo for five years. There was no difference in the mortality rates in the vitamin vs. placebo groups (14.1% vs. 13.5%). There were also no differences in rates of heart attacks (10.4% vs. 10.2%), stroke, cancer, or any other health outcome assessed.[13] In the Primary Prevention Project Study, 4,495 patients were randomized to vitamin E, aspirin, or no treatment. Although aspirin decreased the rate of heart attacks, vitamin E had no effect.[14]

The Gruppo Italiano per lo Studio della Sopravvivenza nell'Infarto Miocardico (GISSI) Prevenzione Trial assessed 11,324 Italians after a heart attack and randomly assigned them to take polyunsaturated fatty acids, vitamin E, both, or neither.[15] The polyunsaturated fatty acids led to a reduction in heart attacks and related events, but vitamin E had no effect. The ATBC study showed an increase in strokes with vitamin E. Three other studies, involving observations of tens of thousands of people, the Cambridge Heart Association AntiOxidant Study (CHAOS),[16] the Heart Outcomes Prevention Evaluation (HOPE) study,[17] and the Women's Health Study,[18] also failed to find a protective effect for vitamin E on heart disease. When Vivekananthan and colleagues looked at all of the published studies, they found that overall there were no heart-protective effects of vitamin E. In fact, if anything, there was a tendency to *increase* mortality, although only about 2%, which is less than that for vitamin A and beta-carotene.

One study of vitamin E combined with vitamin C showed that vitamins actually accelerated the progression of thickening of the coronary arteries and doubled the risk of dying of heart disease.[19] Another study of a combination of antioxidants, including vitamins E, C, beta-carotene, and selenium, showed that vitamins actually blocked the effects of anticholesterol treatment (simvastatin plus niacin) on reducing atherosclerosis and preventing heart attacks and strokes.[20] The vitamins in this study interfered with the ability of the other medications to raise HDL (good) cholesterol. When Bjelakovich and colleagues looked at all the studies combined in which vitamin E was given with beta-carotene, there was a 10% overall increase in mortality. Nobody knows why.

A 2005 analysis of all the published studies of the effects of vitamin E on health[21] found that nine out of eleven studies surveyed showed an increase in mortality with high-dose vitamin E treatment that was statistically significant. In short, there is no reason to add extra vitamin E in the form of supplements and vitamins to your diet; what you get in food is enough.

FOLIC ACID

The most practical reason for women of childbearing age to take multivitamins with folic acid supplements is the prevention of neural tube–related birth defects like spina bifida. Prevention of neural-tube birth defects is accomplished with 400 mcg of folic acid daily, obtained from food and/or vitamin supplements. Foods high in folate include leafy vegetables like lettuce and spinach as well as asparagus, broccoli, cauliflower, beets, and lentils. Folate is routinely added to a variety of food products because it has been shown to reduce the number of birth defects related to neural-tube defects when given to pregnant mothers. Folate is required at the time of conception, so if you wait until after you find out that you are pregnant it may be too late to add folate to your diet. However, this effect is related to the fact that a small fraction (<1%) of women have antibodies to folate that can cause birth defects in their babies. Is it safe and effective to give extra amounts of folate to everyone to prevent this problem in this small number of women with antibodies to folate? The answer is probably not.

Although the effects of massive administration of folate to the general population are not fully known, studies from animals are worrisome. David

Schwartz, M.D., MPH, director of the National Institute of Environmental Health, in a lecture to the Emory Predictive Health Symposia, talked about his unpublished research showing that animals who were chronically administered folate early in development developed constriction of the airways. The implications of this research is that folate in fortified foods like bread and cereals may be related to the increase in asthma in children that has occurred over the past few decades, although no one has shown a direct link so far.

Low folate in the blood has been linked to depression. However, obtaining adequate folate in the diet should be enough to prevent depression as well as problems related to birth defects in pregnant women.

There is a small fraction of the population of women who have antibodies to folate. For them, taking dietary folate *before* they get pregnant will prevent spina bifida in their offspring (a tragic condition involving abnormality of the spinal cord that leads to death and/or neurological impairment of the infant). Given the small risk that you may be one of these women I recommend taking folate *before* you conceive (the only time I will tell you to take vitamins or supplements).

STEROIDS

Several steroids are sold over the counter as supplements, although they probably should be classified as drugs because they have potentially dangerous side effects. Steroids are produced by the body and promote secondary sexual characteristics and reproduction (androgenic effects) as well as increases in muscle mass (anabolic). They are often marketed as antiaging pills or as energy and libido enhancers. All steroids are synthesized from cholesterol. Cholesterol is converted to pregnenolone, progesterone, dehydroepiandrosterone (DHEA), androstenedione, and testosterone. Progesterone is combined with estrogen for hormone replacement therapy to treat hot flashes and depression in postmenopausal women.

TESTOSTERONE

Several anabolic steroids are used by bodybuilders to artificially build up muscle mass. These drugs are sold over the counter as "pro-hormone" supplements. They are, however, converted into androgens in the body and should be considered such since they have potentially dangerous side effects. The U.S. is the only country in the world where these compounds are not regulated and controlled. These supplements include oxymethalone, stanozolol, oxandrolone, nandrolone phenproprionate, and nandrolone decanoate, which are all derived from testosterone. Anabolic steroids promote the hormone erythropoietin, which is responsible for the production of red blood cells, and they are therefore useful in the treatment of some anemias. They are mostly used by bodybuilders, and can cause hepatitis, loss of sperm, liver tumor, atherosclerosis, increased lipids, masculinization, and birth defects.

Androstenedione, a precursor of testosterone that is marketed over the counter as Andro, is promoted as an energy booster but is actually used by many athletes to build muscle mass. Andro can cause a loss of fertility and other side effects similar to those of the other anabolic steroids.

Testosterone and its precursors and derivatives are anabolic steroids that promote the buildup of muscle mass. Testosterone is used to treat decreased libido and to increase muscle mass in athletes. Taking testosterone supplements, however, can actually depress libido, and shuts off sperm production, causing infertility that can take months to recover from. In some cases recovery does not occur. Testosterone also leads to psychiatric side effects, including suicide. Other side effects are hypertension, tendon ruptures, liver tumors, and development of male characteristics in women. Based on these potential side effects and the lack of any good reason to take these steroids I do not recommend taking them.

DHEA

Dehydroepiandrosterone (DHEA) is marketed as an antiaging pill, which, thanks to some fancy footwork in Congress (the DSHEA, or the Dietary

Supplement Health and Education Act, as explained earlier), is available over the counter. DHEA declines with normal aging. Since DHEA blocks the effects of stress hormones like cortisol and has a protective effect on neurons in animal models, it has been described as an antistress and antiaging hormone. DHEA, since it is a precursor of testosterone, is being used by athletes to build muscle mass, but it is not very effective for this purpose. DHEA is also promoted for the prevention of normal aging. Studies have not shown that DHEA prevents the changes in body mass and chemistry that occur with normal aging. DHEA does not have effects on measures of body composition affected by aging, like muscle strength, insulin sensitivity, and oxygen consumption or on quality of life.[22] Studies *have* shown that DHEA improves feelings of well-being and is useful in the treatment of depression. However, DHEA does not work better than antidepressants. I do not recommend DHEA for the treatment of depression or for any other indication.

CREATINE

Creatine, an oral supplement that increases muscle phosphocreatine, a molecule that stores energy in muscle, is commonly used by high school athletes to enhance their athletic performance. The use of supplemental creatine speeds up regeneration of adenosine triphosphate, which increases energy availability during exercise, thereby buffering lactate and reducing muscle pain. The main side effect of chronic use is weight gain.

Herbs and Other Plant Life

One of the most popular means of self-medication is the use of herbs and other plant products that are sold over the counter as supplements. Some medications, like digitalis, which is used in the treatment of heart failure, are derived from plants whose beneficial properties have been known for many centuries. Another example is red rice yeast extract, which contains natural forms of statins. Clinical trials have shown that St.-John's-wort is as effective for the treatment of depression as antidepressants like Prozac. However, for every plant or herb product that has some utility in the treatment of a specific condition, there are another ten that are actively marketed but are in fact useless or potentially harmful.

ALPHA LIPOIC ACID

Alpha lipoic acid (ALA) (sold as Juvenon, or as ALA, from a number of supplement makers) is found in liver, potatoes, and broccoli. It is also naturally found in the body and can be synthesized in the brain. ALA is a natural cofactor for a number of enzyme complexes involved in energy transfer. It is promoted in the U.S. as an antioxidant that can help prevent everything from cancer to heart disease, and is prescribed as a supplement for diabetic neuropathy in Germany. Alpha lipoic acid has no effect on glucose levels, but one study has shown it to decrease pain in patients with diabetic neuropathy. ALA does not have known major toxicities.

CHROMIUM

Chromium is an essential metal whose exact mechanism of action is unknown. Chromium is present in foods, and although the prevalence of chromium deficiency in humans is unknown, it is thought to be rare. Based on animal studies of chromium deficiency showing the development of insulin resistance, chromium has been advocated as a supplement for the treatment of diabetes. Some studies have shown some improvement with chromium, although these were mostly uncontrolled trials. Randomized controlled trials have not shown definitive efficacy for chromium in diabetics. In addition, excess doses can cause renal failure.

CHOLESTIN

Cholestin has been used in Chinese medicine for centuries for the treatment of heart problems. It is derived from yeast found on red rice and is marketed under the name "red rice yeast extract." This extract has eight statin compounds that are HMG coenzymeA reductase inhibitors and, just like statins, have been shown to reduce cholesterol. However, since the active ingredients of this supplement are chemically identical to those of the statins, they also have the same side effects. Some of these side effects (as described in Chapter 4) are sufficiently severe that treatment requires monitoring by a doctor; but if you want to work with your doctor and take red rice yeast extract, that is a reasonable course of action.

ECHINACEA

Echinacea is the name of a plant native to North America that has been used by Native Americans for centuries to treat infections. Echinacea is used now for the treatment of colds and other upper-respiratory-tract infections. Echinacea has been shown in animal studies to increase immunologic activity. Results of randomized, double-blind trials, however, have not shown echinacea to be useful in the prevention of upper respiratory tract infections. Echinacea and infection are reviewed in more detail in Chapter 10.

GARLIC

Garlic has been shown to improve glucose control in rat models of diabetes; studies in humans, however, have not shown the same result. Although garlic was initially promoted for cholesterol reduction, subsequent research has not confirmed that garlic has a beneficial effect for this purpose. Studies have shown, however, that daily ingestion of a garlic supplement reduces the number of colds. Garlic is also promoted for the prevention of a number of infections. It is thought that the chemical allicin, which is present in garlic, breaks down to sulfur, which has antibiotic properties. However, sulfur-containing antibiotic drugs can be substituted for the daily ingestion of garlic.

GINGER

Ginger (*Zingiber officinale*), which is obtained from the root of the ginger flower, is believed to have anti-inflammatory properties, and is used in Ayurvedic medicine for the treatment of inflammation and rheumatism. A recent treatment study of patients with osteoarthritis showed better efficacy for ibuprofen than ginger and no difference between ginger and placebo. There are no risks or major side effects from taking ginger.

GINKGO

People have long believed that *ginkgo biloba,* a supplement derived from the ancient ginkgo tree of China, increases memory, energy, and concentration. It is used to treat tinnitus (ringing in the ears) and vascular disease, and is believed to be a neuroprotective agent and antioxidant. In Germany more than 5 million prescriptions are written for ginkgo every year, and sales in the U.S. are $240 million per year. Studies of the effects of ginkgo on patients with dementia have shown some benefit, although the effects on cognitive tests were no greater than the modest effects of anticholinesterase inhibitors, and it is not associated with a subjective impression of improvement by families and doctors.

Manufacturers, however, also promote gingko for the enhancement of memory in normal individuals, or for prevention of the normal decline of memory with aging. A recent large controlled trial using a large battery of tests of normal individuals found that ginkgo had no effect on memory function. Ginkgo can have serious side effects, including coma, bleeding, and seizures. It should not be used with medications like Warfarin, which causes thinning of the blood. Minor but more common side effects are nausea, vomiting, diarrhea, headaches, and dizziness.

GINSENG

Ginseng products are derived from the roots of several plant species in the Araliaceae plant family, which is indigenous to Asia. Ginseng has been promoted as a "tonic" or "adaptogen" that promotes energy and endurance. Controlled studies have not found that ginseng promotes physical endurance, although some studies suggest an increase in feelings of well-being. So if you want to drink some ginseng tea to make yourself feel better, go ahead and enjoy it. There are no adverse effects of ginseng tea to worry about.

GREEN TEA

Widely consumed in Asian countries, green tea is believed to have antioxidant and anticancer effects. Steeping fresh leaves in very hot (not quite boiling) water makes green tea, which inactivates oxidizing enzymes and leaves intact polyphenols, which have been shown to have anti-inflammatory and anticancer properties in animal models. Based on this evidence, many consider green tea to be healthful, and many Japanese drink large quantities of it. Green tea extracts sold as supplements in the U.S. are promoted as having cancer-prevention properties. One study that examined the risk of stomach cancer in Japanese men found that drinking green tea conferred no protective effect.[23] In fact, there was a greater incidence of cancer among smokers who drank a lot of green tea than among those who drank less tea, which was of borderline statistical significance, although this might have been caused by the fact that people who smoke also tend to drink green tea.

Another study followed 40,530 Japanese adults for eleven years to measure mortality and green tea consumption. The authors found a significant inverse correlation between consumption of green tea and death from all causes (more green tea, fewer deaths) and death from heart disease (but not cancer).[24] This study was an observational study, however, and it may be that green-tea drinkers do other things that are good for their health and it is not the green tea itself that is helpful.

J. DOUGLAS BREMNER

HYDROXYCITRIC ACID

Hydroxycitric acid, a natural product that comes from the rind of the Indian brindle berry (*Garcinia*), is sold as the natural product garcinia and is promoted to aid weight loss and relieve gastrointestinal discomfort. It has been shown to inhibit the enzymes that convert compounds into coenzyme A, thereby blocking the storage of energy as fat. There is no good evidence to support its claimed ability to promote weight loss.

KAVA

Kava, derived from the plant *Piper methysticum,* is used in the South Pacific as a recreational drink. The kavapyrones it contains have a number of active ingredients that have muscle-relaxant properties and may act centrally in the brain. There is also some evidence from controlled trials that kava can reduce anxiety. However, kava can cause irreversible liver damage and death. Because of the risk of death from liver failure, kava should not be taken.

MA HUANG

The Chinese plant ma huang, one of the most popular supplements, contains ephedra, a compound similar to ephedrine (see Chapter 6 for more information, page 123). Ephedra is one of the most dangerous over-the-counter supplements available today. It is associated with a two- to three-fold increase in psychiatric, autonomic, heart-related, and gastrointestinal side effects. Eighty-seven episodes of heart attack, stroke, seizures, and high blood pressure have been reported to the FDA.[25] It has been associated with several deaths, including that of a pitcher for the Baltimore Orioles, which led the FDA to take the unusual step of banning it in 1994. The FDA, perhaps because of political pressure, has since revoked the ban.

Ephedra increases heart rate, blood pressure, and energy expenditure by stimulating beta-1 and beta-2 adrenergic receptors. It is often combined with caffeine as a weight-loss supplement. Ma huang is also combined with guarana, a Brazilian plant with a high caffeine concentration, and promoted as a weight-loss supplement. A recent meta-analysis showed that ephedra-containing products result in a weight loss of two pounds per month, although no information is available for treatment longer than six months.

I recommend avoiding it.

ST.-JOHN'S-WORT

St.-John's-wort (*Hypericum perforatum*) is a popular medication for the over-the-counter treatment of mild depression (see page 302 for additional information related to depression); 12% of Americans report using it at least once a year. The chemical action of St.-John's-wort is similar to that of antidepressants, including monoamine oxidase inhibition, serotonin reuptake inhibition, and actions on sigma receptors. Some earlier controlled studies have shown St.-John's-wort to be better than placebo and as effective as tricyclic antidepressants in the treatment of depression. Most of these earlier studies, however, were poorly controlled and did not use standard definitions of depression, which makes it difficult to draw accurate conclusions about the efficacy of St.-John's-wort.

More recently there have been several large controlled trials as well as meta-analyses that have provided information on the efficacy of St.-John's-wort. A large placebo-controlled randomized trial using appropriate methodology in patients with severe cases of major depression showed no difference between St.-John's-wort and placebo.[26] However, a direct head-to-head comparison of St.-John's-wort to the SSRI paroxetine showed that it was better in reducing symptoms of depression in patients with severe major depression: 71% of St.-John's-wort–treated patients experienced a 50% reduction in symptoms compared with 60% of those on paroxetine.[27]

Headache was the only side effect with St.-John's-wort that was more common than with placebo. A second study funded by the NIH and performed by the Hypericum Depression Trial Study Group (HDTSG) showed that St.-John's-wort was no more effective than placebo but no worse than an antidepressant comparison.[28] Response was 32% for placebo, 25% for sertraline, and 24% for St.-John's-wort. St.-John's-wort caused an increase in swelling, frequent urination, and sexual dysfunction, while sertraline caused more diarrhea, nausea, sexual dysfunction, forgetfulness, frequent urination, and sweating than placebo. My recommendation is that if you want to try St.-John's-wort for depression, it is okay to try. You may get some help and avoid the hassle of going to the doctor, and the potential risks and side effects are low.

SAW PALMETTO

Saw palmetto is a supplement derived from the fruit of *Serenoa repens* or *Sabal serrulatum,* the American dwarf palm, which is native to the Southeast U.S. Saw palmetto is marketed for the treatment of benign prostatic hypertrophy (BPH), a hardening of the prostate gland that is associated with problems with urination, and is used by 2 million men in the U.S. for that purpose. Saw palmetto is often mixed with nettle root in a formulation for the prostate. It is promoted as having anti-inflammatory properties as well as blocking conversion of testosterone to dihydrotestosterone, with resultant shrinkage of prostate tissue. The primary side effect is stomach upset, which can be reduced by taking it with food.

In an initial controlled trial saw palmetto was shown to be efficacious in the treatment of BPH. However, a more recent double-blind placebo-controlled trial failed to show any effects of saw palmetto on symptoms of BPH, objective measures of BPH, or quality of life.[29] I think that the patients in earlier trials may have been able to smell the saw palmetto, thus breaking the blind. I therefore do not think that saw palmetto is very helpful for BPH, although it is free of risk, and if you want to try it, you are free to do so.

SOY

Substitution of soy protein for animal protein is associated with a reduction in LDL cholesterol[30] that is primarily related to the reduction of animal-fat intake rather than any direct effect of soy itself. Soy extracts have been promoted for the treatment of hot flashes in postmenopausal women. Although some studies have found a reduction in hot flashes, other placebo-controlled trials have not found any efficacy of soy extract. Therefore I do not recommend the use of soy extract for hot flashes. If you want to eat less animal protein and more soy, it is probably a good idea, but you can substitute beans, lentils, and other legumes for animal protein just as effectively and get the same cholesterol-lowering effects. However, if you want to use soy, it is free of bad side effects, so feel free to use it.

VALERIAN

A wide variety of herbs and supplements have been marketed for insomnia, most of which have not been thoroughly evaluated and compared to placebo or have not been shown to be effective for sleep. These include almonds, chamomile, catmint, fennel, hops, lettuce, lime, marjolaine, may blossom, mullein, oats, orange flower, passionflower, rosemary, and willow. Some plants are known to have psychoactive properties, like poppy seed and Indian hemp. Growing these plants in the U.S. for consumption is, however, illegal.

Valerian, a supplement available in the U.S., is an extract of the valerian root (*Valeriana officinalis*), a perennial plant native to North America, Asia, and Europe, and widely prescribed in Europe for the treatment of insomnia. The composition of valerian includes sesquiterpenes of the volatile oil (including valeric acid), iridoids (valepotriates), alkaloids, furanofuran lignans, and free amino acids such as γ-aminobutyric acid (GABA), tyrosine, arginine, and glutamine. Valerian administered to animals shows sedative effects.

Valerian is often combined with passionflower and St.-John's-wort for treating anxiety or sleeplessness. A number of studies in humans have shown that it significantly decreases the time it takes to fall asleep and improves sleep quality when compared to a placebo. Other studies have shown it to be as effective as the benzodiazepine oxazepam and with fewer side effects: Patients were less sleepy the next day with valerian than with oxazepam.[31] Valerian seems to be most effective when used daily rather than as an acute sleep aid. Other uncontrolled studies have shown that valerian decreases the heart-rate response to stress.[32] Like pharmaceuticals with sedative effects, however, discontinuation of valerian can be associated with withdrawal symptoms. For more information on valerian, see Chapter 16. My recommendation is to take it if you want, although there still is not enough information to know for sure if it is useful for insomnia. I remind you, however, of the fact that any efficacious medication of insomnia will have a drawback. You should try to find a nondrug (or herb) way to fall asleep.

OTHER HERBAL REMEDIES

Finally, other lesser-known plants whose efficacy is not well enough known to recommend them are also available. For example, the plant hawthorn has been used to treat heart failure. Although some studies show efficacy, no formal research has been done outside of Germany. Fenugreek is a dried seed that contains fiber and steroid saponins that decrease glucose levels and cholesterol as demonstrated by clinical trials. Gugulipid (Guggul gum) is a natural product from India that is derived from resin of the mukul myrrh tree. Gugulipid has also been shown to reduce cholesterol. None of these products has been assessed for its ability to prevent or treat heart disease.

Other Naturally Occurring Supplements

A variety of compounds occurring naturally in the human body have been promoted for specific conditions. Often the logic behind this is that if a compound occurs naturally in the body, then adding more of it will be even better. Unfortunately, however, this type of reasoning does not always correspond to reality. Other supplements are derived from nonhuman animal products.

S-ADENOSYLMETHIONINE (SAME)

SAMe is a molecule found in all human cells that is also promoted as a supplement for the treatment of depression. It plays a role in methylation reactions, including gene expression, maintenance of cell membranes, and neurotransmitter synthesis. Administration of SAMe has been shown to increase levels of serotonin in the brain. Uncontrolled studies have shown efficacy for SAMe in the treatment of depression, but inadequate controlled studies with long-term follow-up have been performed to recommend usage of this supplement for depression. See Chapter 15.

COENZYME Q10

Coenzyme Q10 is an enzyme occurring naturally in the body that is involved in energy transfer in the mitochondria. Since coenzyme Q10 decreases naturally with aging, and since the risk of heart disease increases with aging, this has led to the conclusion that supplementation with coenzyme Q10 will prevent heart disease or prevent recurrence of heart attacks. Studies of coenzyme Q10, however, have shown only modest changes in measures of cardiovascular function that were not directly related to clinical function.[33] No studies have shown clinical improvement related to heart-disease treatment or prevention with coenzyme Q10. See Chapter 4.

GLUCOSAMINE AND CHONDROITIN

Glucosamine, a product derived from the shells of crabs and oysters, is widely promoted for the treatment of arthritis and joint pain. Glucosamine is felt to be a precursor of proteoglycans, which are thought to be instrumental in helping cartilage retain water and in promoting formation of an elastic layer that may improve the functional characteristics of cartilage. Chondroitin, a product derived from the cartilage of sharks and cows, is promoted for the prevention of arthritis and the treatment of joint pain. Chondroitin stimulates the production of proteoglycans and hyaluronic acid and inhibits proteolytic enzymes, which destroy cartilage. Glucosamine and chondroitin are often combined and sold in health-food stores.

One placebo-controlled study in older males with osteoarthritis of the knee showed no difference in pain ratings between patients treated with glucosamine and those treated with placebo.[34] Glucosamine was also associated with more side effects, including loose stools, nausea, heartburn, and headache. Other studies found it beneficial in patients with less-severe osteoarthritis,[35] suggesting that more-severe disease may not respond because the cartilage is already damaged.

Another study showed efficacy with glucosamine-chondroitin combinations compared to placebo.[36] The Glucosamine/chondroitin Arthritis Intervention Trial (GAIT) was a multisite placebo-controlled study in which 1,583 arthritis patients were randomly assigned to glucosamine, chondroitin, Celebrex, combination glucosamine/chondroitin, or a placebo. Although glucosamine and chondroitin (alone or in combination) did not result in a statistically significant reduction in pain, combination therapy was superior to placebo (but not to Celebrex) in a subset of patients with moderate to severe arthritis pain.

Overall the studies of glucosamine and chondroitin show some evidence for efficacy of the combination, although the results are not definitive. These supplements do not have potentially dangerous side effects, unlike other medications for arthritis, like Celebrex. Therefore I would not try to dissuade you from taking glucosamine and chondroitin for arthritis pain. See Chapter 2 for more information on arthritis treatments.

The Bottom Line

We often look to and depend on government experts to accurately tell us how to eat healthy and live right. The primary source of government information on eating healthy is its widely distributed food pyramid, which is constructed by the U.S. Department of Agriculture (USDA). More recently, the USDA has created a new food plan called MyPyramid, which is an improvement over earlier versions that were heavy on meat and dairy, and complicated to use. Because the pyramid plans are so widely known in this country, many consumers see the agency's primary function as developing a food plan for the nation. However, the USDA's *raison d'etre* is to promote the interests of agribusiness, cattlemen, and dairy farmers, *not* to promote sound nutrition.

That has always been the problem with USDA recommendations, particularly regarding the food pyramid. The USDA's interest in promoting agribusiness is at odds with its attempts to recommend a healthful diet. Historically, lobbyists for the dairy and cattle industries have pressured the USDA to include recommendations for dietary intakes of meat and dairy products that are not always in the best interests of our health.

The Recommended Daily Allowance (RDA) recommendations made by the USDA and the "bigger is better" attitude that prevails in our country have created an opening for many vitamin and supplement producers to recommend taking very high doses of vitamins, sometimes up to 1,000 times the already-high recommended daily dose! Many vitamins, like B_{12}, aren't stored in the body, so if you take megadoses they will all just be expelled in your urine in the next few hours. Talk about throwing money down the toilet! Fat-soluble vitamins A, D, E, and K are stored in the fat and liver, which means that even if you are temporarily deficient, you have enough stored in your liver to last you until you can replenish the vitamins with your next meal. However, with megadoses, those concentrations build up and can become toxic, sometimes with devastating effects, as I have explained in this chapter.

My advice is to discard your vitamins and instead eat a wide variety of fresh vegetables, fruits, whole grains, lean protein, nuts, and legumes. If you want a pyramid, I personally recommend the Mediterranean Diet Pyramid, which provides all the nutrition that you require, along with a more healthy balance of fats, carbohydrates, and protein (http://oldwayspt.org). Colleagues at the Emory University School of Medicine, Department of Cardiology, also recommend the Mediterranean Diet Pyramid. That kind of healthy (and delicious) diet combined with a little bit of time in the sun (about ten to fifteen minutes a day), and you will get all the vitamins and minerals you need.

So spend your vitamin money on something else, like a vacation. Rest and relaxation will do more for you than a bottle of letters.

Drug	Use	Common, Benign Side Effects	Serious Side Effects	Life-threatening Side Effects	Reasons Not to Take
Vitamins					
Low Risk					
Vitamin C (Ascorbic Acid)	Cold prevention	Nausea, diarrhea, stomach cramps	No definitive evidence	Kidney stones (high doses)	History of kidney stones
Medium Risk					
Vitamin E	Vitamin E deficiency, putative cancer prevention	Dizziness, diarrhea, headache, weakness	Blurred vision	Heart disease; bleeding	Should not be taken by anyone without proven vitamin E deficiency

Drug	Use	Common, Benign Side Effects	Serious Side Effects	Life-threatening Side Effects	Reasons Not to Take
Folate (Folic Acid, Vitamin B₉)	Pernicious anemia, birth-defect prevention	Stomach problems, sleep problems	Rash	Allergic reaction, seizures (megadose)	None
Vitamin D (Cholecalciferol)	Putative osteo-porosis prevention, rickets prevention	Thirst, metal taste, weight loss, vomiting, diarrhea	Mood changes	Allergic reaction, kidney damage (high dose)	Heart or kidney disease, hyper-calcemia
High Risk					
Vitamin A (or Beta-carotene)	Vitamin A deficiency, putative antioxidant effects	Skin dryness, headache	Bone and joint pain, colonic ulcers	Cancer, heart disease, osteoporotic fracture, birth defects, psychosis and depression, brain swelling	Should not be taken by anyone without a proven vitamin A deficiency
Minerals					
Low Risk					
Calcium	Putative osteo-porosis prevention	Constipation	Gastritis	Alkalosis, kidney stones	History of hyper-calcemia or kidney stones, kidney disease
Chromium	Putative type 2 diabetes	Stomach upset	Memory loss	Anemia, kidney damage	Insulin-dependent diabetes

Drug	Use	Common, Benign Side Effects	Serious Side Effects	Life-threatening Side Effects	Reasons Not to Take
Steroids					
High Risk					
Testosterone	Testosterone deficiency, body-building, loss of libido	Acne	Secondary male sexual characteristics, infertility, loss of libido, ruptured tendons	Suicidal thinking, depression, hypertension, liver tumors, hypercholesterol	Not recommended
Androstene-dione (Andro)	Body-building	Acne	Secondary male sexual characteristics, infertility, loss of libido, ruptured tendons	Suicidal thinking, depression, hypertension, liver tumors, hypercholesterol	Not recommended
Oxymethalone	Body-building	Acne	Secondary male sexual characteristics, infertility, loss of libido, ruptured tendons	Suicidal thinking, depression, hypertension, liver tumors, hypercholesterol	Not recommended
Stanozolol	Body-building	Acne	Secondary male sexual characteristics, infertility, loss of libido, ruptured tendons	Suicidal thinking, depression, hypertension, liver tumors, hypercholesterol	Not recommended
Oxanderolone	Body-building	Acne	Secondary male sexual characteristics, infertility, loss of libido, ruptured tendons	Suicidal thinking, depression, hypertension, liver tumors, hypercholesterol	Not recommended

Drug	Use	Common, Benign Side Effects	Serious Side Effects	Life-threatening Side Effects	Reasons Not to Take
Nandrolone Phenproprionate	Body-building	Acne	Secondary male sexual characteristics, infertility, loss of libido, ruptured tendons	Suicidal thinking, depression, hypertension, liver tumors, hypercholesterol	Not recommended
Nandrolone Decanoate	Body-building	Acne	Secondary male sexual characteristics, infertility, loss of libido, ruptured tendons	Suicidal thinking, depression, hypertension, liver tumors, hypercholesterol	Not recommended
Dehydroepiandrosterone (DHEA)	"Anti-aging"	Acne, headache	Insomnia, masculinization, insulin resistance	Arrhythmias, blood clots, liver damage	Not recommended

Supplements: Natural Compounds

Low Risk

SAMe	Depression	Anxiety, constipation, headache, insomnia, dry mouth	Confusion, restlessness, vomiting	Hallucinations	Depression

Medium Risk

Coenzyme Q10	Heart disease	Nausea, vomiting, stomach upset, insomnia, headache	Dizziness, irritability, light sensitivity	Decreased platelets (rare), hypotension, liver damage	Diabetes, bleeding disorders
Creatine	Exercise endurance	Nausea, vomiting, diarrhea, muscle cramps	Weight gain	Kidney damage, liver damage	Not recommended

Drug	Use	Common, Benign Side Effects	Serious Side Effects	Life-threatening Side Effects	Reasons Not to Take
Herbal Supplements					
Low Risk					
Alpha Lipoic Acid (ALA)	Antioxidant (heart disease, cancer), diabetic nephropathy	Stomach upset	Skin rash	Allergic reaction	History of allergic reaction to ALA
Garcinia	Weight loss	Stomach pain, vomiting	None	None	None
Garlic	Colds, infections	Nausea, diarrhea	None	Allergic reactions, bleeding	History of allergy
Ginger	Inflammation, arthritis	Stomach upset, heartburn	Mood changes, drowsiness	Irregular pulse, kidney damage	Gallstones, neurological disorder
Ginseng	Fatigue	Headache, anxiety, insomnia	Skin rash, hypertension	None	None
St.-John's-wort	Depression	Headache, frequent urination	Swelling, sexual dysfunction	None	None
Saw Palmetto	Benign prostatic hypertrophy (BPH)	Stomach upset	None	None	None
Soy Extract	High cholesterol, hot flashes	None	None	None	None
Valerian	Insomnia	Headache, restlessness	Withdrawal	Irregular heartbeat, allergic reaction	History of allergic reaction

Drug	Use	Common, Benign Side Effects	Serious Side Effects	Life-threatening Side Effects	Reasons Not to Take
Medium Risk					
Red rice Yeast Extract	High cholesterol	Dizziness, constipation, nausea, vomiting	Myopathy, joint pain, memory impairment, impotence, stomach pain	Long-term cancer risk possible, liver damage, rhabdomyolysis with kidney damage (may be fatal)	Liver disease, pregnancy, breast-feeding; men over 70, women without heart disease
Echinacea	Colds	Upset stomach, nausea, constipation	Worsening of asthma, dizziness	Allergic reactions, asthmatic attack	Asthmatics, history of plant allergies
Ginkgo Biloba	Memory, tinnitus, energy	Upset stomach, diarrhea, headache	Muscle cramps, skin problems	Bleeding, seizures	Bleeding disorder, taking blood thinner, epilepsy
High Risk					
Ephedra (Ma Huang)	Weight loss	Jitteriness, anxiety, insomnia	Increased blood pressure, heart rate	Heart attacks, stroke	Not recommended
Kava	Anxiety	Acne, skin rash, headaches, constipation, nausea, vomiting, stomach pain	Confusion	Liver damage	Liver disease

Drug	Use	Common, Benign Side Effects	Serious Side Effects	Life-threatening Side Effects	Reasons Not to Take
Supplements: Minerals					
Low Risk					
Chondroitin	Arthritis	Diarrhea, constipation	Stomach pain, hair loss	Swelling in the eyelids and limbs; heart arrhythmia (rare)	Recommend
Glucosamine	Arthritis	Loose stools, nausea, heartburn, headache	None	Insulin resistance	Recommend (unless you have a sea-food allergy)

19.

Medications for Children

I have a close friend whose son (I'll call him Jack, although that is not his name) was having trouble concentrating in school. He and his wife spent hours helping the young boy with work that he was unable to complete at school because of this inability to pay attention and focus in the classroom. Finally, after a lot of soul-searching and frustration, they agreed with their pediatrician's recommendation to give Jack a medication called Adderall. As the dosage was increased the boy began to experience the jitters and a racing heart. His appetite vanished and he lost ten pounds in spite of his parents doing everything they could to entice him to eat.

After Jack developed a series of odd tics, including flicking his tongue over his lips or continuously scrunching up his nose, his parents went to the Internet to look for information on Adderall's side effects (the doctor had not reviewed anything remotely like what Jack was experiencing) but found only that the drug could possibly accentuate preexisting tics. While on vacation his parents stopped giving him the drug to try and get him to eat. After his first day back at school and back on his meds, his body had not adjusted to the full dose, and he ended up sleepless, rapidly flicking his tongue over his lips. Enough was enough. Jack was switched to another medication (Ritalin) that had fewer side effects, even though it was not as effective for treating his concentration problems. The good news is that the side effects have subsided, Jack's eating a healthy diet, and he's doing better at school; the family is managing well.

Children and Attention Deficit Hyperactivity Disorder

The story I just told is not uncommon. If you have children, you might even have had a firsthand experience just like this one or know someone who has. An entire generation of kids who cannot pay attention is being diagnosed more and more frequently (and sometimes inaccurately) with Attention Deficit Hyperactivity Disorder, or ADHD.

It seems strange that it has been increasing so dramatically over the past few years. Certainly in the last generation many children with concentration problems were simply labeled unintelligent or "problem kids." However, with current competition for children to excel in school having reached such a fever pitch, it is no longer acceptable to let children fall behind. The elimination of recess, the lengthening of the school year, and the insistence that children remain rigidly fixed in their chairs without making a peep flies in the face of the realities of normal childhood. That said, we have to do our best to help our children move ahead in the world as it exists.

Children with ADHD can't pay attention in class, are easily distracted, tend to be in constant motion, and do poorly in school. Some scientists think that ADHD is related to alterations in the dopamine brain chemical that modulates attention. Prescriptions for Ritalin, the popular drug for ADHD, increased threefold in a four-year period from 1991 to 1995. Ten percent of boys in America are prescribed some kind of stimulant for the treatment of ADHD or other mental condition.

ADHD Drugs

AMPHETAMINE STIMULANTS

Ritalin, Adderall, and Strattera currently dominate the ADHD market. Ritalin (methylphenidate, Methylin), the first medication shown to be useful in the treatment of ADHD, works by increasing the release of dopamine, which helps kids concentrate. Ritalin needs to be taken a couple of times or more a day, but many children don't like having to take a medication at school, which has led to a decline in its use. Ritalin suppresses growth in children; other side effects include palpitations, nervousness, rapid heart rate, loss of appetite, increased blood pressure, headache, upset stomach, and mood changes. High doses can cause psychosis. It can also interact with a number of antidepressant and antihypertensive medications by decreasing elimination of these drugs and therefore increasing their concentrations in the blood and causing toxic side effects. You should not be on an Ritalin and MAOI at the same time (see Chapter 15). Extended-release forms of methylphenidate, which include Concerta, Metadate, and dexmethylphenidate (Focalin), are essentially identical to Ritalin and have no demonstrated difference in efficacy.

Another stimulant medication used in the treatment of ADHD is the amphetamine Adderall (mixed amphetamine salts), a mixture of two forms of amphetamine, which is marketed as a medication that has to be taken only once a day. Adderall now dominates the market, with a half billion dollars a year in sales. Dextroamphetamine (Dexedrine) is composed of one of the forms of amphetamine but is essentially the same thing as Adderall. Because of some well-publicized cases of abuse in the past, however, it has gotten bad publicity and therefore is rarely prescribed anymore. Ironically, socialite, hotel heiress, and tabloid favorite Paris Hilton recently admitted during a post-jail interview with Larry King that she takes Adderall for ADHD.

Adderall has some serious side effects, however. Amphetamines are also used as diet pills, and as a consequence Adderall often has serious appetite-suppression effects: Remember that Jack lost ten pounds when he was taking the drug, a substantial loss for a young boy. Like Ritalin, Adderall probably has some long-term growth-suppression effects, either directly or through its effects on appetite suppression and consequent decreased food intake. Other side effects are palpitations, nervousness, rapid heart rate, and upset stomach.

Adderall has also been linked to rare cases of sudden death. About fifteen cases of sudden death have been reported to the FDA over the past ten years. This has prompted Canada to take it off the market. Children with heart defects are particularly at risk. The other cases of sudden death occurred in children on multiple medications who were engaged in strenuous activities. The mechanism is probably the increase in catecholamines (chemical messengers in the body that send signals to the heart, increasing the heart rate and influencing electrical activity of the heart) caused by Adderall, which affects the function of the heart and leads to cardiac arrest.

All of the amphetaminelike stimulants, including Ritalin and Adderall, have been linked to approximately a doubling of heart-related deaths in children. This has recently prompted the FDA to put a black-box warning on these medications. Death from heart disease is rare in children, however, so a doubling of heart-disease deaths should not necessarily completely preclude use of these medications.

NOREPINEPHRINE REUPTAKE INHIBITORS
AND OTHER STIMULANTS

Atomoxetine (Strattera), which blocks uptake of norepinephrine into the neurons, is also used in the treatment of ADHD, but unlike Adderall and Ritalin it is not a stimulant and is therefore not associated with cardiac side effects. It does, however, have other side effects, including indigestion, fatigue, dizziness, decreased appetite, and mood swings. Like Adderall, Strattera can inhibit growth in children.

Pemoline (Cylert), another medication that is sometimes used to treat ADHD, has been associated with liver toxicity that led to nine documented deaths in children, and for this reason it was removed from the market in the U.K. in 1997. It remains on the market in the U.S., although it is not commonly prescribed. Its mechanism of action is unknown, but it is thought to act on dopaminergic systems. It should not be used as a first-line treatment for ADHD. Since it has not been shown to be efficacious in patients not responsive to first-line drugs, its use is questionable.

Kids and Depression

Diagnosis of depression in children is a problem. Before adolescence there is no consensus that depression exists in the same form as adult depression. Adolescence is a stormy period when children's moods are frequently changing. It is not clear that depression in this phase of development is equivalent to adult depression. Epidemiological data show that depression increases from adolescence to the early adult years, after which it remains stable, until increasing in late life (probably related to vascular-related depression) (www.cdc.gov). The much-quoted fact that "suicide is the third leading cause of death in adolescents" ignores the fact that depression is half as common in fourteen-year-olds as it is in twenty-five-year olds.

However, kids are being given a host of drugs to treat depression. This is another example of a generational shift in the way kids are treated for their problems. In fact, as reported in the June 19, 2004, edition of *BMJ* ("Bush Plans to Screen Entire U.S. Population for Mental Illness"), the president's New Freedom Commission Report of 2003 recommended that *all* children receive mandatory screening for mental disorders and that those who are diagnosed with a psychiatric disorder should receive "state-of-the-art treatments" using "specific medications for specific conditions." The Texas Medication Algorithm Project (TMAP), which was developed while President Bush was governor of Texas, was cited as a model.

Developed in 1995 by a consortium of pharmaceutical-industry representatives, state mental-health facilities, and the University of Texas, TMAP recommends first-line use of patented medications for treatment of mental disorders in spite of the fact that there is no evidence that they are better than older medications. A program in Indiana modeled after TMAP, called TeenScreen, used passive screening, where schools were allowed to test children for mental disorders if the parents did *not* return a form to the school specifically asking them not to. This outraged many of the parents who did not feel they had provided consent.

The 2002 Best Pharmaceuticals for Children Act also had a significant impact on how drugs are now tested and administered to children in this country. The act stipulates that pharmaceutical companies can extend the patents on their drugs by six months if they do studies on their effectiveness in children. This was and is an important incentive for companies to do research studies on their drugs in children, even if no rationale exists for using the drugs for children. Often these studies are done quickly and are not carefully designed, and their results are not published. This has become a particular issue in the case of treating childhood depression with SSRIs.

Parents may take their kids into the general practitioner if they are sad about a breakup with a boyfriend or girlfriend or are having trouble fitting in at school. The doctor's natural response these days, more frequently than not, may be to get out a prescription pad and write a scrip for an SSRI. In the past decade there has been a dramatic shift from the psychiatrist and appropriate therapy to Prozac as the "mind drug" of the general practitioner. Clearly there are a number of situations where a wait-and-see approach or a referral for counseling or psychotherapy would be the preferred approach.

Dr. Andrew Mosholder, a psychiatrist at the FDA who reviewed data collected from SSRI trials in childhood depression, became concerned about an increase in suicidal thoughts, but was specifically excluded by his superiors at the FDA from attending an FDA advisory panel meeting on drug treatment of childhood depression. As described in *The Lancet* (April 24, 2004, "Depressing Research"), after reviewing the evidence from clinical trials conducted by the drug companies, the Medicines and Healthcare Products Regulatory Agency (MHRA) of the United Kingdom (U.K.) quickly decided that all SSRIs, with the exception of fluoxetine, did not have efficacy for the treatment of childhood depression and that they were associated with a doubling of suicidal thoughts. The FDA then sent its data to Columbia University, which came to the same conclusions. At that point, the FDA responded with a black-box warning related to suicidal ideation with the SSRIs.

As I mentioned, one of the issues that came out of this controversy was nonpublication of trials. In this case it was found that there were more unpublished than published studies and that the unpublished studies tended to show less efficacy for the SSRIs. The FDA requires that two multisite placebo-controlled studies show superiority to placebo in order to approve a drug for a specific indication. In the case of the SSRIs, companies plan on doing eight studies in order to get two out of eight to show efficacy.

Dr. Craig Whittington and colleagues from the Centre for Outcomes Research and Effectiveness at University College London reviewed all published studies of SSRIs vs. placebo in children, plus some unpublished reports. Fluoxetine (Prozac) was shown to have a modest effect on depressive symptoms compared to placebo, with no increase in suicidal thoughts. (See Chapter 15 for more on antidepressants in general.) Paroxetine (Paxil), sertraline (Zoloft), citalopram (Celexa), and venlafaxine (Effexor) were associated with a two- to threefold or greater increase in suicidal thoughts. None of these studies were associated with an increase in completed suicide, although these events are relatively rare. Only Prozac was shown to have efficacy without the risk of increased suicidal ideation. A recent meta-analysis showed a 59% increase overall in suicidal thoughts in children who are prescribed SSRIs compared to those who are prescribed tricyclics.

Some children develop racing thoughts, "electric head," or a feeling of lightning bolts in the head several weeks into treatment with SSRIs. This side effect can be associated with suicidal thoughts, and appears to be more common in children and young adults. It may be a form of what is called akathisia, an internal restlessness associated with psychotropic medication use, which can be treated successfully with benzodiazepine medications like diazepam (Valium). Children and young adults treated with SSRIs should be watched carefully for signs of suicidal thoughts or akathisia, and a one-week course of benzodiazepines should be started if necessary.

Antipsychotic Medications and Children

Over the past two decades there has been a stunning increase in the use of antipsychotic medications for children. In the U.S., doctor visits for antipsychotic treatment increased from 201,000 in 1993 to 1,224,000 in 2002. Eighteen percent of youth visits to psychiatrists involved antipsychotic treatment; 92% of the antipsychotics prescribed were second generation (from 1993 to 2002). Antipsychotic drugs are approved by the FDA for use in children with schizophrenia, bipolar disorder, and Tourette's syndrome; the only approved antipsychotics for children, however, are Haldol (haloperidol), generic thioridazine, and Orap (pimozide, for Tourette's), which are first-generation antipsychotic drugs. Doctors do have the discretion to prescribe drugs for indications other than those approved by the FDA. Doctors treating children with mental disorders often do just that, prescribing psychotropic drugs for children for uses not approved by the FDA, in many cases cheered on by representatives of the companies that make the drugs that the doctors are prescribing.

A study of children in Tennessee's Managed Care program for Medicare showed that the number of prescriptions for antipsychotics doubled in a five-year period ending in 2001. During this time, one in every one hundred children became a new user of an antipsychotic. The proportion of atypical (newer and more expensive) antipsychotics went from 7% to 96% of antipsychotic prescriptions. The number of children treated for psychotic disorders or Tourette's did not change; the increase was accounted for by children treated with attention deficit disorder, conduct disorder, and affective disorders.

In my opinion a lot of these children suffer from abuse, neglect, and other family disruptions and traumas, not psychotic disorders that need antipsychotic medications. Antipsychotics should be used for what they are approved for: psychosis and Tourette's. There is no reason to use the newer atypical antipsychotics, which are not approved by the FDA for use in children, and which can cause obesity and diabetes—certainly things you do not want to stimulate in children. Many of the symptoms that children are medicated for are more appropriately dealt with by treating the root causes, such as childhood abuse and other traumas, lack of appropriate two-family parenting, lack of supervision, lack of role models, exposure to violence in the schools, and the failure of social service agencies to appropriately provide for these children.

Diet and Behavior

The topic of children and nutrition is a huge one that is beyond the scope of this book. I urge you to seek out credible nutritional information if you have a child, particularly one who has behavior problems. There has been some promising research in the area of children with ADHD and nutrition. For example, English researchers at the University of Southampton studied more than 1,800 three-year-old children, some with and some without ADHD and some with and some without allergies. The results were published in the June 2004 *Archives of Diseases in Childhood.* Removing artificial colors and preservatives from the diet was dramatically effective at reducing hyperactivity, somewhere between the effectiveness of clonidine and Ritalin.

After initial behavioral testing and diagnosis, all of the children were fed a diet of whole, fresh foods with no artificial food colorings or chemical preservatives for one week, after which their behavior improved significantly. The next week the researchers continued the whole-food diet but also gave the children capsules containing a mixture of artificial colorings, the preservative benzoate, or nothing. The behavior of the children who consumed the artificial colors or the preservative was substantially worse than when they were eating only the whole-food diet. This behavior was the same across the board in the children who had ADHD, those who had allergies, and those with neither of those diagnoses.

The Bottom Line

If your child does have a learning or concentration problem, the first step is to work with his or her teacher to improve concentration and attention in the classroom. Have the teacher send home work that was not completed in school. Sit with your child in an environment free of distractions and help him or her focus on the work. Give rewards and credit for work successfully completed, such as playing a favorite game, awarding prizes, and so on. Even something as simple as a gold star or a special handmade plaque is a great incentive for a young person.

Try changes in diet. Reductions in sugary foods and foods with artificial colors and preservatives have been shown in scientific studies to help ADHD. Get your kid involved in athletics. If after several months there is no improvement, you may need to try alternatives. Many schools offer team appointments with your child's teacher, social worker, and psychologist. In public schools that kind of intervention can take years. You don't want to wait until your child is in the third or fourth grade, has become frustrated with school, and is already on a bad track; take charge and ask for a meeting if you think your child's attention span and schoolwork problems have lasted longer than a day or a week.

Some children may still need medicine, but a healthy diet could lower the dosage. Sugar has also been associated with hyperactivity and should be avoided in hyperactive kids. Getting your kids involved in an exercise program can be helpful; it burns off their energy, helps them stay fit, and lifts their mood. Obviously, you should ensure that your kids aren't using alcohol and/or other drugs.

The next step is to get an evaluation by a psychologist or psychiatrist as well as an appointment with a neuropsychologist. They will do a number of tests, like Intelligence Quotient (IQ) testing, which involves solving mental problems, and tests of writing and reading. They are well equipped to assess your child's needs. Based on the results of these tests, your child may be eligible for special schooling. You will have to weigh the benefits of the intervention against the potential stigma of being in "special" classes. However, children in first or second grade usually don't notice things like kids being pulled out of the classroom for special tutoring.

Finally, the best way to determine whether a child has an ADHD is with a *trial* of an appropriate medication. If there is an improvement in concentration with one of the ADHD drugs and it helps your child achieve and be happy, that is what is most important.

Drug	Use	Common, Benign Side Effects	Serious Side Effects	Life-threatening Side Effects	Reasons Not to Take
Stimulants					
Moderate Risk					
Methylpheni-date (Ritalin, Methylin, Concerta, Metadate)	ADHD	Palpitations, stomach upset, nervousness, headache	Loss of appetite, tics, psychosis, hallucinations	Heart disease, growth inhibition, high blood pressure, cardiovascular events	History of heart disease, glaucoma, high blood pressure, addictions, on an MAOI
Dexmethyl-phenidate (Focalin)	ADHD	Palpitations, stomach upset, nervousness, headache	Weight loss, tics, psychosis, hallucinations	Heart disease, growth inhibition, high blood pressure, cardiovascular events	History of heart disease, glaucoma, high blood pressure, addictions

Drug	Use	Common, Benign Side Effects	Serious Side Effects	Life-threatening Side Effects	Reasons Not to Take
Adderall (Amphetamine Salts)	ADHD	Nervousness, headache, rapid heart rate, upset stomach	Weight loss, tics	Heart disease, growth inhibition, high blood pressure, cardiovascular events	History of heart disease, glaucoma, high blood pressure, addictions
Dextroamphet-amine (Dexedrine)	ADHD	Nervousness, headache, rapid heart rate, upset stomach	Weight loss, tics	Heart disease, growth inhibition, high blood pressure, cardiovascular events	History of heart disease, glaucoma, high blood pressure, addictions
Norepinephrine Reuptake Inhibitors					
Low Risk					
Atomoxetine (Strattera)	ADHD	Indigestion, fatigue, dizziness	Decreased appetite, mood swings	Growth inhibition	History of heart disease or defect
Stimulants—Other Mechanism					
High Risk					
Pemoline (Cylert)	ADHD	Insomnia, headache, dizziness	Movements of tongue and lips, hallucinations, convulsions	Liver damage	Use only as last resort

Conclusion:
How Do You Keep Yourself and Your Family Safe?

In the future, controlling medical costs will be just as important, if not more so, than halting global warming and finding a way to pay for our aging baby-boomer population. If we don't find a way to inject rational thinking into our approach to health care soon, the bankruptcy of our society may find a way for us. Clearly the system is broken, and it needs to be fixed.

Sadly, in spite of all the energy that has gone into pharmaceutical development, the future of our health looks bleak. Gains in life expectancy made since the nineteenth century have slowed considerably in recent years, largely as a result of the surge in obesity. Obesity has increased by 50% over the last couple of decades, and now two thirds of Americans are obese or overweight. It has been predicted that this increase in obesity will lead to a blunting or decline in life expectancy in the twenty-first century.

It should be clear by now that there are simply too many medications being needlessly taken in the U.S. and that it is costing us too much money for too little benefit. How else can you keep your family and yourself safe? You can start by choosing the drugs you take very carefully in terms of cost, safety, and effectiveness. But there are many other things we can do that can have a dramatic impact on our health and our health costs.

First of all, I recommend that you not go to the doctor unless you are sick. Not even for an annual checkup. Most Americans don't know this, but the American Medical Association and other medical organizations worldwide, including the Canadian Medical Association, have recommended *against* getting annual physical and blood work *unless* you have a disease. This is based on scientific evidence that screening normal people with annual laboratory tests and physical exams does not improve health-care outcomes. The reasons doctors give for the annual checkup are that it promotes a closer doctor-patient relationship, which is useful for when something does go wrong, and that it can promote healthy behaviors. But with HMO-style care, how much time do you really spend with your doctor during an exam anyway? As for the lab tests, doctors say "patients like it." Why? The only screening you really need on an annual basis if you're healthy is that for high blood pressure, which can be done in any drugstore.

Some aspects of the annual GYN checkups are also overdone. For instance, PAP screens for cervical cancer in women can be done every three years if a woman has had two consecutive negative tests; after the age of thirty-five they can be done every five years. However, women who are sexually active and do not use barrier protection should have yearly PAP screens. The annual gynecological exam is not efficient at the diagnosis of ovarian and uterine cancer and thus is superfluous. Women ages fifty to fifty-nine are encouraged to have an annual breast exam and mammography.

Second, doctors themselves acknowledge that they often treat a disease with a medication even if they know it won't help because they would rather do something than just stand by. Or they may take the position that the medicine "might help, and couldn't hurt." Unfortunately, many times a drug that won't help you may indeed hurt you. In the past twenty years the length of time it takes to review a medication for approval has gone from a few years to six months. This was in response to complaints (from HIV patients and others) that the FDA "bureaucrats" were keeping "lifesaving medicines" from getting to patients in need. After reading this book it should be clear that the rush to bring medicines to market may be putting you and your family at risk.

The good news is that negative publicity about drug safety and the FDA led to the 2006 Institute of Medicine Report, which included a number of recommendations for the future, including increased monitoring of drugs after approval, increased regulatory powers for the FDA, and increased transparency for studies performed by drug companies. This report has led to further congressional activity regarding the FDA and drug safety.

Third, we need to change our focus from medication (including vitamins and supplements) to treatment and prevention, and concentrate on the things that will make a bigger impact, like diet, exercise, and smoking. One of the best things you can do for yourself is to eat less and move more. Exercise has no side effects; it is free (actually saves money); and it has a good long-term outcome. Unlike drugs, it has also been shown to prolong your life and prevent negative health outcomes like stroke, heart attack, and hypertension.

Exercise can be as simple as walking briskly for twenty to thirty minutes a day. How hard is that? Doubling the amount of time you spend walking to ten thousand steps a day (counted with a step counter on your belt) can lead to significant improvements in health (www.10k-steps.com). Find something you like to do. Walk to the post office or store. Swim laps. Ride your bike. Take up tennis. Grab your spouse or a friend and go out dancing every night. Exercise improves cognitive function (not to mention your sex life), reduces depression and the stresses of daily life, and can even help you become more successful in your career.

Don't eat in restaurants all the time, especially fast-food establishments. When you shop, stay on the periphery of your supermarket, where the fresh foods are found. Then look for fresh, whole food—organic when possible—not processed food filled with additives and chemicals. Eat lots of wild-caught fish. Once or twice a week replace beef with beans. Take a walk in the sunshine (vitamin D) every day for at least thirty minutes. Don't drink beverages with added sugar.

Specific diets may promote weight loss as well as good health. The Mediterranean diet is healthy and nutritious, lowers cholesterol, reduces heart attacks, lengthens your life, and tastes good.[1] And you can (and should, if you are of legal drinking age and do not have an addiction problem) have a glass of wine with your meals as well. What more do you want? This diet is better than medications for the treatment of heart disease, obesity, and diabetes.[2] People who followed this diet cut their mortality in half over a four-year period. Unsaturated fats are substituted for saturated fats (butter, animal fat).

At Emory University in Atlanta, Georgia, we have started the Institute for Predictive Health and the Center for Health Discovery and Well-Being, whose goal is to promote healthy behaviors rather than merely to react once disease develops, when it may be too late.

Of course, there are times when you will need to take medicine, and I have provided some guidelines for common meds in this book. I hope you use it to make informed decisions. If, however, you have a life-threatening illness, such as cancer or type 1 diabetes, you should see a doctor and review all your treatment options.

Finally, become an active health-care consumer. Question your doctors, other health-care providers, insurance companies, your senators, and your Congresspeople. Become a vigorous participant in your own health and don't just mindlessly follow "doctor's orders." We have a lot more control over our health and well-being than we've been led to believe. Taking the reins of our own well-being brings us one step closer to unraveling a health-care status quo that has not been serving us well.

ACKNOWLEDGMENTS

A number of people made this book possible. Karen Kelly did an amazing job helping me to write this book and was a constant source of inspiration and ideas. I couldn't have pulled it off without her. My agent, Susan Arellano, kept with me through the long and strange journey that was the passage of this book from an idea to a reality. Lucia Watson, editor at Avery, was always patient and helped point me in the direction that led to the final goal. I would also like to thank my wife, Viola, who was another patient source of support and who provided invaluable feedback as a reader and a doctor on drafts of the book. Pina Emperatore, M.D., is a friend who provided feedback on the diabetes chapter.

I would also like to acknowledge my dog, Julius, a Cavalier King Charles Spaniel, who sat on my lap while I wrote this book, and who runs round and round the house, barking at every passerby, and therefore does *not* need doggie diet pills, and my cat, Arianna, who is looking forward to the spring, when we will buy some valerian root, but *not* for insomnia, since she sleeps twenty-three hours a day (and begs for milk the other hour), but rather for the pungent odor that cats supposedly love. And to my dentist, Nancy Stewart (I think you *should* go to the dentist, even if you are normal, but not the doctor unless you are sick), who somehow managed to put a prescription for Zovirax cream in my hands when I had a cold sore (it was not filled), and again to my wife, Viola, who wakes up with hot flashes but does not take Prempro, and who has occasional bouts of anxiety but is not ingesting kava root.

My sources of disclosure are on my Web site, www.dougbremner.com. Citations and book references not included in this book are at www.beforeyoutake thatpill.com.

NOTES

INTRODUCTION

1. Bremner, J.D., Fani, N., Ashraf, A., Votaw, J.R., Brummer, M.E., Cummins, R., Vaccarino, V., Goodman, M.M., Reed, R., Siddiq, S., Nemeroff, C.B. Functional brain imaging alterations in acne patients with isotretinoin. *American Journal of Psychiatry.* 2005; 162:983–91.

CHAPTER 2

1. Bombardier, C., Laine, L., Reicin, A., Shapiro, D., Burgos-Vargas, R., Davis, B., Day, R., Bosi Ferraz, M., Hawkey, C.J., Hochberg, M.C., Kvien, T.K., Schnitzer, T.J. Comparison of upper gastrointestinal toxicity of Rofecoxib and Naproxen in patients with rheumatoid arthritis. *New England Journal of Medicine.* 2000; 343:1520–28.

2. Bresalier, R.S., Sandler, R.S., Quan, H., Bolognese, J.A., Oxenius, B., Horgan, K., Lines, C., Riddell, R., Morton, D., Lanas, A., Konstam, M.A., Baron, J.A. Cardiovascular events associated with Rofecoxib in a colorectal adenoma chemoprevention trial. *New England Journal of Medicine.* 2005; 352:2–11.

3. Lisse, J.R., Perlman, M., Johansson, G., Shoemaker, J.R., Schechtman, J., Skalky, C.S., Dixon, M.E., Polis, A.B., Mollen, A.J., Geba, G.P. Gastrointestinal tolerability and effectiveness of rofecoxib versus naproxen in the treatment of osteoarthritis. *Annals of Internal Medicine.* 2003; 139(7):539–46.

4. Graham, D.J., Campen, D., Hui, R., Spence, M., Cheetham, C., Levy, G., Shoor, S.,

Ray, W.A. Risk of acute myocardial infarction and sudden cardiac death in patients treated with cyclo-oxygenase 2 selective and non-selective non-steroidal anti-inflammatory drugs: nested case-control study. *The Lancet.* 2005; 365(9450):475–81.

5. Nussmeier, N., Whelton, A.A., Brown, M.T., Langford, R.M., Hoeft, A., Parlow, J.L., Boyce, S.W., Verburg, K.M. Complications of the COX-2 inhibitors paracoxib and valdecoxib after cardiac surgery. *New England Journal of Medicine.* 2005; 352:1081–91.

6. Furberg, C.D., Psaty, B.M., FitzGerald, G.A. Parecoxib, valdecoxib, and cardiovascular risk. *Circulation.* 2005; 111:249–51.

7. Silverstein, F.E., Faich, G., Goldstein, J.L., Simon, L.S., Pincus, T., Whelton, A., Makuch, R., Eisen, G., Agrawal, N.M., Stenson, W.F., Burr, A.M., Zhao, W.W., Kent, J.D., Lefkowith, J.B., Verburg, K.M., Geis, G.S. Gastrointestinal toxicity with celecoxib vs nonsteroidal anti-inflammatory drugs for osteoarthritis and rheumatoid arthritis: The CLASS study: a randomized controlled trial. *Journal of the American Medical Association.* 2000; 284(10):1247–55.

8. Solomon, S.D., McMurray, J.J.V., Pfeffer, M.A., Wittes, J., Fowler, R., Finn, P., Anderson, W.F., Zauber, A., Hawk, E., Bertagnolli, M. Cardiovascular risk associated with celecoxib in a clinical trial for colorectal adenoma prevention. *New England Journal of Medicine.* 2005; 352:1071–80.

9. Bertagnolli, M.M., Eagle, C.J., Zauber, A.G., Redston, M., Solomon, S.D., Kim, K., Tang, J., Rosenstein, R.B., Wittes, J., Corle, D., Hess, T.M., Woloj, G.M., Boisserie, F., Anderson, W.F., Viner, J.L., Bagheri, D., Burn, J., Chung, D.C., Dewar, T., Foley, T.R., Hoffman, N., Macrae, F., Pruitt, R.E., Saltzman, J.R., Salzberg, B., Sylwestrowicz, T., Gordon, G.B., Hawk, E.T. Celecoxib for the prevention of sporadic colorectal adenomas. *New England Journal of Medicine.* Aug. 31, 2006; 355(9):873–74.

10. Arber, N., Eagle, C.J., Spicak, J., Racz, I., Dite, P., Hajer, J., Zavoral, M., Lechuga, M.J., Gerletti, P., Tang, J., Rosenstein, R.B., Macdonald, K., Bhadra, P., Fowler, R., Wittes, J., Zauber, A.G., Solomon, S.D., Levin, B. Celecoxib for the prevention of colorectal adenomatous polyps. *New England Journal of Medicine.* Aug. 31, 2006; 355:885–95.

11. Pfizer. A double-blind placebo-controlled comparison study of celecoxib (SC-58635) for the inhibition of progression of Alzheimer's Disease, protocol IQ5-97-02-001. Available at: http://www.clinicalstudyresults.org/documents/companystudy__76__0.pdf. Accessed Jan. 5, 2007.

12. Schnitzer, T.J., Burmester, G.R., Mysler, E., Hochberg, M.C., Doherty, M., Ehrsam, E., Gitton, X., Krammer, G., Mellein, B., Matchaba, P., Gimona, A., Hawkey, C.J. Comparison of lumiracoxib with naproxen and ibuprofen in the Therapeutic Arthritis Research and Gastrointestinal Event Trial (TARGET), reduction in ulcer complications: Randomised controlled trial. *The Lancet.* 2004; 364:665–74.

13. Farkouh, M., Kirshner, H., Harrington, R.A., Ruland, S., Verheugt, F.W.A., Schnitzer, T.J., Burmester, G.R., Mysler, E., Hochberg, M.C., Doherty, M., Ehrsam, E., Gitton,

X., Krammer, G., Mellein, B., Gimona, A.P.M., Hawkey, C.J., Chesebro, J.H. Comparison of lumiracoxib with naproxen and ibuprofen in the Therapeutic Arthritic Research and Gastrointestinal Event Trial (TARGET), cardiovascular outcomes: randomised controlled trial. *The Lancet.* 2004; 364:675–84.

14. Kearney, P.M., Baigent, C., Godwin, J., Halls, H., Emberson, J.R., Patrono, C. Do selective cyclo-oxygenase-2 inhibitors and traditional non-steroidal anti-inflammatory drugs increase the risk of atherothrombosis? Meta-analysis of randomised trials. *British Medical Journal* June 3, 2006; 332(7553):1302–08.

15. Furberg, C.D., Psaty, B.M., Fitzgerald, G.A. Parecoxib Valdecoxib and cardiovascular risk. *Circulation.* 2005; 111: 249–51.

16. McAlindon, T.E., LaValley, M.P., Gulin, J.P., Felson, D.T. Glucosamine and chondroitin for treatment of osteoarthritis: A systematic quality assessment and meta-analysis. *Journal of the American Medical Association.* 2000; 283(11):1469–75.

17. *Ibid.*

18. Reginster, J.-Y., Deroisy, R., Rovati, L.C., Lee, R.L., Lejeune, E., Bruyere, O., Giacovelli, G., Henrotin, Y., Dacre, J.E., Gossett, C. Long-term effects of glucosamine sulphate on osteoarthritis progression: a randomised, placebo-controlled clinical trial. *The Lancet.* 2001; 357:251–56.

19. Rindone, J.P., Hiller, D., Collacott, E., Nordhaugen, N. Randomized, controlled trial of glucosamine for treating osteoarthritis of the knee. *Western Journal of Medicine.* 2000; 172(2):91–94.

20. Lefler, C.T., Philippi, A.F., Leffler, S.G. Glucosamine, chondroitin, and manganese ascorbate for degenerative joint disease of the knee or low back: a randomized, double-blind, placebo-controlled pilot study. *Military Medicine.* 1999; 164:85–91.

21. Clegg, D.O., Reda, D.J., Harris, C.L., Klein, M.A., O'Dell, J.R., Hooper, M.M., Bradley, J.D., Bingham, C.O., 3rd, Weisman, M.H., Jackson, C.G., Lane, N.E., Cush, J.J., Moreland, L.W., Schumacher, H.R., Jr., Oddis, C.V., Wolfe, F., Molitor, J.A., Yocum, D.E., Schnitzer, T.J., Furst, D.E., Sawitzke, A.D., Shi, H., Brandt, K.D., Moskowitz, R.W., Williams, H.J. Glucosamine, chondroitin sulfate, and the two in combination for painful knee osteoarthritis. *New England Journal of Medicine.* Feb. 23, 2006; 354(8):795–808.

22. Bliddal, H., Rosetzsky, A., Schlichting, P., Weidner, M.S., Andersen, L.A., Ibfelt, H.H. A randomized, placebo-controlled, cross-over study of ginger extracts and ibuprofen in osteoarthritis. *Osteoarthritis Cartilage.* 2000; 8:9–12.

CHAPTER 3

1. Meynadier, J. Efficacy and safety of two zinc gluconate regimens in the treatment of inflammatory acne. *European Journal of Dermatology.* 2000;10: 269–73.

2. Middelkoop, T. Roaccutane. (Isotretinoin) and the risk of suicide: Case report and a

review of the literature and pharmacovigilance reports. *Journal of Pharmacy Practice.* 1999; 12:374–378.

3. Bremner, J.D., Fani, N., Ashraf, A., Votaw, J.R., Brummer, M.E., Cummins, T., Vaccarino, V., Goodman, M.M., Reed, R., Siddiq, S., Nemeroff, C.B. Functional brain imaging alterations in acne patients treated with isotretinoin. *American Journal of Psychiatry.* 2005; 162:983–91.

CHAPTER 4

1. Huttunen, J.K., Heinonen, O.P., Manninen, V., Koskinen, P., Hakulinen, T., Teppo, L., Mänttäri, M., Frick, M.H. The Helsinki Heart Study: an 8.5-year safety and mortality follow-up. *Journal of Internal Medicine.* 1994; 235:31–39.

2. ALLHAT. Major outcomes in moderately hypercholesterolemic, hypertensive patients randomized to pravastatin vs. usual care: The Antihypertensive and Lipid-Lowering Treatment to Prevent Heart Attack Trial (ALLHAT-LLT). *Journal of the American Medical Association.* 2002; 288(23):2998–3007.

3. Colhoun, H.M., Betteridge, D.J., Durrington, P.N., Hitman, G.A., Neil, H.A.W., Livingstone, S.J., Thomason, M.J., Mackness, M.I., Charlton-Menys, V., Fuller, J.H. Primary prevention of cardiovascular disease with atorvastatin in type 2 diabetes in the Collaborative Atorvastatin Diabetes Study (CARDS): multicentre randomised placebo-controlled trial. *The Lancet.* 2004; 364:685–96.

4. Downs, J.R., Clearfield, M., Weis, S., Whitney, E., Shapiro, D.R., Beere, P.A., Langerdorfer, A., Stein, E.A., Kruyer, W., Gotto, A.M. Primary prevention of acute coronary events with lovastatin in men and women with average cholesterol levels: Results of AFCAPS/TexCAPS. *Journal of the American Medical Association.* 1998; 279(20):1615–22.

5. Shepherd, J., Cobbe, S.M., Ford, I., Isles, C.G., Lorimer, A.R., Macfarlane, P.W., McKillop, J.H., Packard, C.J. Prevention of coronary heart disease with Pravastatin in men with hypercholesterolemia. *New England Journal of Medicine.* 1995; 333:1301–07.

6. Sever, P.S., Dahlof, B., Poulter, N.R., Wedel, H., Beevers, G., Caulfield, M., Collins, R., Kjeldsen, S.E., Kristinsson, A., McInnes, G.T., Mehlsen, J., Nieminen, M., O'Brien, E., Ostergren, J. Prevention of coronary and stroke events with Atorvastatin in hypertensive patients who have average or lower-than-average cholesterol concentrations, in the Anglo-Scandinavian Cardiac Outcomes Trial-Lipid Lowering Arm (ASCOT-LLA): a multicentre randomised controlled trial. *The Lancet.* 2003; 361:1149–58.

7. HPS. MRC/BHF Heart Protection Study of cholesterol lowering with simvastatin in 20,563 high-risk individuals: a randomised placebo-controlled trial. *The Lancet.* 2002; 360:7–22.

8. LIPID. Prevention of cardiovascular events and death with Pravastatin in patients with coronary heart disease and a broad range of initial cholesterol levels. *New England Journal of Medicine.* 1998; 339:1349–57.

9. Sacks, F.M., Pfeffer, M.A., Moye, L.A., Rouleau, J.L., Rutherford, J.D., Cole, T.G., Brown, L., Warnica, J.W., Arnold, J.M.O., Wun, C.C., Davis, B.R., Braunwald, E. The effect of Pravastatin on coronary events after myocardial infarction in patients with average cholesterol levels. *New England Journal of Medicine.* 1996; 335(14):1001–09.

10. Schwartz, G.G., Olsson, A.G., Ezekowitz, M.D., Ganz, P., Oliver, M.F., Waters, D., Zeiher, A., Chaitman, B.R., Leslie, S., Stern, T. Effects of Atorvastatin on early recurrent ischemic events in acute coronary syndromes: The MIRACL study: A randomized controlled trial. *Journal of the American Medical Association.* 2001; 285(13):1711–18.

11. Serruys, P.W.J.C., de Feyter, P., Macaya, C., Kokott, N., Puel, J., Vrolix, M., Branzi, A., Bertolami, M.C., Jackson, G., Strauss, B., Meier, B. Fluvastatin for prevention of cardiac events following successful first percutaneous coronary intervention: A randomized controlled trial. *Journal of the American Medical Association.* 2002; 287(24):3215–22.

12. Shepherd, J., Cobbe, S.M., Ford, I., Isles, C.G., Lorimer, A.R., Macfarlane, P.W., McKillop, J.H., Packard, C.J. Prevention of coronary heart disease with Pravastatin in men with hypercholesterolemia. *New England Journal of Medicine.* 1995; 333:1301–07.

13. SSSS(4S). Randomised trial of cholesterol lowering in 4444 patients with coronary heart disease: The Scandinavian Simvastatin Survival Study (4S). *The Lancet.* 1994; 344:1383–89.

14. SPARCL. High-dose atorvastatin after stroke or transient ischemic attack. *New England Journal of Medicine.* Aug. 10, 2006; 355(6):549–59.

15. Shepherd, J., Blauw, G.J., Murphy, M.B., Bollen, E.L.E.M., Buckley, B.M., Cobbe, S.M., Ford, I., Gaw, A., Hyland, M., Jukema, J.W., Kamper, A.M., Macfarlane, P.W., Meinders, A.E., Norrie, J., Packard, C.J., Perry, I.J., Stott, D.J., Sweeney, B.J., Twomey, C., Westendorp, R.G.J. Pravastatin in elderly individuals at risk of vascular disease (PROSPER): a randomised controlled trial. *The Lancet.* 2002; 360:1623–30.

16. Walsh, J.M., Pignone, M. Drug treatment of hyperlipidemia in women. *Journal of the American Medical Association.* 2004; 291:2243–52.

17. Mosca, L., Appel, L.J., Benjamin, E.J., Berra, K., Chandra-Strobos, N., Fabunmi, R.P., Grady, D., Haan, C.K., Hayes, S.N., Judelson, D.R., Keenan, N.L., McBride, P., Oparil, S., Ouyang, P., Oz, M.C., Mendelsohn, M.E., Pasternak, R.C., Pinn, V.W., Robertson, R.M., Schenck-Gustafsson, K., Sila, C.A., Smith, S.C., Jr., Sopko, G., Taylor, A.L., Walsh, B.W., Wenger, N.K., Williams, C.L. Evidence-based guidelines for cardiovascular disease prevention in women. American Heart Association scientific statement. *Arterioscler Thromb Vasc Biol.* Mar. 2004; 24(3):e29–50.

18. Keech, A., Colquhoun, D., Best, J., Kirby, A., Simes, R.J., Hunt, D., Hague, W., Beller, E., Arulchelvam, M., Baker, J., Tonkin, A. Secondary prevention of cardiovascular events with long-term pravastatin in patients with diabetes or impaired fasting glucose: Results from the LIPID trial. *Diabetes Care.* 2003; 26:2713–21.

19. Newman, T.B., Hulley, S.B. Carcinogenicity of lipid-lowering drugs. *Journal of the American Medical Association.* 1996; 275(1):55–60.

20. Baigent, C., Keech, A., Kearney, P.M., Blackwell, L., Buck, G., Pollicino, C., Kirby, A., Sourjina, T., Peto, R., Collins, R., Simes, R. Efficacy and safety of cholesterol-lowering treatment: prospective meta-analysis of data from 90,056 participants in 14 randomised trials of statins. *The Lancet.* Oct. 8, 2005; 366(9493):1267–78.

21. Steffens, D.C., McQuoid, D.R., Krishnan, K.R.R. Cholesterol-lowering medication and relapse of depression. *Psychopharmacology Bulletin.* 2003; 37(4):92–98.

22. Hayward, R.A., Hofer, T.P., Vijan, S. Narrative review: Lack of evidence for recommended low-density lipoprotein treatment targets: a solvable problem. *Annals of Internal Medicine.* Oct. 3, 2006; 145(7):520–30.

23. Berger, J.S., Roncaglioni, M.C., Avanzini, F., Pangrazzi, I., Tognoni, G., Brown, D.L. Aspirin for the primary prevention of cardiovascular events in women and men: A sex-specific meta-analysis of randomized controlled trials. *Journal of the American Medical Association.* Jan. 18, 2006; 295:306–13.

24. ATC. Antithrombotic Trialists' Collaboration: Collaborative meta-analysis of randomised trials of antiplatelet therapy for prevention of death, myocardial infarction, and stroke in high risk patients. *British Medical Journal.* 2002; 324:71–86.

25. Esprit. Aspirin plus dipyridamole versus aspirin alone after cerebral ischaemia of arterial origin (ESPRIT): randomised controlled trial. *The Lancet.* 2006; 367:1665–73.

26. CAPRIE. A randomised, blinded trial of Clopidogrel versus Aspirin in Patients At Risk of Ischaemic Events (CAPRIE). *The Lancet.* 1996; 348(9038):1329–39.

27. Bhatt, D., Fox, K.A.A., Hacke, W., Berger, P.B., Black, H.R., Boden, W.E., Cacoub, P., Cohen, E.A., Creager, M.A., Easton, J.D., Flather, M.D., Haffner, S.M., Hamm, C.W., Hankey, G.J., Claiborne Johnston, S., Mak, K.-H., Mas, J.-L., Montalescot, G., Pearson, T.A., Steg, P.G., Steinhubl, S.R., Weber, M.A., Brennan, D.M., Fabry-Ribaudo, L., Booth, J., Topol, E.J. Clopidogrel and aspirin versus aspirin alone for the prevention of atherothrombotic events. *New England Journal of Medicine.* Apr. 20, 2006; 354:1706–17.

28. COMMIT. Addition of clopidogrel to aspirin in 45,852 patients with acute myocardial infarction: randomised placebo-controlled trial. *The Lancet.* Nov. 5, 2006; 366:1607–21.

29. Diener, H.-C., Bogousslavsky, J., Cimminiello, C., Csiba, L., Kaste, M., Leys, D., Matias-Guiu, J., Rupprecht, H.-J. Aspirin and clopidogrel compared with clopidogrel alone after recent ischaemic stroke or transient ischaemic attack in high-risk patients (MATCH): randomised, double-blind, placebo-controlled trial. *The Lancet.* July 24, 2004; 364:331–37.

30. Chan, F.K.L., Ching, J.Y.L., Hung, L.C.T., Wong, V.W.S., Leung, V.K.S., Kung, N.N.S., Hui, A.J., Wu, J.C.Y., Leung, W.K., Lee, V.W.Y., Lee, K.K.C., Lee, Y.T., Lau, J.Y.W., To, K.F., Chan, H.L.Y., Chung, S.C.S., Sung, J.J.Y. Clopidogrel versus aspirin and esomeprazole to prevent recurrent ulcer bleeding. *New England Journal of Medicine.* Jan. 20, 2005; 352(3):238–44.

31. Vivekananthan, D.P., Penn, M.S., Sapp, S.K., Hsu, A., Topol, E.J. Use of antioxidant

vitamins for the prevention of cardiovascular disease: Meta-analysis of randomised trials. *The Lancet.* 2003; 361:2017–23.

32. Hennekens, C.H., Buring, J.E., Manson, J.E., Stampfer, M., Rosner, B., Cook, N.R., Belanger, C., LaMotte, F., Gaziano, J.M., Ridker, P.M., Willett, W., Peto, R. Lack of effect of long-term supplementation with beta carotene on the incidence of malignant neoplasms and cardiovascular disease. *New England Journal of Medicine.* 1996; 334(18):1145–49.

33. Omenn, G.S., Goodman, G.E., Thornquist, M.D., Balmes, J., Cullen, M.R., Glass, A., Keogh, J.P., Meyskens, F.L.J., Valanis, B., Williams, J.H., Barnhart, S., Hammar, S. Effects of a combination of beta carotene and Vitamin A on lung cancer and cardiovascular disease. *New England Journal of Medicine.* 1996; 334(18):1150–55.

34. ATBC. The Alpha-Tocopherol, Beta Carotene Cancer Prevention Study Group. The effect of vitamin E and beta carotene on the incidence of lung cancer and other cancers in male smokers. *New England Journal of Medicine.* 1994; 330:1029–35.

35. Rapola, J.M., Virtamo, J. Randomised trial of alpha-tocopherol and beta-carotene supplements on incidence of major coronary events in men with previous myocardial infarction. *The Lancet.* 1997; 349:1715–20.

36. Bjelakovic, G., Nikolova, D., Simonetti, R.G., Gluud, C. Antioxidant supplements for prevention of gastrointestinal cancers: a systematic review and meta-analysis. *The Lancet.* 2004; 364:1219–28.

37. MRC/BHF. Heart Protection Study of antioxidant vitamin supplementation in 20,536 high-risk individuals: a randomised placebo-controlled trial. *The Lancet.* 2002; 360:23–33.

38. Collaborative Group of the Primary Prevention Project (PPP). Low-dose aspirin and Vitamin E in people at cardiovascular risk: a randomised trial in general practice. *The Lancet.* 2001; 357:89–95.

39. HOPE. The Heart Outcomes Prevention Evaluation Study Investigators. Vitamin E supplementation and cardiovascular events in high-risk patients. *New England Journal of Medicine.* 2000; 342:154–160.

40. GISSI. GISS-Prevenzione Investigators (Gruppo Italiano per lo Studio della Sopravvivenza Nell'Infarto Miocardio). Dietary supplementation with n-2 polyunsaturated fatty acids and vitamin E after myocardial infarction: results of the GISSI-Prevenzione Trial. *The Lancet.* 1999; 354:447–55.

41. Stephens, N.G., Parsons, A., Schofield, P.M., Kelly, F., Cheeseman, K., Mitchinson, M.J. Randomised controlled trial of Vitamin E in patients with coronary disease: Cambridge Heart Association Antioxidant Study (CHAOS). *The Lancet.* 1996; 347:781–86.

42. Waters, D.D., Alderman, E.L., Hsia, J., Howard, B.V., Cobb, F.R., Rogers, W.J., Ouyang, P., Thompson, P., Tardif, J.C., Higginson, L., Bittner, V., Steffes, M., Gordon, D.J., Proschan, M., Younes, N., Verter, J.I. Effects of hormone replacement therapy and antioxidant vitamin supplements on coronary atherosclerosis in postmenopausal

women: A randomized controlled trial. *Journal of the American Medical Association.* 2002; 288(19):2432–40.

43. Brown, B.G., Zhao, X.-Q., Chait, A., Fisher, L.D., Cheung, M.C., Morse, J.S., Dowdy, A.A., Marino, E.K., Bolson, E.L., Alaupovic, P., Frohlich, J., Albers, J.J. Simvastatin and niacin, antioxidant vitamins, or the combination for the prevention of coronary disease. *New England Journal of Medicine.* 2001; 345(22):1583–92.

44. Manson, J.E., Hsiao, J., Johnson, K.C., Rossouw, J.E., Assaf, A.R., Lasser, N.L., Trevisan, M., Black, H.R., Heckbert, S.R., Detrano, R., Strickland, O.L., Wong, N.D., Crouse, J.R., Stein, E., Cushman, M. Estrogen plus progestin and the risk of coronary heart disease. *New England Journal of Medicine.* 2003; 349(6):523–34.

45. Grady, D., Herrington, D.M., Bittner, V., Blumenthal, R., Davidson, M., Hlatky, M., Hsia, J., Hudley, S., Herd, A., Khan, S., Newby, L.K., Waters, D., Vittinghoff, E., Wenger, N. Cardiovascular disease outcomes during 6.8 years of hormone therapy: Heart and Estrogen/Progesterone Replacement Study Follow-up (HERS II). *Journal of the American Medical Association.* 2002; 288(1):49–57.

46. Hulley, S., Grady, D., Bush, T., Furberg, C., Herrington, D., Riggs, B., Vittinghoff, E. Randomized trial of estrogen plus progestin for secondary prevention of coronary heart disease in postmenopausal women. *Journal of the American Medical Association.* 1998; 280(7):605–13.

47. Chlebowski, R.T., Hendrix, S.L., Langer, R.D., Stefanick, M.L., Gass, M., Lane, D., Rodabough, R.J., Gilligan, M.A., Cyr, M.G., Thomson, C.A., Khandekar, J., Petrovitch, H., McTiernan, A. Influence of estrogen plus progestin on breast cancer and mammography in healthy postmenopausal women: The Women's Health Initiative Randomized Trial. *Journal of the American Medical Association.* 2003; 289(24):3243–53.

48. WGWHII. Writing Group for the Women's Health Initiative Investigators. Risks and benefits of estrogen plus progestin in healthy postmenopausal women: Principal results from the Women's Health Initiative Randomized Controlled Trial. *Journal of the American Medical Association.* 2002; 288(3):321–33.

49. Hulley, S., Furberg, C., Barrett-Connor, E., Cauley, J., Grady, D., Haskell, W., Knopp, R., Lowery, M., Satterfield, S., Schrott, H., Vittinghoff, E., Hunninghake, D. Noncardiovascular disease outcomes during 6.8 years of hormone therapy: Heart and Estrogen/Progesterone Replacement Study Follow-up (HERS II). *Journal of the American Medical Association.* 2002; 288(1):58–66.

50. Anderson, J.W., Johnstone, B.M., Cook-Newell, M.E. Meta-analysis of the effects of soy protein intake on serum lipids. *New England Journal of Medicine.* 1995; 333:276–82.

51. Burr, M.L., Fehily, A.M., Gilbert, J.F., Rogers, S., Holliday, R.M., Sweetnam, P.M. Effects of changes in fat, fish, and fibre intakes on death and myocardial reinfarction. *The Lancet.* 1989; 2:757–61.

52. Hooper, L., Thompson, R.L., Harrison, R.A., Summerbell, C.D., Ness, A.R., Moore, H.J., Worthington, H.V., Durrington, P.N., Higgins, J.P., Capps, N.E., Riemersma,

R.A., Ebrahim, S.B., Davey Smith, G. Risks and benefits of omega 3 fats for mortality, cardiovascular disease, and cancer: systematic review. *British Medical Journal.* Apr. 1, 2006; 332(7544):752–760.

53. Brouwer, I.A., Zock, P.L., Camm, A.J., Bocker, D., Hauer, R.N.W., Wever, E.F.D., Dullemeijer, C., Ronden, J.E., Katan, M.B., Lubinski, A., Buscler, H., Schouten, E.G. Effect of fish oil on ventricular tachyarrhythmia and death in patients with implantable cardioverter defibrillators: The study on Omega-3 fatty acids and ventricular arrhthmia (SOFA) randomized trial. *Journal of the American Medical Association.* June 14, 2006; 295(22):2613–19.

54. Burr, M.L., Ashfield-Watt, P.A.L., Dunstan, F.D.J., Fehily, A.M., Breay, P., Ashton, T. Lack of benefit of dietary advice to men with angina: results of a controlled trial. *European Journal of Clinical Nutrition.* 2003; 57:193–200.

55. Leaf, A., Kang, J.X., Xiao, Y.-F., Billman, G.E. Clinical presentation of sudden cardiac death by n-3 polyunsaturated fatty acids and mechanism of prevention of arrhythmias by n-3 fish oils. *Circulation.* 2003; 107:2646–52.

56. Kuriyama, S., Shimazu, T., Ohmori, K., Kikuchi, N., Nakaya, N., Nishino, Y., Tsubono, Y., Tsuji, I. Green tea consumption and mortality due to cardiovascular disease, cancer, and all causes in Japan: The Ohsaki Study. *Journal of the American Medical Association.* Sept. 13, 2006; 296(10):1255–65.

57. Jenkins, D.J., Kendall, C.W., Marchie, A., Faulkner, D.A., Wong, J.M., de Souza, R., Emam, A., Parker, T.L., Vidgen, E., Trautwein, E.A., Lapsley, K.G., Josse, R.G., Leiter, L.A., Singer, W., Connelly, P.W. Direct comparison of a dietary portfolio of cholesterol-lowering foods with a statin in hypercholesterolemic participants. *American Journal of Clinical Nutrition.* 2005; 81(2):380–87.

58. Trichopoulou, A., Orfanos, P., Norat, T., Bueno-de-Mesquita, B., Ocke, M.C., Peeters, P.H.M., van der Schouw, Y.T., Boeing, H., Hoffmann, K., Boffetta, P., Nagel, G., Masala, G., Krogh, V., Panico, S., Tumino, R., Vineis, P., Bamia, C., Naska, A., Benetou, V., Ferrari, P., Slimani, N., Pera, G., Martinez-Garcia, C., Navarro, C., Rodriguez-Barranco, M., Dorronsor, M., Spencer, E.A., Key, T.J., Bingham, S., Khaw, K.-T., Kesse, E., Clavel-Chapelon, F., Boutron-Ruault, M.-C., Berglund, G., Wirfalt, E., Hallmans, G., Johansson, I., Tjonneland, A., Olsen, A., Overvad, K., Hundborg, H.H., Riboli, E., Trichopoulos, D. Modified Mediterranean diet and survival: EPIC-elderly prospective cohort study. *British Medical Journal.* 2005; 330:991–98.

59. de Lorgeril, M., Salen, P., Martin, J.L., Monjaud, I., Delaye, J., Mamelle, N. Mediterranean diet, traditional risk factors, and the rate of cardiovascular complications after myocardial infarction: Final report of the Lyon Diet Heart Study. *Circulation.* 1999; 99:779–85.

60. Howard, B.V., Van Horn, L., Hsia, J., et al., Low-fat dietary pattern and risk of cardiovascular disease: The Women's Health Initiative randomized controlled dietary modification trial. *Journal of the American Medical Association.* 2006; 295(6):655–66.

61. Halton, T.L., Willett, W.C., Liu, S., Manson, J.E., Albert, C.M., Rexrode, K., Hu, F.B. Low-carbohydrate-diet score and the risk of coronary heart disease in women. *New England Journal of Medicine.* Nov. 9, 2006; 355(19):1991–2002.

CHAPTER 5

1. Davis, B.R. Major cardiovascular events in hypertensive patients randomized to doxazosin versus chlorthalidone: The Antihypertensive and Lipid-Lowering Treatment to Prevent Heart Attack Trial (ALLHAT). *Journal of the American Medical Association.* 2000; 283(15):1967–75.

2. Brown, M.J., Palmer, C.R., Castaigne, A., de Leeuw, P.W., Mancia, G., Rosenthal, T., Ruilope, L.M. Morbidity and mortality in patients randomised to double-blind treatment with long-acting calcium-channel blocker or diuretic in the International Nifedipine GITS study: Intervention as a Goal in Hypertension Treatment (INSIGHT). *The Lancet.* 2000; 356:366–72.

3. Lindberg, G., Bingefors, K., Ranstam, J., Rastam, L., Melander, A. Use of calcium channel blockers and risk of suicide: Ecological findings confirmed in population based cohort study. *British Medical Journal.* 1998; 316:741–45.

4. BPLTTC. Blood Pressure Lowering Treatment Trialists' Collaboration. Effects of different blood-pressure-lowering regimens on major cardiovascular events: results of prospectively-designed overviews of randomised trials. *The Lancet.* 2003; 362:1527–35.

5. Hansson, L., Hedner, T., Lund-Johansen, P., Kjeldsen, S.E., Lindholm, L.H., Syvertsen, J.O., Lanke, J., de Faire, U., Karlberg, B.E. Randomised trial of effects of calcium antagonists compared with diuretics and beta blockers on cardiovascular morbidity and mortality in hypertension: the Nordic Diltiazem (NORDIL) study. *The Lancet.* 2000; 356:359–65.

6. Black, H.R., Elliott, W.J., Grandits, G., Brambsch, P., Lucent, T., White, W.B., Neaton, J.D., Grimm, R.H., Hansson, L., Lacourciere, Y., Muller, J., Sleight, P., Weber, M.A., Williams, G., Wittes, J., Zanchetti, A., Anders, R.J. Principal results of the Controlled Onset Verapamil Investigation of Cardiovascular End Points (CONVINCE) Trial. *Journal of the American Medical Association.* 2003; 289(16):2073–82.

7. Poole-Wilson, P.A., Lubsen, J., Kirwan, B.-A., van Dalen, F.J., Danchin, N., Just, H., Fox, K.A.A., Pocock, S.J., Clayton, T.C., Motro, M., Parker, J.D., Bourassa, M.G., Hildebrandt, P., Hjalmarson, A., Kragten, J.A., Molhoek, G.P., Otterstad, J.-K., Seabra-Gomes, R., Soler-Soler, J., Weber, S. Effect of long-acting nifedipine on mortality and cardiovascular morbidity in patients with stable angina requiring treatment (ACTION): randomised controlled trial. *The Lancet.* 2004; 364:849–57.

8. BPLTTC. Blood Pressure Lowering Treatment Trialists Collaboration. Effects of ACE inhibitors, calcium antagonists, and other blood-pressure-lowering drugs: results

of prospectively designed overviews of randomised trials. *The Lancet.* 2000; 355: 1955–64.

9. Pahor, M., Psaty, B.M., Alderman, M.H., Applegate, W.B., Williamson, J.D., Cavazzini, C., Furberg, C.D. Health outcomes associated with calcium antagonists compared with other first-line antihypertensive therapies: a meta-analysis of randomised controlled trials. *The Lancet.* 2000; 356:1949–54.

10. ALLHAT: Major outcomes in high-risk hypertensive patients randomized to angiotensin-converting enzyme inhibitor or calcium channel blocker vs diuretic: The antihypertensive and lipid-lowering treatment to prevent heart attack trial (ALLHAT). *Journal of the American Medical Association* 2002; 288(23):2981–97.

11. Pepine, C.J., Handberg, E.M., Cooper-DeHoff, R.M., Marks, R.G., Kowey, P., Messerli, F.H., Mancia, G., Cangiano, J.L., Garcia-Barreto, D., Keltai, H., Erdine, S., Bristol, H.A., Kolb, H.R., Bakris, G.L., Cohen, J.D., Parmley, W.W. A calcium antagonist vs a non-calcium antagonist hypertension treatment strategy for patients with coronary artery disease: The International Verapamil-Trandolapril Study (INVEST): A randomized controlled trial. *Journal of the American Medical Association.* 2003; 21:2805–16.

12. Hansson, L., Lindholm, L.H., Ekborn, T., Dahlof, B., Lanke, J., Schersten, B., Wester, P.-O., Hender, T., de Faire, U. Randomised trial of old and new antihypertensive drugs in elderly patients: cardiovascular mortality and morbidity: the Swedish Trial in Old Patients with Hypertension-2 study. *The Lancet.* 1999; 354:1751–56.

13. Hansson, L., Lindholm, L.H., Niskanen, L., Lanke, J., Hender, T., Niklason, A., Luomanmaki, K., Dahlof, B., de Faire, U., Morlin, C., Karlberg, B.E., Wester, P.-O., Bjorck, J.-E. Effect of angiotensin-converting-enzyme inhibition compared with conventional therapy on cardiovascular morbidity and mortality in hypertension: the Captropril Prevention Project (CAPP) randomised trial. *The Lancet.* 1999; 353:611–16.

14. HOPE. Effects of an angiotensin-converting-enzyme inhibitor, ramipril, on cardiovascular events in high-risk patients. The Heart Outcomes Prevention Evaluation Study Investigators. *New England Journal of Medicine.* 2000; 342(3):145–53.

15. PEACE. The PEACE Trial Investigators. Angiotensin-Converting Enzyme inhibition in stable coronary artery disease. *New England Journal of Medicine.* 2004; 351(20):2058–68.

16. Julius, S., Kjeldsen, S.E., Weber, B., Brunner, H.R., Ekman, S., Hansson, L., Hua, T., Laragh, J., McInnes, G.T., Mitchell, L., Plat, F., Schork, A., Smith, B., Zanchetti, A. Outcomes in hypertensive patients at high cardiovascular risk treated with regimens based on valsartan or amlodipine: the VALUE randomised trial. *The Lancet.* 2004; 363:2022–31.

17. Borhani, N., Mercuir, M., Borhani, P.A., Buckalew, V.M., Canossa-Terris, M., Carr, A.A., Kappagoda, T., Rocca, M.V., Schnaper, H.W., Sowers, J.R., Bond, M.G. Final outcome results of the Multicenter Isradipine Diuretic Atherosclerosis Study (MIDAS):

A randomized controlled trial. *Journal of the American Medical Association.* 1996;
276(10):785–91.

18. Dahlof, B., Sever, P.S., Poulter, N.R., Wedel, H., Beevers, D.G., Caulfield, M., Collins, R., Kjeldsen, S.E., Kristinsson, A., McInnes, G.T., Mehlsen, J., Nieminen, M., O'Brien, E., Ostergren, J. Prevention of cardiovascular events with an antihypertensive regimen of amlodipine adding perindopril as required versus atenolol adding bendroflumethiazide as required, in the Anglo-Scandinavian Cardiac Outcomes Trial-Blood Pressure Lowering Arm (ASCOT-BBLA): A multicentre randomised controlled trial. *The Lancet.* 2005; 366:895–906.

19. Carlberg, B., Samuelsson, O., Lindholm, L.H. Atenolol in hypertension: is it a wise choice? *The Lancet.* Nov. 6–12, 2004; 364(9446):1684–89.

20. Freemantle, N., Cleland, J., Young, P., Mason, J., Harrison, J. Beta blocker after myocardial infarction: systematic review and meta regression analysis. *British Medical Journal.* June 26, 1999; 318:1730–31.

21. Psaty, B.M., Lumley, T., Furberg, C.D., Schellenbaum, G., Pahor, M., Alderman, M.H., Weiss, N.S. Health outcomes associated with various antihypertensive therapies used as first-line agents: A network meta-analysis. *Journal of the American Medical Association.* May 21, 2003; 289(19):2534–44.

22. Wassertheil-Smoller, S., Psaty, B., Greenland, P., Oberman, A., Kotchen, T., Mouton, C., Black, H., Aragaki, A., Trevisan, M. Association between cardiovascular outcomes and antihypertension drug treatment in older women. *Journal of the American Medical Association.* 2004; 292(23):2849–59.

23. Dahlof, B., Devereux, R.B., Kjeldsen, S.E., Julius, S., Beevers, G., de Faire, U., Fyhrquist, F., Ibsen, H., Kristiansson, K., Lederballe-Pedersen, O., Lindholm, L.H., Nieminen, M.S., Omvik, P., Oparil, S., Wedel, H. Cardiovascular morbidity and mortality in the Losartan Intervention for Endpoint reduction in hypertension study (LIFE): a randomised trial against atenolol. *The Lancet.* 2002; 359:995–1003.

24. Wing, L.M.H., Reid, C.M., Ryan, P., Beilin, L.J., Brown, M.A., Jennings, G.L.R., Johnston, C.I., McNeil, J.J., Macdonald, G.J., Marley, J.E., Morgan, T.O., West, M. J. A comparison of outcomes with angiotensin-converting-enzyme inhibitors and diuretics for hypertension in the elderly. *New England Journal of Medicine.* 2003; 348(7):583–92.

25. Lindholm, L.H., Ibsen, H., Dahlof, B., Devereux, R.B., Beevers, G., de Faire, U., Fyhrquist, F., Julius, S., Kjeldsen, S.E., Kristiansson, K., Lederballe-Pedersen, O., Nieminen, M.S., Omvik, P., Oparil, S., Wedel, H., Aurup, P., Edelman, J., Snapinn, S. Cardiovascular morbidity and mortality in patients with diabetes in the Losartan Invervention for Endpoint reduction in hypertension study (LIFE): a randomised trial against atenolol. *The Lancet.* 2002; 359:1004–10.

26. Cohn, J.N., Tognoni, G. A randomized trial of the angiotensin-receptor blocker valsartan in chronic heart failure. *New England Journal of Medicine.* 2001; 345:1667–75.

27. Pitt, B., Poole-Wilson, P.A., Segal, R. Effect of losartan compared with captopril on mortality in patients with symptomatic heart failure: Randomised trial—the Losartan Heart Failure Survival Study ELITE II. *The Lancet.* 2000; 355:1582–87.

28. Hippisley-Cox, J., Coupland, C. Effect of combinations of drugs on all cause mortality in patients with ischaemic heart disease: Nested case-control analysis. *British Medical Journal.* 2005; 330:1059–63.

29. Raina Elley, C., Arroll, B. Refining the exercise prescription for hypertension. *The Lancet.* Oct. 8, 2005; 366:1248–49.

CHAPTER 6

1. Li, Z., Maglione, M., Tu, W., Mojica, W., Arterbum, D., Shugarman, L.R., Hilton, L., Suttorp, M., Solomon, V., Shekelle, P.G., Morton, S.C. Meta-analysis: Pharmacological treatment of obesity. *Annals of Internal Medicine.* 2005; 142:532–46.

2. Godoy-Matos, A., Carraro, L., Vieira, A., Oliveira, J., Guedes, E.P., Mattos, L., Rangel, C., Moreira, R.O., Coutinho, W., Appolinario, J.C. Treatment of obese adolescents with sibutramine: A randomized, double-blind, controlled study. *Journal of Clinical Endocrinology & Metabolism.* 2005; 90(3):1460–65.

3. Torgerson, J.S., Hauptman, J., Boldrin, M.N., Sjostrom, L. Xenical in the prevention of diabetes in obese subjects (XENDOS) study: A randomized study of orlistat as an adjunct to lifestyle changes for the prevention of type 2 diabetes in obese patients. *Diabetes Care.* 2004; 27(1):155–61.

4. Shekelle, P.G., Hardy, M.L., Morton, S.C., Maglione, M., Mojica, W.A., Suttorp, M.J., Rhodes, S.L., Jungvig, L., Gagne, J. Efficacy and safety of ephedra and ephedrine for weight loss and athletic performance: a meta-analysis. *Journal of the American Medical Association.* 2003; 289:1537–45.

5. de Lorgeril, M., Salen, P., Martin, J.L., Monjaud, I., Delaye, J., Mamelle, N. Mediterranean diet, traditional risk factors, and the rate of cardiovascular complications after myocardial infarction: Final report of the Lyon Diet Heart Study. *Circulation.* 1999; 99:779–85.

6. Trichopoulou, A., Orfanos, P., Norat, T., Bueno-de-Mesquita, B., Ocke, M.C., Peeters, P.H.M., van der Schouw, Y.T., Boeing, H., Hoffmann, K., Boffetta, P., Nagel, G., Masala, G., Krogh, V., Panico, S., Tumino, R., Vineis, P., Bamia, C., Naska, A., Benetou, V., Ferrari, P., Slimani, N., Pera, G., Martinez-Garcia, C., Navarro, C., Rodriguez-Barranco, M., Dorronsor, M., Spencer, E.A., Key, T.J., Bingham, S., Khaw, K.-T., Kesse, E., Clavel-Chapelon, F., Boutron-Ruault, M.-C., Berglund, G., Wirfalt, E., Hallmans, G., Johansson, I., Tjonneland, A., Olsen, A., Overvad, K., Hundborg, H.H., Riboli, E., Trichopoulos, D. Modified Mediterranean diet and survival: EPIC-elderly prospective cohort study. *British Medical Journal.* 2005; 330:991–98.

7. de Lorgeril et al., 1999.

CHAPTER 7

1. Boushey, H.A., Sorkness, C.A., King, T.S., Sullivan, S.D., Fahy, J.V., Lazarus, S.C., Chinchilli, V.M., Craig, T.J., Dimango, E.A., Deykin, A., Fagan, J.K., Fish, J.E., Ford, J.G., Kraft, M., Lemanske, R.F., Leone, F.T., Martin, R.J., Mauger, E.A., Pesola, G.R., Peters, S.P., Rollings, N.J., Szefler, S.J., Wechsler, M.E., Israel, E. Daily versus as-needed corticosteroids for mild persistent asthma. *New England Journal of Medicine.* 2005; 325(15):1519–28.

2. www.fda.gov/ohrms/codkets/ac/05/briefing/2005–4148B1_03_02-FDA-Smart-Study.pdf. Accessed Jan. 8, 2007.

3. Salpeter, S.R., Buckley, N.S., Ormiston, T.M., Salpeter, E.E. Meta-analysis: effect of long-acting beta-agonists on severe asthma exacerbations and asthma-related deaths. *Annals of Internal Medicine.* June 20, 2006; 144(12):904–12.

4. Lucas, S.R., Platts-Mills, T.A.E. Physical activity and exercise in asthma: Relevance to etiology and treatment. *Journal of Allergy and Clinical Immunology.* May, 2005; 115(5):928–34.

CHAPTER 8

1. Nickel, J.C., Fradet, Y., Boake, R.C., Pommerville, P.J., Perreault, J.P., Afridi, S.K. Efficacy and safety of finasteride therapy for benign prostatic hyperplasia: results of a 2-year randomized controlled trial (the PROSPECT study). PROscar Safety Plus Efficacy Canadian Two-year Study. *Canadian Medical Association Journal.* 1996; 348:602–06.

2. Lepor, H., Williford, W.O., Barry, M.J. The efficacy of terazosin, finasteride, or both in benign prostatic hyperplasia. Veterans Affairs Cooperative Studies Benign Prostatic Hyperplasia Study Group. *New England Journal of Medicine.* 1996; 335:533–39.

3. McConnell, J.D., Roehrborn, C.G., Bautista, O.M. The long-term effect of doxazosin, finasteride, and combination therapy on the clinical progression of benign prostatic hyperplasia. *New England Journal of Medicine.* 2003; 349:2387–98.

4. Bent, S., Kane, C., Shinohara, K., Neuhaus, J., Hudes, E.S., Goldberg, H., Avins, A.L. Saw palmetto for benign prostatic hyperplasia. *New England Journal of Medicine.* Feb. 9, 2006; 354(6):557–66.

CHAPTER 9

1. Salas, M., Ward, A., Caro, J. Are proton pump inhibitors the first choice for acute treatment of gastric ulcers? A meta analysis of randomized clinical trials. *BMC Gastroenterology.* 2002; 2(17):1–7.

2. Leontiadis, G.I., Sharma, V.K., Howden, C.W. Systematic review and meta-analysis of proton pump inhibitor therapy in peptic ulcer bleeding. *British Medical Journal.* Jan. 31, 2005; 330:568–72.

3. Camilleri, M., Northcutt, A.R., Kong, S., Dukes, G.E., McSorley, D., Mangel, A.W. Efficacy and safety of alosetron in women with irritable bowel syndrome: a randomised, placebo-controlled trial. *The Lancet.* Mar. 25, 2000; 355:1035–40.

4. Lunardi, C., Bambara, L.M., Biasi, D. Double-blind crossover trial of oral sodium cromoglycate in patients with irritable bowel syndrome due to food intolerance. *Clinical & Experimental Allergy.* 1991; 21(5):569–72.

5. Holtmann, G., Talley, N.J., Liebregts, T., Adam, B., Parow, C. A placebo-controlled trial of itopride in functional dyspepsia. *New England Journal of Medicine.* 2006; 354(8):832–40.

6. Odes, H.S., Madar, Z. A double-blind trial of a celandin, aloe vera, and psyllium laxative preparation in adult patients with constipation. *Digestion.* 1991; 49(2):65–71.

7. Liu, J.H., Chen, G.H., Yeh, H.Z., Huang, C.K., Poon, S.K. Enteric-coated peppermint-oil capsules in the treatment of irritable bowel syndrome: A prospective, randomized trial. *Journal of Gastroenterology.* 1997; 32:765–68.

8. Dew, M.J., Evans, B.K., Rhodes, J. Peppermint oil for the irritable bowel syndrome: A multicentre trial. *British Journal of Clinical Practice.* 1984; 38:394–98.

9. Bensoussan, A., Talley, N.J., Hing, M., Menzies, R., Guo, A., Ngu, M. Treatment of irritable bowel syndrome with Chinese herbal medicine: A randomized controlled trial. *Journal of the American Medical Association.* 1998; 280:1585–89.

10. O'Sullivan, M.A., O'Morain, C.A. Bacterial supplementation in the irritable bowel syndrome. A randomised double-blind placebo-controlled crossover study. *Digestive & Liver Diseases.* 2000; 32:294–301.

11. D'Souza, A.L., Rajkumar, C., Cooke, J., Bulpitt, C.J. Probiotics in prevention of antibiotic associated diarrhoea: A meta-analysis. *British Medical Journal.* 2002; 324:1361–64.

CHAPTER 10

1. Little, P., Gould, C., Williamson, I., Moore, M., Warner, G., Dunleavey, J. Pragmatic randomised controlled trial of two prescribing strategies for childhood acute otitis media. *British Medical Journal.* Feb. 10, 2001; 322:336–42.

2. Spiro, D.M., Tay, K.Y., Arnold, D.H., Dziura, J.D., Baker, M.D., Shapiro, E.D. Wait-and-see prescription for the treatment of acute otitis media: a randomized controlled trial. *Journal of the American Medical Association.* Sept. 13 2006; 296(10):1235–41.

3. Damoiseaux, R.A.M.J., van Balen, F.A.M., Hoes, A.W., Verheij, T.J.M., de Melker, R.A. Primary care based randomised, double blind trial of amoxicillin versus placebo for acute otitis media in children aged under 2 years. *British Medical Journal.* Feb. 5, 2000; 320(7231):350–54.

4. Little, P., Gould, C., Moore, M., Warner, G., Dunleavey, J., Williamson, I. Predictors of poor outcome and benefit from antibiotics in children with acute otitis media: Pragmatic randomised trial. *British Medical Journal.* July 6, 2002; 325(7354):22.

5. Jefferson, T. Influenza vaccination: policy versus evidence. *British Medical Journal.* 2007; 333:912–15.

6. van Riemsdijk, M.M., Ditters, J.M., Sturkenboom, M.C.J.M., Tulen, J.H.M., Ligthelm, R.J., Overbosch, D., Stricker, B.H. Neuropsychiatric events during prophylactic use of mefloqine before travelling. *European Journal of Clinical Pharmacology.* 2002; 58:441–45.

7. Karlowski, T.R., Chalmers, T.C., Frenkel, L.D., Kapikian, A.Z., Lewis, T.L., Lynch, J.M. Ascorbic acid for the common cold. A prophylactic and therapeutic trial. *Journal of the American Medical Association.* 1975; 231(10):1038–42.

8. El-Kadiki, A., Sutton, A.J. Role of multivitamins and mineral supplements in preventing infections in elderly people: systematic review and meta-analysis of randomised controlled trials. *British Medical Journal.* 2005; 330:871–76.

9. Barrett, B.P., Brown, R.L., Locken, K., Maberry, R., Bobula, J.A., D'Alessio, D. Treatment of the common cold with unrefined echinacea: A randomized, double-blind, placebo-controlled trial. *Annals of Internal Medicine.* Dec. 17, 2002; 137(12):939–46.

10. Taylor, J.A., Weber, W., Standish, L., Quinn, H., Goesling, J., McGann, M., Calabrese, C. Efficacy and safety of echinacea in treating upper respiratory tract infections in children: A randomized controlled trial. *Journal of the American Medical Association.* Dec. 2, 2003; 290(21):2824–30.

11. Szajewska, H., Ruszcynski, M., Radzikowski, A. Probiotics in the prevention of antibiotic-associated diarrhea in children: A meta-analysis of randomized controlled trials. *Journal of Pediatrics.* 2006; 149:367–72.

12. D'Souza, A.L., Rajkumar, C., Cooke, J., Bulpitt, C.J. Probiotics in prevention of antibiotic associated diarrhoea: A meta-analysis. *British Medical Journal.* 2002; 324:1361–64.

13. Szajewska, H., Kotowska, M., Mrukowicz, J.Z., Armanska, M., Mikolajczyk, W. Efficacy of *Lactobacillus* GG in prevention of nosocomial diarrhea in infants. *Journal of Pediatrics.* 2001; 138:361–65.

14. Ouwenhand, A.C., Lagstrom, H., Suomalainen, T., Salminen, S. Effect of probiotics on constipation, fecal azoreductase activity and fecal mucin content in the elderly. *Annals of Nutrition & Metabolism.* 2002; 46:159–62.

15. Banaszkiewicz, A., Szajewska, H. Ineffectiveness of *Lactobacillus* GG as an adjunct to lactulose for the treatment of constipation in children: A double-blind placebo-controlled randomized trial. *Journal of Pediatrics.* 2005; 146:364–69.

16. Szajewska et al., 2006.

CHAPTER 11

1. Liberman, U.A., Weiss, S.R., Broll, J., Minne, H.W., Quan, H., Bell, N.H., Rodriguez-Portales, J., Downs, R.W., Dequeker, J., Favus, M., Seeman, E., Recker, R.R., Capizzi, T., Santora, A.C., Lombardi, A., Shah, R.V., Hirsch, L.J., Karpf, D.B. Effect of

oral alendronate on bone mineral density and the incidence of fractures in postmenopausal osteoporosis. *New England Journal of Medicine.* November 30, 1995; 333(22): 1437–44.

2. Cummings, S.R., Black, D.M., Thompson, D.E., Applegate, W.B., Barrett-Connor, E., Musliner, T.A., Palermo, L., Prineas, R., Rubin, S.M., Scott, J.C., Vogt, T., Wallace, R., Yates, A.J., LaCroix, A.Z. Effect of alendronate on risk of fracture in women with low bone density but without vertebral fractures: Results from the fracture intervention trial. *Journal of the American Medical Association.* 1998; 280(24):2077–82.

3. Black, D.M., Cummings, S.R. Randomised trial of effect of alendronate on risk of fracture in women with existing vertebral fractures. *The Lancet.* 1996; 348(9041):1535–41.

4. Pols, H.A.P., Felsenberg, D., Hanley, D.A., Stepan, J., Munoz-Torres, M., Wilkin, T.J., Quin-sheng, G., Galich, A.M., Vandormael, K., Yates, A.J., Stych, B. Multinational placebo-controlled randomized trial of the effects of alendronate on bone density and fracture risk in postmenopausal women with low bone mass: results of the FOSIT study. *Osteoporosis International.* 1999; 9:461–68.

5. Harris, S.T., Watts, N.B., Genant, H.K., McKeever, C.D., Hangartner, T., Keller, M., Chestnut, C.H., Brown, J., Eriksen, E.F., Hoseyni, H.S., Axelrod, D.W., Miller, P.D. Effects of risedronate treatment on vertebral and nonvertebral fractures in women with postmenopausal osteoporosis: A randomized controlled trial. *Journal of the American Medical Association.* 1999; 282(14):1344–52.

6. McClung, M.R., Geusens, P., Miller, P.D., Zippel, H., Bensen, W.G., Roux, C., Adami, S., Fogelman, I., Diamond, T., Eastell, R., Meunier, P.J., Reginster, J.-Y. Effect of risedronate on the risk of hip fracture in elderly women. *New England Journal of Medicine.* 2001; 344(5):333–40.

7. Orwoll, E., Ettinger, M., Weiss, S., Miller, P., Kendler, D., Graham, J., Adami, S., Weber, K., Lorenc, R., Pietschmann, P., Vandormael, K., Lombardi, A. Alendronate for the treatment of osteoporosis in men. *New England Journal of Medicine.* 2000; 343:604–10.

8. Tonino, R.P., Meunier, P.J., Emkey, R.D., Rodriguez-Portales, J.A., Menkes, C.-J., Wasnich, R.D., Bone, H.G., Santora, A.C., Wu, M., Desai, R., Ross, P.D. Skeletal benefits of alendronate: 7-year treatment of postmenopausal osteoporotic women. *Journal of Clinical Endocrinology & Metabolism.* 2000; 85:3109–15.

9. Bone, H.G., Hosking, D., Devogelaer, J.-P., Tucci, J.R., Emkey, R.D., Tonino, R.P., Rodriguez-Portales, J.A., Downs, R.W., Gupta, J., Santora, A.C., Liberman, U.A. Ten years' experience with alendronate for osteoporosis in postmenopausal women. *New England Journal of Medicine.* 2004; 350(12):1189–99.

10. Black, D.M., Schwartz, A.V., Ensrud, K.E., Cauley, J.A., Levis, S., Quandt, S.A., Satterfield, S., Wallace, R.B., Bauer, D.C., Palermo, L., Wehren, L.E., Lombardi, A., Santora, A.C., Cummings, S.R. Effects of continuing or stopping alendronate after 5 years of treatment: The Fracture Intervention Trial Long-term Extension (FLEX): A

randomized trial. *Journal of the American Medical Association.* Dec. 27, 2006; 296(24):2927–38.

11. Migliatori, C. Bisphosphonates and oral cavity avascular bone necrosis (letter). *Journal of Clinical Oncology.* Nov. 15, 2003; 21(22):4253–54.

12. Ettinger, B., Black, D.M., Mitlak, B.H., Knickerbocker, R.K., Nickelsen, T., Genant, H.K., Christiansen, C., Delmas, P.D., Zanchetta, J.R., Stakkestad, J., Gluer, C.C., Krueger, K., Cohen, F.J., Eckert, S., Ensrud, K.E., Avioli, L.V., Lips, P., Cummings, S.R. Reduction of vertebral fracture risk in postmenopausal women with osteoporosis treated with raloxifene: Results from a 3-year randomized clinical trial. *Journal of the American Medical Association.* 1999; 282(7):637–45.

13. Barrett-Connor, E., Mosca, L., Collins, P., Geiger, M.J., Grady, D., Kornitzer, M., McNabb, M.A., Wenger, N.J. Effects of raloxifene on cardiovascular events and breast cancer in postmenopausal women. *New England Journal of Medicine.* July 13, 2006; 355(2):125–37.

14. WGWHII. Writing Group for the Women's Health Initiative Investigators. Risks and benefits of estrogen plus progestin in healthy postmenopausal women: Principal results from the Women's Health Initiative Randomized Controlled Trial. *Journal of the American Medical Association.* 2002; 288(3):321–33.

15. Wassertheil-Smoller, S., Hendrix, S.L., Limacher, M., Heiss, G., Kooperberg, C., Baird, A., Kotchen, T., Curb, J.D., Black, H., Rossouw, J.E., Aragaki, A., Safford, M., Stein, E., Laowattana, S., Mysiw, W.J. Effect of estrogen plus progestin on stroke in postmenopausal women: The Women's Health Initiative: A randomized trial. *Journal of the American Medical Association.* 2003; 289(20):2673–84.

16. Dawson-Hughes, B., Harris, S.S., Krall, E.A., Dallal, G.E. Effect of calcium and vitamin D supplementation on bone density in men and women 65 years of age or older. *New England Journal of Medicine.* 1997; 337:670–76.

17. Chapuy, M.C., Arlot, M.E., Delmans, P.D., Meunier, P.J. Effect of calcium and cholecalciferol treatment for three years on hip fractures in elderly women. *British Medical Journal.* 1994; 308:1081–82.

18. Porthouse, J., Cockaynes, S., King, C., Saxon, L., Steele, E., Aspray, T., Baverstock, M., Birks, Y., Dumville, J., Francis, R., Iglesius, C., Puffer, S., Sutcliffe, A.A.W., Torgerson, D.J. Randomised controlled trial of calcium and supplementation with cholecalciferol (vitamin D 3) for prevention of fractures in primary care. *British Medical Journal.* 2005; 330:1–6.

19. RECORD. Oral vitamin D3 and calcium for secondary prevention of low-trauma fractures in elderly people (Randomised Evaluation of Calcium Or vitamin D, RECORD): a randomised placebo-controlled trial. *The Lancet.* 2005; 365:1621–28.

20. Jackson, R.D., LaCroix, A.Z., Gass, M., Wallace, R.B., Robbins, J., Lewis, C.E., Bassford, T., Beresford, S.A., Black, H.R., Blanchette, P., Bonds, D.E., Brunner, R.L., Brzyski, R.G., Caan, B., Cauley, J.A., Chlebowski, R.T., Cummings, S.R., Granek, I.,

Hays, J., Heiss, G., Hendrix, S.L., Howard, B.V., Hsia, J., Hubbell, F.A., Johnson, K.C., Judd, H., Kotchen, J.M., Kuller, L.H., Langer, R.D., Lasser, N.L., Limacher, M.C., Ludlam, S., Manson, J.E., Margolis, K.L., McGowan, J., Ockene, J.K., O'Sullivan, M.J., Phillips, L., Prentice, R.L., Sarto, G.E., Stefanick, M.L., Van Horn, L., Wactawski-Wende, J., Whitlock, E., Anderson, G.L., Assaf, A.R., Barad, D. Calcium plus vitamin D supplementation and the risk of fractures. *New England Journal of Medicine.* Feb. 16 2006; 354(7):669–83.

CHAPTER 12

1. Chlebowski, R.T., Hendrix, S.L., Langer, R.D., Stefanick, M.L., Gass, M., Lane, D., Rodabough, R.J., Gilligan, M.A., Cyr, M.G., Thomson, C.A., Khandekar, J., Petrovitch, H., McTiernan, A. Influence of estrogen plus progestin on breast cancer and mammography in healthy postmenopausal women: The Women's Health Initiative Randomized Trial. *Journal of the American Medical Association.* 2003; 289(24):3243–53.

2. WGWHII. Writing Group for the Women's Health Initiative Investigators. Risks and benefits of estrogen plus progestin in healthy postmenopausal women: Principal results from the Women's Health Initiative Randomized Controlled Trial. *Journal of the American Medical Association.* 2002; 288(3):321–33.

3. Wassertheil-Smoller, S., Hendrix, S.L., Limacher, M., Heiss, G., Kooperberg, C., Baird, A., Kotchen, T., Curb, J.D., Black, H., Rossouw, J.E., Aragaki, A., Safford, M., Stein, E., Laowattana, S., Mysiw, W.J. Effect of estrogen plus progestin on stroke in postmenopausal women: The Women's Health Initiative: A randomized trial. *Journal of the American Medical Association.* 2003; 289(20):2673–84.

4. Grady, D., Herrington, D.M., Bittner, V., Blumenthal, R., Davidson, M., Hlatky, M., Hsia, J., Hudley, S., Herd, A., Khan, S., Newby, L.K., Waters, D., Vittinghoff, E., Wenger, N. Cardiovascular disease outcomes during 6.8 years of hormone therapy: Heart and Estrogen/Progesterone Replacement Study Follow-up (HERS II). *Journal of the American Medical Association.* 2002; 288(1):49–57.

5. Hulley, S., Grady, D., Bush, T., Furberg, C., Herrington, D., Riggs, B., Vittinghoff, E. Randomized trial of estrogen plus progestin for secondary prevention of coronary heart disease in postmenopausal women. *Journal of the American Medical Association.* 1998; 280(7):605–13.

6. Hulley, S., Furberg, C., Barrett-Connor, E., Cauley, J., Grady, D., Haskell, W., Knopp, R., Lowery, M., Satterfield, S., Schrott, H., Vittinghoff, E., Hunninghake, D. Noncardiovascular disease outcomes during 6.8 years of hormone therapy: Heart and Estrogen/Progesterone Replacement Study Follow-up (HERS II). *Journal of the American Medical Association.* 2002; 288(1):58–66.

7. Waters, D.D., Alderman, E.L., Hsia, J., Howard, B.V., Cobb, F.R., Rogers, W.J., Ouyang, P., Thompson, P., Tardif, J.C., Higginson, L., Bittner, V., Steffes, M., Gordon,

D.J., Proschan, M., Younes, N., Verter, J.I. Effects of hormone replacement therapy and antioxidant vitamin supplements on coronary atherosclerosis in postmenopausal women: A randomized controlled trial. *Journal of the American Medical Association.* 2002; 288(19):2432–40.

8. Rapola, J.M., Virtamo, J. Randomised trial of alpha-tocopherol and beta-carotene supplements on incidence of major coronary events in men with previous myocardial infarction. *The Lancet.* 1997; 349:1715–20.

9. Shumaker, S.A., Legault, C., Rapp, S.R., Thal, L., Wallace, R.B., Ockene, J.K., Hendrix, S.L., Jones, B.N., Assaf, A.R., Jackson, R.D., Kotchen, J.M., Wassertheil-Smoller, S., Wactawski-Wende, J. Estrogen plus progestin and the incidence of dementia and mild cognitive impairment in postmenopausal women: The Women's Health Initiative Memory Study: A randomized controlled trial. *Journal of the American Medical Association.* 2003; 289(20):2651–62.

10. Rapp, S.R., Espeland, M.A., Shumaker, S.A., Henderson, V.W., Brunner, R.L., Manson, J.E., Gass, M.L.S., Stefanick, M.L., Lane, D.S., Hays, J., Johnson, K.C., Coker, L.H., Dailey, M., Bowen, D. Effect of estrogen plus progestin on global cognitive function in postmenopausal women: The Women's Health Initiative Memory Study: A randomized controlled trial. *Journal of the American Medical Association.* 2003; 289(20):2663–72.

11. Hays, J., Ockene, J.K., Brunner, R.L., Kotchen, J.M., Manson, J.E., Patterson, R.E., Aragaki, A.K., Shumaker, S.A., Brzyski, R.G., LaCroix, A.Z., Granek, I.A., Valanis, B.G. Effects of estrogen plus progestin on health-related quality of life. *New England Journal of Medicine.* 2003; 348(19):1839–54.

12. Shumaker, S.A., Legault, C., Kuller, L., Rapp, S.R., Thal, L., Lane, D.S., Fillit, H., Stefanick, M.L., Lewis, C.E., Masaki, K., Coker, L.H. Conjugated equine estrogens and incidence of probable dementia and mild cognitive impairment in postmenopausal women: Women's Health Initiative Memory Study. *Journal of the American Medical Association.* 2004; 291(24):2947–58.

13. Soares, C.N., Almeida, O.P., Joffe, H., Cohen, L.S. Efficacy of estradiol for the treatment of depressive disorders in perimenopausal women: a double-blind, randomized, placebo-controlled trial. *Archives of General Psychiatry.* 2001; 58(6):529–34.

14. Steffen, A.M., Thompson, L.W., Gallagher-Thompson, D., Koin, D. Physical and psychosocial correlates of hormone replacement therapy with chronically stressed postmenopausal women. *Journal of Aging & Health.* 1999; 11(1):3–26.

CHAPTER 13

1. Hauber, A., Gale, E.A.M. The market in diabetes. *Diabetologia.* 2006; 49:247–252.

2. DPPRG. Prevention of type 2 diabetes with troglitazone in the Diabetes Prevention Program. The Diabetes Prevention Program Research Group. *Diabetes.* 2005; 54:1150–56.

3. Nissen, S.E., Wolski, K., Topol, E.J. Effect of muraglitazar on death and major adverse cardiovascular events in patients with type 2 diabetes mellitus. *Journal of the American Medical Association.* 2005; 294(20):2581–86.

4. Kahn, S.E., Haffner, S.M., Heise, M.A., Herman, W.H., Holman, R.R., Jones, N.P., Kravitz, B.G., Lachin, J.M., O'Neill, M.C., Zinman, B., Viberti, G. Glycemic durability of rosiglitazone, metformin, or glyburide monotherapy. *New England Journal of Medicine.* Dec. 7, 2006; 355(23):2427–42.

5. Dormandy, J.A., Charbonnel, B., Eckland, D.J.A., Erdmann, E., Massi-Benedetti, M., Moules, I.K., Skene, A.M., Tan, M.H., Lefebure, P.J., Murray, G.D., Standl, E., Wilcox, R.G., Wilhelmsen, L., Betteridge, J., Birkeland, K., Golay, A., Heine, R.J., Koranyi, L., Laakso, M., Mokan, M., Norkus, A., Pirags, V., Podar, T., Scheen, A.J., Scherbaum, W., Schernthaner, G., Schmitz, O., Skrha, J., Smith, U., Taton, J. Secondary prevention of macrovascular events in patients with type 2 diabetes in the PROactive study (PROspective pioglitAzone Clinical Trial In macroVascular Events): a randomised controlled trial. *The Lancet.* 2005; 366:1279–89.

6. Raskin, P., Rendell, M., Riddle, M.C., Dole, J.F., Freed, M.I., Rosenstock, J. A randomized trial of rosiglitazone therapy in patients with inadequately controlled insulin-treated type 2 diabetes. *Diabetes Care.* 2001; 24:1226–32.

7. HPS. MRC/BHF Heart Protection Study of cholesterol lowering with simvastatin in 20,563 high-risk individuals: a randomised placebo-controlled trial. *The Lancet.* 2002; 360:7–22.

8. Colhoun, H.M., Betteridge, D.J., Durrington, P.N., Hitman, G.A., Neil, H.A.W., Livingstone, S.J., Thomason, M.J., Mackness, M.I., Charlton-Menys, V., Fuller, J.H. Primary prevention of cardiovascular disease with atorvastatin in type 2 diabetes in the Collaborative Atorvastatin Diabetes Study (CARDS): multicentre randomised placebo-controlled trial. *The Lancet.* 2004; 364:685–96.

9. ALLHAT. Major outcomes in moderately hypercholesterolemic, hypertensive patients randomized to pravastatin vs usual care: The Antihypertensive and Lipid-Lowering Treatment to Prevent Heart Attack Trial (ALLHAT-LLT). *Journal of the American Medical Association.* 2002; 288(23):2998–3007.

10. Sever, P.S., Dahlof, B., Poulter, N.R., Wedel, H., Beevers, G., Caulfield, M., Collins, R., Kjeldsen, S.E., Kristinsson, A., McInnes, G.T., Mehlsen, J., Nieminen, M., O'Brien, E., Ostergren, J. Prevention of coronary and stroke events with Atorvastatin in hypertensive patients who have average or lower-than-average cholesterol concentrations, in the Anglo-Scandinavian Cardiac Outcomes Trial-Lipid Lowering Arm (ASCOT-LLA): a multicentre randomised controlled trial. *The Lancet.* 2003; 361:1149–58.

11. Shepherd, J., Blauw, G.J., Murphy, M.B., Bollen, E.L.E.M., Buckley, B.M., Cobbe, S.M., Ford, I., Gaw, A., Hyland, M., Jukema, J.W., Kamper, A.M., Macfarlane, P.W., Meinders, A.E., Norrie, J., Packard, C.J., Perry, I.J., Stott, D.J., Sweeney, B.J., Twomey,

C., Westendorp, R.G.J. Pravastatin in elderly individuals at risk of vascular disease (PROSPER): a randomised controlled trial. *The Lancet.* 2002; 360:1623–30.

12. LIPID. Prevention of cardiovascular events and death with pravastatin in patients with coronary heart disease and a broad range of initial cholesterol levels. *New England Journal of Medicine.* 1998; 339:1349–57.

13. Sacks, F.M., Pfeffer, M.A., Moye, L.A., Rouleau, J.L., Rutherford, J.D., Cole, T.G., Brown, L., Warnica, J.W., Arnold, J.M.O., Wun, C.C., Davis, B.R., Braunwald, E. The effect of pravastatin on coronary events after myocardial infarction in patients with average cholesterol levels. *New England Journal of Medicine.* 1996; 335(14):1001–09.

14. Keech, A., Colquhoun, D., Best, J., Kirby, A., Simes, R.J., Hunt, D., Hague, W., Beller, E., Arulchelvam, M., Baker, J., Tonkin, A. Secondary prevention of cardiovascular events with long-term pravastatin in patients with diabetes or impaired fasting glucose: Results from the LIPID trial. *Diabetes Care.* 2003; 26:2713–21.

15. DPPRG. Reduction in the incidence of type 2 diabetes with lifestyle intervention or metformin. Diabetes Prevention Program Research Group. *New England Journal of Medicine.* 2002; 346(6):393–403.

CHAPTER 14

1. Knapp, M.J., Knopman, D.S., Solomon, P.R., Pendlebury, W.W., Davis, C.S., Gracon, S.I. A 30-week randomized trial of high-dose tacrine in patients with Alzheimer's disease. *Journal of the American Medical Association.* 1994; 271(13):985–91.

2. Knopman, D., Schneider, L., Davis, K., Talwalker, S., Smith, F., Hoover, T., Gracon, S.I. Long-term tacrine (Cognex) treatment: Effects on nursing home placement and mortality. *Neurology.* 1996; 47(1):166–77.

3. Watkins, P.B., Zimmerman, H.J., Knapp, M.J., Gracon, S.I., Lewis, K.W. Hepatoxic effects of tacrine administration in patients with Alzheimer's disease. *Journal of the American Medical Association.* 1994; 271(13):992–98.

4. Mohs, R.C., Doody, R.S., Morris, R.C., Ieni, J.R., Rogers, S.L., Perdomo, C.A., Pratt, R.D. A 1-year, placebo-controlled preservation of function survival of donepezil in AD patients. *Neurology.* 2001; 57:481–88.

5. Winblad, B., Engedal, K., Soininen, H., Verhey, F., Waldemar, G., Wimo, A., Wetterholm, A.-L., Zhang, R., Haglund, A., Subbiah, P. A 1-year, randomized placebo-controlled study of donepezil in patients with mild to moderate AD. *Neurology.* 2001; 57:489–95.

6. Feldman, H., Gauthier, S., Hecker, J., Vellas, B., Subbiah, P., Whalen, E. A 24-week, randomized, double-blind study of donepezil in moderate to severe Alzheimer's Disease. *Neurology.* 2001; 57:613–20.

7. Rogers, S.L., Friedhoff, L.T. Long-term efficacy and safety of donepezil in the treat-

ment of Alzheimer's disease: An interim analysis of the results of the US multicentre open label extension study. *European Neuropsychopharmacology.* 1998; 8:67–75.

8. Petersen, R.C., Thomas, R.G., Grundman, M., Bennett, D., Doody, R., Ferris, S., Galasko, D., Jin, S., Kaye, J., Levey, A., Pfeiffer, E., Sano, M., van Dyck, C.H., Thal, L.J. Vitamin E and donepezil for the treatment of mild cognitive impairment. *New England Journal of Medicine.* 2005; 352(23):2379–88.

9. Winblad, B., Kilander, L., Eriksson, S., Minthon, L., Batsman, S., Wetterholm, A.L., Jansson-Blixt, C., Haglund, A. Donepezil in patients with severe Alzheimer's disease: double-blind, parallel-group, placebo-controlled study. *The Lancet.* Apr. 1, 2006; 367 (9516):1057–65.

10. Farlow, M., Anand, R., Messina, J., Hartman, R., Veach, J. A 52-week study of the efficacy of rivastigmine in patients with mild to moderately severe Alzheimer's disease. *European Neurology.* 2000; 44:236–41.

11. Tariot, P.N., Solomon, P.R., Morris, J.C., Kershaw, P., Lilienfeld, S., Ding, C. A 5-month, randomized, placebo-controlled trial of galantamine in AD. *Neurology.* 2000; 54(12):2269–76.

12. Raskind, M.A., Peskind, E.R., Wessel, T., Yuan, W. Galantamine in AD: A 6-month randomized, placebo-controlled trial with a 6-month extension. *Neurology.* 2000; 54(12):2261–68.

13. Kaduszkiewicz, H., Zimmermann, T., Beck-Bornholdt, H.-P., van den Bussche, H. Cholinesterase inhibitors for patients with Alzheimer's disease: systematic review of randomised clinical trials. *British Medical Journal.* 2005; 331:321–27.

14. Shumaker, S.A., Legault, C., Rapp, S.R., Thal, L., Wallace, R.B., Ockene, J.K., Hendrix, S.L., Jones, B.N., Assaf, A.R., Jackson, R.D., Kotchen, J.M., Wassertheil-Smoller, S., Wactawski-Wende, J. Estrogen plus progestin and the incidence of dementia and mild cognitive impairment in postmenopausal women: The Women's Health Initiative Memory Study: A randomized controlled trial. *Journal of the American Medical Association.* 2003; 289(20):2651–62.

15. Hays, J., Ockene, J.K., Brunner, R.L., Kotchen, J.M., Manson, J.E., Patterson, R.E., Aragaki, A.K., Shumaker, S.A., Brzyski, R.G., LaCroix, A.Z., Granek, I.A., Valanis, B.G. Effects of estrogen plus progestin on health-related quality of life. *New England Journal of Medicine.* 2003; 348(19):1839–54.

16. Rapp, S.R., Espeland, M.A., Shumaker, S.A., Henderson, V.W., Brunner, R.L., Manson, J.E., Gass, M.L.S., Stefanick, M.L., Lane, D.S., Hays, J., Johnson, K.C., Coker, L.H., Dailey, M., Bowen, D. Effect of estrogen plus progestin on global cognitive function in postmenopausal women: The Women's Health Initiative Memory Study: A randomized controlled trial. *Journal of the American Medical Association.* 2003; 289(20):2663–72.

17. Shumaker, S.A., Legault, C., Kuller, L., Rapp, S.R., Thal, L., Lane, D.S., Fillit, H., Stefanick, M.L., Lewis, C.E., Masaki, K., Coker, L.H. Conjugated equine estrogens

and incidence of probable dementia and mild cognitive impairment in postmenopausal women: Women's Health Initiative Memory Study. *Journal of the American Medical Association.* 2004; 291(24):2947–58.

18. Espeland, M.A., Rapp, S.R., Shumaker, S.A., Brunner, R.L., Manson, J.E., Sherwin, B.B., Hsia, J., Margolis, K.L., Hogan, P.E., Wallace, R., Dailey, M., Freeman, R., Hays, J. Conjugated equine estrogens and global cognitive function in postmenopausal women. *Journal of the American Medical Association.* 2004; 291(24):2959–68.

19. Newcomer, J.W. Abnormalities of glucose metabolism associated with atypical antipsychotic drugs. *Journal of Clinical Psychiatry.* 2004; 18:36–46.

20. Sernyak, M.J., Leslie, D.L., Alarcon, R.D., Losonczy, M.F., Rosenheck, R. Association of diabetes mellitus with use of atypical neuroleptics in the treatment of schizophrenia. *American Journal of Psychiatry.* 2002; 159(4):561–66.

21. McMahon, J.A., Green, T.J., Skeaff, C.M., Knight, R.G., Mann, J.I., Williams, S.M. A controlled trial of homocysteine lowering and cognitive performance. *New England Journal of Medicine.* June 29, 2006; 354(26):2764–72.

22. LeBars, P.L., Katz, M.M., Berman, N. A placebo-controlled, double-blind, randomized trial of an extract of *Ginkgo biloba* for dementia. *Journal of the American Medical Association.* 1997; 278:1327–32.

23. Solomon, P.R., Adams, F., Silver, A., Zimmer, J., DeVeaux, R. Ginkgo for memory enhancement: A randomized controlled trial. *Journal of the American Medical Association.* 2002; 288(7):835–40.

CHAPTER 15

1. DUAG. Danish University Antidepressant Group: Paroxetine: a selective serotonin reuptake inhibitor showing better tolerance, but weaker antidepressant effect than clomipramine in a controlled multicenter study. *Journal of Affective Disorders.* 1990; 18(4):289–99.

2. Kirsch, I., Moore, T.J., Scoboria, A., Nicholls, S.S. The emperor's new drugs: An analysis of antidepressant medication data submitted to the U.S. Food and Drug Administration. Available at: http://www.journals.aoa.org/prevention/volume5/pre 0050023a.html. Accessed Nov. 7, 2005.

3. Moncrieff, J., Kirsch, I. Efficacy of antidepressants in adults. *British Medical Journal.* July 16, 2005; 331:155–59.

4. Shelton, R.C., Keller, M.B., Gelenberg, A., Dunner, D.L., Hirschfeld, R., Thase, M.E., Russell, J., Lydiard, R.B., Crits-Cristoph, P., Gallop, R., Todd, L., Hellerstein, D., Goodnick, P., Keitner, G., Stahl, S.M., Halbreich, U. Effectiveness of St John's Wort in major depression: A randomized controlled trial. *Journal of the American Medical Association.* 2001; 285(15):1978–86.

5. Szegedi, A., Kohnen, R., Dienel, A., Kieser, M. Acute treatment of moderate to severe

depression with hypericum extract WS 5570 (St. John's wort): Randomised controlled double blind non-inferiority trial versus paroxetine. *British Medical Journal*. 2005; 330:503–08.

6. HDTSG. Hypericum Depression Trial Study Group: Effect of Hypericum perforatum (St Joh's Wort) in major depressive disorder: A randomized controlled trial. *Journal of the American Medical Association*. 2002; 287(14):1807–14.

7. Stoll, A.L., Severus, E., Freeman, M.P., Rueter, S., Zboyan, H.A., Diamond, E., Cress, K.K., Marangell, L.B. Omega 3 fatty acids in bipolar disorder: A preliminary double-blind, placebo-controlled trial. *Archives of General Psychiatry*. 1999; 56:407–12.

8. Blumenthal, J.A., Bayak, M.A., Moore, K.A. Effects of exercise training on older patients with major depression. *Archives of Internal Medicine*. 1999; 159:2349–56.

CHAPTER 16

1. Barbone, F., McMahon, M.D., Davey, P.G., Morris, A.D., Reid, I.C., McDevitt, D.G., MacDonald, T.M. Association of road-traffic accidents with benzodiazepine use. *The Lancet*. 1998; 352(9137):1331–36.

2. Sivertsen, B., Omvik, S., Pallesen, S., Bjorvatn, B., Havik, O.E., Kvale, G., Nielsen, G.H., Nordhus, I.H. Cognitive behavioral therapy vs zopiclone for treatment of chronic primary insomnia in older adults: a randomized controlled trial. *Journal of the American Medical Association*. June 28, 2006; 295(24):2851–58.

3. Kripke, D.F., Garfinkel, L., Wingard, D.L., Klauber, M.R., Marler, M.R. Mortality associated with sleep duration and insomnia. *Archives of General Psychiatry*. 2002; 59:131–36.

4. *Ibid.*

CHAPTER 17

1. Goldstein, I., Lue, T.F., Padma-Nathan, H., Rosen, R.C., Steers, W.D., Wicker, P.A. Oral sildenafil in the treatment of erectile dysfunction. *New England Journal of Medicine*. 1998; 338(20):1397–1404.

2. Esposito, K., Giugliano, F., Di Palo, C., Giugliano, G., Marfella, R., D'Andrea, F., D'Armiento, M., Giugliano, D. Effect of lifestyle changes on erectile dysfunction in obese men: A randomized controlled trial. *Journal of the American Medical Association*. 2004; 291(24):2978–84.

CHAPTER 18

1. Vivekananthan, D.P., Penn, M.S., Sapp, S.K., Hsu, A., Topol, E.J. Use of antioxidant vitamins for the prevention of cardiovascular disease: Meta-analysis of randomised trials. *The Lancet*. 2003; 361:2017–23.

2. Feskanich, D., Singh, V.B., Willett, W.C. Vitamin A intake and hip fracture among postmenopausal women. *Journal of the American Medical Association.* 2002; 287:47–54.

3. Hennekens, C.H., Buring, J.E., Manson, J.E., Stampfer, M., Rosner, B., Cook, N.R., Belanger, C., LaMotte, F., Gaziano, J.M., Ridker, P.M., Willett, W., Peto, R. Lack of effect of long-term supplementation with beta carotene on the incidence of malignant neoplasms and cardiovascular disease. *New England Journal of Medicine.* 1996; 334(18):1145–49.

4. Omenn, G.S., Goodman, G.E., Thornquist, M.D., Balmes, J., Cullen, M.R., Glass, A., Keogh, J.P., Meyskens, F.L.J., Valanis, B., Williams, J.H., Barnhart, S., Hammar, S. Effects of a combination of beta carotene and vitamin A on lung cancer and cardiovascular disease. *New England Journal of Medicine.* 1996; 334(18):1150–55.

5. ATBC. The Alpha-Tocopherol, Beta Carotene Cancer Prevention Study Group. The effect of vitamin E and beta carotene on the incidence of lung cancer and other cancers in male smokers. *New England Journal of Medicine.* 1994; 330:1029–35.

6. Rapola, J.M., Virtamo, J. Randomised trial of alpha-tocopherol and beta-carotene supplements on incidence of major coronary events in men with previous myocardial infarction. *The Lancet.* 1997; 349:1715–20.

7. Bjelakovic, G., Nikolova, D., Simonetti, R.G., Gluud, C. Antioxidant supplements for prevention of gastrointestinal cancers: a systematic review and meta-analysis. *The Lancet.* 2004; 364:1219–28.

8. Dawson-Hughes, B., Harris, S.S., Krall, E.A., Dallal, G.E. Effect of calcium and vitamin D supplementation on bone density in men and women 65 years of age or older. *New England Journal of Medicine.* 1997; 337:670–76.

9. Chapuy, M.C., Arlot, M.E., Delmans, P.D., Meunier, P.J. Effect of calcium and cholecalciferol treatment for three years on hip fractures in elderly women. *British Medical Journal.* 1994; 308:1081–82.

10. Shea, B., Wells, G., Cranney, A., Zytaruk, N., Robinson, V., Griffith, L., Guyatt, G., Hamel, C., Ortiz, Z., Peterson, J., Robinson, V.A., Tugwell, P., Wells, G., Zytaruk, N. Calcium supplementation on bone loss in postmenopausal women. *Cochrane Database Systematic Review.* 2004:CD004526.

11. Porthouse, J., Cockaynes, S., King, C., Saxon, L., Steele, E., Aspray, T., Baverstock, M., Birks, Y., Dumville, J., Francis, R., Iglesius, C., Puffer, S., Sutcliffe, A.A.W., Torgerson, D.J. Randomised controlled trial of calcium and supplementation with cholecalciferol (vitamin D 3) for prevention of fractures in primary care. *British Medical Journal.* 2005; 330:1–6.

12. Jackson, R.D., LaCroix, A.Z., Gass, M., Wallace, R.B., Robbins, J., Lewis, C.E., Bassford, T., Beresford, S.A., Black, H.R., Blanchette, P., Bonds, D.E., Brunner, R.L., Brzyski, R.G., Caan, B., Cauley, J.A., Chlebowski, R.T., Cummings, S.R., Granek, I., Hays, J., Heiss, G., Hendrix, S.L., Howard, B.V., Hsia, J., Hubbell, F.A., Johnson, K.C., Judd, H., Kotchen, J.M., Kuller, L.H., Langer, R.D., Lasser, N.L., Limacher,

M.C., Ludlam, S., Manson, J.E., Margolis, K.L., McGowan, J., Ockene, J.K., O'Sullivan, M.J., Phillips, L., Prentice, R.L., Sarto, G.E., Stefanick, M.L., Van Horn, L., Wactawski-Wende, J., Whitlock, E., Anderson, G.L., Assaf, A.R., Barad, D. Calcium plus vitamin D supplementation and the risk of fractures. *New England Journal of Medicine.* Feb. 16 2006; 354(7):669–83.

13. MRC/BHF. Heart Protection Study of antioxidant vitamin supplementation in 20,536 high-risk individuals: a randomised placebo-controlled trial. *The Lancet.* 2002; 360:23–33.

14. PPP. Collaborative Group of the Primary Prevention Project (PPP). Low-dose aspirin and vitamin E in people at cardiovascular risk: a randomised trial in general practice. *The Lancet.* 2001; 357:89–95.

15. GISSI. GISS-Prevenzione Investigators (Gruppo Italiano per lo Studio della Sopravvivenza Nell'Infarto Miocardio). Dietary supplementation with n-2 polyunsaturated fatty acids and vitamin E after myocardial infarction: results of the GISSI-Prevenzione Trial. *The Lancet.* 1999; 354:447–55.

16. Stephens, N.G., Parsons, A., Schofield, P.M., Kelly, F., Cheeseman, K., Mitchinson, M.J. Randomised controlled trial of Vitamin E in patients with coronary disease: Cambridge Heart Antioxidant Study (CHAOS). *The Lancet.* 1996; 347:781–86.

17. HOPE. The Heart Outcomes Prevention Evaluation Study Investigators. Vitamin E supplementation and cardiovascular events in high-risk patients. *New England Journal of Medicine.* 2000; 342:154–60.

18. Lee, I.-M., Cook, N.R., Gaziano, J.M., Gordon, D., Ridker, P.M., Manson, J.E., Hennekens, C.H., Buring, J.E. Vitamin E in the primary prevention of cardiovascular disease and cancer: The Women's Health Study: A randomized controlled trial. *Journal of the American Medical Association.* 2005; 294(1):56–65.

19. Waters, D.D., Alderman, E.L., Hsia, J., Howard, B.V., Cobb, F.R., Rogers, W.J., Ouyang, P., Thompson, P., Tardif, J.C., Higginson, L., Bittner, V., Steffes, M., Gordon, D.J., Proschan, M., Younes, N., Verter, J.I. Effects of hormone replacement therapy and antioxidant vitamin supplements on coronary atherosclerosis in postmenopausal women: A randomized controlled trial. *Journal of the American Medical Association.* 2002; 288(19):2432–40.

20. Brown, B.G., Zhao, X.-Q., Chait, A., Fisher, L.D., Cheung, M.C., Morse, J.S., Dowdy, A.A., Marino, E.K., Bolson, E.L., Alaupovic, P., Frohlich, J., Albers, J.J. Simvastatin and niacin, antioxidant vitamins, or the combination for the prevention of coronary disease. *New England Journal of Medicine.* 2001; 345(22):1583–92.

21. Miller, E.R., Pastor-Barrluso, R., Dalal, D., Rlemersma, R.A., Appel, L.J., Guallar, E. Meta-analysis: High-dosage vitamin E supplementation may increase all-cause mortality. *Annals of Internal Medicine.* 2005; 142:37–46.

22. Nair, K.S., Rizza, R.A., O'Brien, P., Dhatariya, K., Short, K.R., Nehra, A., Vittone, J.L., Klee, G.G., Basu, A., Basu, R., Cobelli, C., Toffolo, G., Dalla Man, C., Tindall,

D.J., Melton, L.J., 3rd, Smith, G.E., Khosla, S., Jensen, M.D. DHEA in elderly women and DHEA or testosterone in elderly men. *New England Journal of Medicine.* Oct. 19, 2006; 355(16):1647–59.

23. Tsubono, Y., Nishino, Y., Komatsu, S., Hsieh, C.-C., Kanemura, S., Tsuji, I., Nakatsuka, H., Fukao, A., Satoh, H., Hisamichi, S. Green tea and the risk of gastric cancer in Japan. *New England Journal of Medicine.* 2001; 344(9):632–36.

24. Kuriyama, S., Shimazu, T., Ohmori, K., Kikuchi, N., Nakaya, N., Nishino, Y., Tsubono, Y., Tsuji, I. Green tea consumption and mortality due to cardiovascular disease, cancer, and all causes in Japan: The Ohsaki Study. *Journal of the American Medical Association.* Sept. 13, 2006; 296(10):1255–65.

25. Shekelle, P.G., Hardy, M.L., Morton, S.C., Maglione, M., Mojica, W.A., Suttorp, M.J., Rhodes, S.L., Jungvig, L., Gagne, J. Efficacy and safety of ephedra and ephedrine for weight loss and athletic performance: a meta-analysis. *Journal of the American Medical Association.* 2003; 289:1537–45.

26. Shelton, R.C., Keller, M.B., Gelenberg, A., Dunner, D.L., Hirschfeld, R., Thase, M.E., Russell, J., Lydiard, R.B., Crits-Cristoph, P., Gallop, R., Todd, L., Hellerstein, D., Goodnick, P., Keitner, G., Stahl, S.M., Halbreich, U. Effectiveness of St John's Wort in major depression: A randomized controlled trial. *Journal of the American Medical Association.* 2001; 285(15):1978–86.

27. Szegedi, A., Kohnen, R., Dienel, A., Kieser, M. Acute treatment of moderate to severe depression with hypericum extract WS 5570 (St. John's wort): Randomised controlled double blind non-inferiority trial versus paroxetine. *British Medical Journal.* 2005; 330:503–08.

28. HDTSG. Hypericum Depression Trial Study Group: Effect of Hypericum perforatum (St Joh's Wort) in major depressive disorder: A randomized controlled trial. *Journal of the American Medical Association.* 2002; 287(14):1807–14.

29. Bent, S., Kane, C., Shinohara, K., Neuhaus, J., Hudes, E.S., Goldberg, H., Avins, A.L. Saw palmetto for benign prostatic hyperplasia. *New England Journal of Medicine.* Feb. 9, 2006;354(6):557–66.

30. Anderson, J.W., Johnstone, B.M., Cook-Newell, M.E. Meta-analysis of the effects of soy protein intake on serum lipids. *New England Journal of Medicine.* 1995; 333:276–82.

31. Ziegler, G., Ploch, M., Miettinen-Baumann, A., Collet, W. Efficacy and tolerability of valerian extract LI 156 compared with oxazepam in the treatment of non-organic insomnia: a randomized double-blind, comparative clinical study. *European Journal of Medical Research.* 2002; 25:480–86.

32. Cropley, M., Cave, Z., Ellis, J., Middleton, R.W. Effect of Kava and Valerian on human physiological and psychological responses to mental stress assessed under laboratory conditions. *Phytotherapy Research.* 2002; 16:23–27.

33. Morisco, C., Trimarco, B., Condorelli, M. Effect of coenzyme Q10 therapy in patients

with congestive heart failure: a long-term multicenter randomized study. *Clinical Investigation.* 1993; 71(8 Suppl.):S134–36.

34. Rindone, J.P., Hiller, D., Collacott, E., Nordhaugen, N. Randomized, controlled trial of glucosamine for treating osteoarthritis of the knee. *Western Journal of Medicine.* 2000; 172(2):91–94.

35. Noak, W., Fisher, M., Forster, K.K. Glucosamine sulfate in osteoarthritis of the knee. *Osteoarthritis and Cartilage.* 1994; 2(1):51–59.

36. Lefler, C.T., Philippi, A.F., Leffler, S.G. Glucosamine, chondroitin, and manganese ascorbate for degenerative joint disease of the knee or low back: a randomized, double-blind, placebo-controlled pilot study. *Military Medicine.* 1999; 164:85–91.

CONCLUSION

1. de Lorgeril, M., Salen, P., Martin, J.L., Monjaud, I., Delaye, J., Mamelle, N. Mediterranean diet, traditional risk factors, and the rate of cardiovascular complications after myocardial infarction: Final report of the Lyon Diet Heart Study. *Circulation.* 1999; 99:779–85.

2. Trichopoulou, A., Orfanos, P., Norat, T., Bueno-de-Mesquita, B., Ocke, M.C., Peeters, P.H.M., van der Schouw, Y.T., Boeing, H., Hoffmann, K., Boffetta, P., Nagel, G., Masala, G., Krogh, V., Panico, S., Tumino, R., Vineis, P., Bamia, C., Naska, A., Benetou, V., Ferrari, P., Slimani, N., Pera, G., Martinez-Garcia, C., Navarro, C., Rodriguez-Barranco, M., Dorronsor, M., Spencer, E.A., Key, T.J., Bingham, S., Khaw, K.-T., Kesse, E., Clavel-Chapelon, F., Boutron-Ruault, M.-C., Berglund, G., Wirfalt, E., Hallmans, G., Johansson, I., Tjonneland, A., Olsen, A., Overvad, K., Hundborg, H.H., Riboli, E., Trichopoulos, D. Modified Mediterranean diet and survival: EPIC-elderly prospective cohort study. *British Medical Journal.* 2005; 330:991–98.

Other citations to material in the book can be found at
www.beforeyoutakethatpill.com.

BOOKS FOR
FURTHER READING

Abramson, J. (2004). *Overdosed America: The Broken Promise of American Medicine: How the Pharmaceutical Companies Distort Medical Knowledge, Mislead Doctors, and Compromise Your Health.* New York, HarperCollins.

Angell, M. (2004). *The Truth About the Drug Companies: How They Deceive Us and What to Do About It.* New York, Random House.

Avorn, J. (2004). *Powerful Medicines: The Benefits, Risks, and Costs of Prescription Drugs.* New York, Alfred A. Knopf.

Bralow, L., Ed. (2003). *The PDR Pocket Guide to Prescription Drugs.* New York, Pocket Books.

Brinker, F. (1998). *Herb Contraindications and Drug Interactions.* Sandy, OR., Eclectic Medical Publications.

Cohen, J. S. (2004). *Overdose: The Case Against the Drug Companies.* New York, Jeremy P. Tarcher/Penguin.

Critser, G. (2003). *Fat Land: How Americans Became the Fattest People in the World.* Boston, Houghton Mifflin.

Goonzer, M. (2004). *The $800 Million Dollar Pill: The Truth Behind the Cost of New Drugs.* Berkeley, CA, University of California Press.

Graedon, J. and T. Graedon (1999). *Dangerous Drug Interactions.* New York, St. Martin's Paperbacks.

Griffith, H. W. (2005). *Complete Guide to Prescription & Nonprescription Drugs.* New York, Perigee.

Hilts, P. J. (2003). *Protecting America's Health: The FDA, Business, and One Hundred Years of Regulation*. New York, Alfred A. Knopf.

Hurley, D. (2006). *Natural Causes: Death, Lies, and Politics in America's Vitamin and Herbal Supplement Industry*. New York, Broadway Books.

Kassirer, J. P. (2005). *On the Take: How Medicine's Complicity with Big Business Can Endanger Your Health*. Oxford, U.K., Oxford University Press.

Lininger, S. W., A.R. Gaby, et al., eds. (1999). *A–Z Guide to Drug-Herb-Vitamin Interactions*. New York, Three Rivers Press.

Nestle, M. (2002). *Food Politics: How the Food Industry Influences Nutrition and Health*. Berkeley, CA, University of California Press.

Pollan, M. (2006). *The Omnivore's Dilemma: A Natural History of Four Meals*. New York, Penguin Press.

Rybacki, J. J. (2004). *The Essential Guide to Prescription Drugs 2004*. New York, Harper-Resource.

Schlosser, E. (2001). *Fast Food Nation: The Dark Side of the All-American Meal*. Boston, Houghton Mifflin.

Silverman, H. M., Ed., (2004). *The Pill Book*. New York, Bantam Books.

Silverman, H. M., J. Romano, et al., eds. (1999). *The Vitamin Book*. New York, Bantam Books.

Spurlock, M. (2005). *Don't Eat This Book: Fast Food and the Supersizing of America*. New York, G. P. Putnam's Sons.

Whitfield, C. L. (2003). *The Truth About Depression*. Deerfield Beach, FL, Health Communications, Inc.

Whitfield, C. L. (2004). *The Truth About Mental Illness*. Deerfield Beach, FL, Health Communications, Inc.

Wolfe, S. M., L. D. Sasich, et al. (2005). *Worst Pills, Best Pills*. New York, Pocket Books.

INDEX